Dementia

Oxford Specialist Handbooks published and forthcoming

Dementia
From advanced disease to bereavement

Edited by

Victor Pace

Consultant in Palliative Medicine
St Christopher's Hospice, London, UK

Adrian Treloar

Consultant and Senior Lecturer in Old Age Psychiatry
Oxleas NHS Foundation Trust, London, UK

Sharon Scott

Senior Research Nurse,
Marie Curie Palliative Care Research Unit
Department of Mental Health Sciences
University College London, UK

Series Editor

Max Watson

Consultant in Palliative Medicine
Northern Ireland Hospice, Belfast, UK, and
Honorary Consultant, The Princess Alice Hospice
Esher, UK

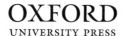

OXFORD
UNIVERSITY PRESS

OXFORD
UNIVERSITY PRESS

Great Clarendon Street, Oxford OX2 6DP

Oxford University Press is a department of the University of Oxford.
It furthers the University's objective of excellence in research, scholarship,
and education by publishing worldwide in

Oxford New York

Auckland Cape Town Dar es Salaam Hong Kong Karachi
Kuala Lumpur Madrid Melbourne Mexico City Nairobi
New Delhi Shanghai Taipei Toronto

With offices in

Argentina Austria Brazil Chile Czech Republic France Greece
Guatemala Hungary Italy Japan Poland Portugal Singapore
South Korea Switzerland Thailand Turkey Ukraine Vietnam

Oxford is a registered trade mark of Oxford University Press
in the UK and in certain other countries

Published in the United States
by Oxford University Press Inc., New York

British Library Cataloguing in Publication Data
Data available

Library of Congress Cataloging in Publication Data
Data available

Typeset by Glyph International, Bangalore, India
Printed in Great Britain by
Ashford Colour Press Ltd, Gosport, Hampshire

ISBN 978–0–19–923780–7

10 9 8 7 6 5 4 3 2 1

Contents

Detailed contents

Contributors

Editors

Dr Victor Pace FRCP
Consultant in Palliative Medicine
St Christopher's Hospice
London

Dr Adrian Treloar MRCPsych FRCP MRCGP
Consultant and Senior Lecturer in Old Age Psychiatry
Oxleas NHS Foundation Trust, London

Sharon Scott MSc, RGN, Dip Ca
Senior Research Nurse
Marie Curie Palliative Care Research Unit
Department of Mental Health Science
UCL Medical School, London

Contributors

Dr Carmelo Aquilina MD FRCPsych FRANZCP
Director of Specialist Mental Health Services for Older People
Western Sydney Local Health Network, Sydney, Australia
Chapter 2: Dementia and its management
Chapter 3: Young-onset dementia (YOD)

Dr Monica Crugel MD, MB BS
Speciality Registrar in Old Age Psychiatry
Oxleas NHS Foundation Trust, London
Chapter 10: Mental distress and psychobehavioural problems
Chapter 16: Communication

Tamsin Dives AGSM DipMT
Music Therapist
St Christopher's Hospice, London
Chapter 23: Some other therapies

Professor Murna Downs PhD
Head of Bradford Dementia Group.
School of Health Studies, University of Bradford, Bradford, UK
Chapter 17: Person-centred dementia care

Dr Gillie Evans BM BCh MRCGP
GP, Jenner Health Centre, Whittlesey, Peterborough
RESEC Research Fellow, Green Templeton College, Oxford
Chapter 20: Provision of appropriate care

Karen Harrison Dening RMN RNMH RGN MA
Lead Practice Development Admiral Nurse
Dementia UK
(GSF Clinical Associate, also seconded to the NCPC and Marie Curie UK)
Chapter 22: Caring for the carers

Dr Karen Le Ball MA FRCP
Consultant Geriatrician South London Healthcare Trust;
Deputy Head of School of Medicine and Medical Specialties
London Deanery
Chapter 12: Intercurrent illness in advanced dementia

Barbara Pointon B.Mus., MBE
Retired lecturer; former
family carer; Ambassador for
the Alzheimer's Society and
Dementia UK; member of the
Standing Commission on Carers
*Chapter 21: A family carer's
perspective*

Dr Sunita Sahu MRCPsych
Consultant in Old Age Psychiatry
Oxleas NHS Foundation Trust,
London
*Chapter 3: Young-onset
dementia (YOD)*

Clare Steves MRCP
Speciality Registrar in Medicine
of the Elderly,
Guy's and St Thomas' NHS
Foundation Trust, London
*Chapter 12: Intercurrent
illness in advanced dementia*

Elaine Syrett RN
Senior Complementary Therapist
St Christopher's Hospice,
London
Chapter 23: Some other therapies

**Dr Amanda
Thompsell MBBS, DRCOG,
DGM, MRCPsych**
Consultant Old Age Psychiatrist,
South London and Maudsley
NHS Foundation Trust;
Clinical Champion for the
Dementia Workstream of the
Modernisation Initiative
End of Life Programme
*Chapter 20: Provision of
appropriate care*

Foreword and acknowledgements

Dementia has replaced cancer (and earlier, tuberculosis) as the most widely-feared disease of the 21st century. Yet our chances of developing it are higher than ever: as we live longer, UK prevalence is doubling every twenty years.

People with advanced dementia depend totally on others' care for survival. Progressive physical frailty coupled with very deranged mental functions often eventually leads to death, contributing to one in eight deaths in the UK—half as many deaths as smoking. But late stage dementia is poorly understood, partly because it belongs to nobody. Old age psychiatry rarely feels it can provide meticulous physical care; palliative care has been little involved so far; old age medicine has become very hospital based. Looking after far advanced dementia forms little part of anybody's training, so end of life care lags far behind that received by cancer patients.

This book, based on the latest evidence, wants to remedy this by providing a practical guide for medical, advanced nursing, other professionals and trainees in these specialties, and others interested in the field, and by encouraging collaboration.

People still die of cancer, and still fear it, but far less than they did thirty years ago. Scientifically based, compassionate, dignity-enhancing care for end-stage dementia is what above all what will take fear out of the illness. We hope this book will help professionals to provide this.

This book received a lot of help from a lot of people. Many, too numerous to mention, helped us develop our ideas and skills over the years. Some had more direct input, not always knowingly. We thank Dame Barbara Monroe, Dr Abigail Wright, Paul Pace SJ and Aida Shoush for reading and commenting on various chapters. Anonymous reviewers from OUP provided invaluable feedback, all the more useful when it was critical. Any remaining errors are our responsibility alone. Professors Malcolm Payne and Matthew Hotopf clarified a number of legal issues. Dr Claud Regnard introduced us to key concepts around symptom assessment in people with learning difficulties; Dr Elizabeth Sampson contributed to our understanding of hospital care for people in late-stage dementia; and Drs Amanda Thompsell and Jo Hockley taught us about care homes and about practical management of difficult behaviour in these settings. Dr Max Watson commissioned this volume and gave much support and encouragement. The long-suffering staff at OUP, in particular Nicola Wilson, Jenny Wright, Victoria Mortimer, Bridget Johnson, and previously Georgia Pinteau and Eloise Moir-Ford, turned an idea into a concrete reality, contributing indispensable advice and support liberally on the way. VP and SS would also like to thank Dr Carmelo Aquilina, who inspired our interest in this area, and worked with us on this and other projects early on.

Above all, we are grateful to our families who put up with prolonged absences from day-to-day family life while working on 'the book'. This book is dedicated to the patients, carers, and our partners in day-to-day clinical work, who day in, day out taught us more than anyone just what constitutes good care.

VP, AT, SS

Symbols and abbreviations

📖	cross reference in this book
AA	Attendance Allowance
ABC chart	antecedents, behaviour, consequences chart
ACh	acetylcholine
AChEI	acetylcholinesterase inhibitor
AD	Alzheimer's disease
ADC	AIDS dementia complex
ADH	antidiuretic hormone
ADL	activities of daily living
ADRT	advance decision to refuse treatment
AIDS	acquired immunodeficiency syndrome
ApOε$_4$	apolipoprotein ε$_4$
APP	amyloid precursor protein
BBB	blood–brain barrier
b.d.	twice a day
BEHAVE-AD	Behavioral Pathology in Alzheimer's Disease Scale
BMA	British Medical Association
BMI	body mass index
b.p.	blood pressure
b.p.m.	beats per minute
BPSD	Behavioural and Psychological Symptoms of Dementia
BSE	bovine spongiform encephalopathy
CA	Carers' Allowance
CADASIL	cerebral autosomal dominant arteriopathy with subcortical infarcts and leukoencephalopathy
CBD	Cortico-basilar degeneration
CDR	Clinical Dementia Rating
CJD	Creutzfeld–Jakob disease
CK	creatine kinase
CMAI	Cohen-Mansfield Agitation Inventory
CNS	central nervous system
COPD	chronic obstructive pulmonary disease
COSHH	control of substances hazardous to health
COX	cyclooxygenase
CPAP	continuous positive airways pressure
CPR	cardiopulmonary resuscitation
CSF	cerebrospinal fluid

CT	computed tomography
CTZ	chemoreceptor trigger zone
CYP450	cytochrome P450
DASNI	Dementia Advocacy and Support Network International
DFG	Disabled Facilities Grant
DisDAT	Disability Distress Assessment Tool
DLA	Disability Living Allowance
DLB	dementia with Lewy bodies
DN	district nurse
DOLS	deprivation of liberty safeguards
DRG	dorsal root ganglion
DS-DAT	Discomfort Scale – Dementia of Alzheimer's Type
DSM-IV TR	Diagnostic and Statistical Manual of the American Psychiatric Association, 4th edition, text revision
DST	decision support tool
DT	delirium tremens
DVLA	Driver and Vehicle Licensing Agency
EAS	external anal sphincter
ECG	electrocardiogram
ECOG	Eastern Cooperative Oncology Group
EEG	electroencephalogram
EMEA	European Medicines Agency
EPA	enduring power of attorney
ESA	Employment and Support Allowance
FAST	Functional Assessment Staging [Scale]
FBC	full blood count
FDA	Food and Drug Administration
fMRI	functional MRI
FPTC	2β-carbomethoxy-3β-(4-chlorophenyl)-8-(-3-fluoropropyl) nortropane
FTLD	frontotemporal lobar degeneration
GABA	Gamma-amino butyric acid
GAD	generalized anxiety disorder
GCS	Glasgow Coma Scale
GDP	gross domestic product
GDS	Global Deterioration Scale
GI	gastrointestinal
GMC	General Medical Council
GP	general practitioner
GSF	Gold Standards Framework

HAART	highly active antiretroviral therapy
HCA	health care assistant
HIV	human immunodeficiency virus
HM3G	hydromorphone-3-glucuronide
^{99m}Tc-HMPAO	Tc-hexamethylpropyleneamine oxime
HONC	hyperosmolar non-ketotic coma
5-HT3	type 3 serotonin
IADLs	instrumental activities of daily living
IAS	internal anal sphincter
IASP	International Association for the Study of Pain
IB	Incapacity Benefit
i.m.	intramuscular
IMCA	independent mental capacity advocate
INR	international normalized ratio
IR	immediate release
i.v.	intravenous
KPS	Karnofsky Performance Status [scale]
LANSS	Leeds Assessment for Neuropathic Symptoms and Signs
LCP	Liverpool Care Pathway
LPA	lasting power of attorney
LRTI	lower respiratory tract infection
M3G	morphine-3-glucuronide
M6G	morphine-6-glucuronide
MAOI	monoamine oxidase inhibitor
MCA	Mental Capacity Act
mcg	microgram
MCMD	minor cognitive motor disorder
MCPCIL	Marie Curie Palliative Care Institute Liverpool
mg	milligram
MHA	Mental Health Act
MMSE	Mini Mental State Examination
MND	motor neuron disease
MR	modified release
MRI	magnetic resonance imaging
MSA	multisystem atrophy
NAA	National Assistance Act (1947, 1951)
NAO	National Audit Office
NaSSA	noradrenergic and specific serotonergic antidepressant
NCPC	National Council for Palliative Care
NGT	nasogastric tube

NHS	(UK) National Health Service
NI	National Insurance
NICE	National Institute for Health and Clinical Excellence
NMDA	N-methyl d-aspartate
NMS	neuroleptic malignant syndrome
NNH	number needed to harm
NNT	number needed to treat
NPI	Neuropsychiatric Inventory
NREM	non-rapid eye movement [sleep]
OBRA	Omnibus Budget Reconciliation Act of 1987 (USA)
OSA	obstructive sleep apnoea
PACSLAC	Pain Assessment Checklist for Seniors with Limited Ability to Communicate
PAINAD	Pain Assessment in Advanced Dementia
PCT	primary care trust
PD	Parkinson's disease
PE	pulmonary embolism
PEG	percutaneous endoscopic gastrostomy
PENS	percutaneous electrical nerve stimulation
p.o.	by mouth
POS	Palliative Care Outcome Scale
PPC	preferred priorities of care
PPI	proton pump inhibitor
p.r.	per rectum
p.r.n.	as needed
PSP	progressive supranuclear palsy
PTH	parathyroid hormone
q.d.s.	four times daily
QOF	Quality and Outcomes Framework
RAID	Rating Anxiety in Dementia Scale
RBD	REM-sleep behaviour disorder
RCN	Royal College of Nursing
RCT	randomized controlled trial
REM	rapid eye movement [sleep]
RIG	radiologically inserted gastrostomy
SARI	serotonin antagonist/reuptake inhibitor
s.c.	subcutaneous
SCIE	Social Care Institute for Excellence
SD	syringe driver
s.l.	sublingual

SLE	systemic lupus erythematosus
SM-EOLD	Symptom Management at End-of-Life in Dementia [scale]
SNRI	selective serotonin/norepinephrine reuptake inhibitor
SPCT	specialist palliative care team
SPECT	single photon emission computed tomography
SSRI	selective serotonin reuptake inhibitor
s.c.	subcutaneous
SWS	slow wave sleep
TCA	tricyclic antidepressant
TD	transdermal
t.d.s.	three times a day
TENS	transcutaneous electrical nerve stimulation
TIA	transient ischaemic attack
UTI	urinary tract infection
VaD	vascular dementia
VAS	visual analogue scale
VPG	vomiting pattern generator
WHO	World Health Organization
YOD	young-onset dementia

Introduction to dementia

Introduction

Dementia is common and becoming commoner. In developed countries the number of people with dementia is doubling every 20 years as a result of an aging population. In developing countries the situation is even worse as their life expectancy is catching up rapidly with richer nations. This has important economic and social consequences for the state, but also huge personal implications for people with dementia and their carers.

An understanding of the nature and epidemiology of dementia is essential for those involved in providing care. A significant number of people die of dementia—as yet few seem to appreciate that it is a terminal illness which can cause death. A much larger number of people die with dementia as a comorbidity to their main illness. And many people with advanced dementia are very frail, often without one predominant illness but with many illnesses which put together account for a lot of disability. In models of care that are diagnosis and hospital based, those who are frail are lost to the system and stay below the radar, and they and their carers suffer grievously as a result.

Definition (see also 📖 Chapter 2)

Dementia, commonly thought of as a disorder of memory, actually involves a much broader deterioration of intellectual function. The latest Diagnostic and Statistical Manual of the American Psychiatric Association (4th edition with text revision) (DSM-IV TR) definition requires memory impairment to be present—without memory impairment there is no dementia. However, memory impairment alone constitutes the dysmnesic syndrome, usually due to chronic alcohol consumption. The memory impairment must be associated with one or more of the following for dementia to exist: aphasia, apraxia, agnosia, or deterioration of executive function (the ability to think abstractly and to plan, initiate, sequence, monitor, and to stop complex behaviour). The condition must be sufficiently severe to interfere with the person's social relationships and work performance, and it must represent a decline from the person's previous level of functioning. Finally the definition requires the deterioration to be progressive.

Such an all-encompassing condition impinges on every aspect of life and calls for management from a holistic and multidisciplinary perspective. That is the perspective this book will take.

Epidemiology

Demographics

- The worldwide population with dementia was estimated in 2010 as around 35 million, expected to double every 20 years (increasing longevity, changes in prevalence of some associated conditions, e.g. vascular disease).
- 61% live in developing countries, rising to 71% by 2040.
- In China and India, the prevalence is likely to increase by 300% by 2040.
- 92% of the global cost (estimated at US$156 billion in 2003) is spent in developed countries. Developing countries have meagre resources to allocate to such a burgeoning problem.
- In the UK, 163,000 new cases occur annually. Currently 750,000 people in the UK have dementia (1.2% of the population), rising to 1.8 million by 2050. In the USA 4–5 million are thought to be affected.
- Disparities in European figures are explained by differing application of the diagnostic criteria.
- Apparent low rates in Africa may be more due to methodological problems in data collection than true differences.

Dementia prevalence

Dementia prevalence increases with age **(Table 2.1)**.

Young-onset dementia (YOD)

YOD is dementia developing in people younger than 65 years (📖 Chapter 3), e.g. frontotemporal dementia, Creutzfeldt–Jakob disease (CJD), human immunodeficiency virus (HIV). It also doubles in prevalence for every 5 year increase in age:

- YOD constitutes 2.2% of all dementias in the UK, though this may be an underestimate.
- This rises to 6.1% in black and ethnic minority groups. The increased frequency in these groups is a reflection of the younger population profile of black and ethnic minority groups in the UK, not of racial differences in susceptibility.

Burden of disease

- Dementia creates an immense burden for people with dementia and their families.
- The World Health Organization (WHO) 2003 World Health Report estimated that dementia accounts for 11.2% of years lived with disability in the over 60s, more than stroke (9.5%), musculoskeletal disease (8.9%), cardiovascular disease (5.0%), or cancer (2.4%). *Dementia carries the highest disability burden after spinal cord injury and terminal cancer.*
- This burden arises out of progressive disability. Those affected become unable to complete complex tasks or self-care, and may exhibit socially inappropriate behaviours. Eventually they may become doubly incontinent, aphasic, immobile, and incapable even of sitting up unassisted.
- In moderately advanced dementia in particular, many exhibit psychobehavioural changes such as depression, wandering, and calling out (📕 Chapter 10). These may prove the most difficult aspects of care for carers (📕 Chapters 21 and 22).
- Most dementias progress relentlessly but slowly. The mean prognosis for Alzheimer's disease (AD) is 4–6 years, but some live for more than twice as long.
- The total dependence of people with moderate or advanced dementia, the long-term nature of the illness, and the psychobehavioural symptoms place a massive burden on carers (📕 Chapters 21 and 22), who are often older and unwell themselves.
- Consequently, more than a third of the population in the UK with dementia live in residential care (Table 1.1). Numbers are imprecise, as many care-home residents have undiagnosed or undeclared dementia.

Economic cost of dementia

In the UK the cost of caring for people aged over 65 with dementia has been calculated to be £17–23 billion annually:

- 55% is due to lost income for informal carers who would otherwise have worked or worked longer hours.
- 40% of this is due to social care.
- 5% to health costs.
- 0.13% due to productivity losses.[1]

This total cost of dementia care in the UK is equivalent to just under a fifth of the UK National Health Service (NHS) budget. The costs per patient according to place of care are shown in Table 1.2. It has been suggested that costs could rise to over £50 billion over the next 30 years, which could have a drastic effect on health economics. By 2031, around 1% of GDP could be taken up by dementia care; even this excludes opportunity cost for informal carers. Projections for dementia care for other developed countries tell a roughly similar story.

1 Luengo-Fernandez R, Leal J, Gray A (2010) *Dementia 2010: the economic burden of dementia and associated research funding in the United Kingdom.* Health Economics Research Centre, University of Oxford, for the Alzheimer's Research Trust, Cambridge.

Table 1.1 Estimated percentage of people with dementia in residential care in the UK

Age (years)	% in residential care
65–74	26.6
75–84	27.8
85–89	40.9
90+	60.8

Source: Knapp M Prince M (2007) *Dementia UK: the full report.* Alzheimer's Society, London.

Table 1.2 Cost of care for a patent with dementia in the UK

People in the community with mild dementia	£16,689
People in the community with moderate dementia	£25,877
People in the community with severe dementia	£37,473
People in care homes with severe dementia	£31,296

Source: Knapp M, Prince M (2007) *Dementia UK: the full report.* Alzheimer's Society, London.

Case example

George, a 73-year-old retired company manager has been noted to be becoming more forgetful. First he got lost when out driving, had a crash, and became involved in a painful and out of character argument with the other driver. He was found to have been caring for himself less well and had also become more irritable at home with his wife. A diagnosis of dementia was made. Two years later he needs the full care of his wife, being unable to wash or dress himself or to be left alone. His wife cares tirelessly and well for him but is exhausted. Carers come in three times a day for washing, dressing and feeding; George has periodic respite care. With that, George continues to live at home and to contribute to family life with his children and grandchildren.

Progression of dementia

- Dementia progression is dealt with in detail in 📖 Chapters 2 and 4.
- People with AD usually spend the last third of their illness heavily dependent on others for care—the definition of advanced dementia.
- While people with dementia lose many cognitive and other skills, and eventually deteriorate physically, they will also retain many aspects of their personality until very late in their illness; frequently their emotional responsiveness and the ability to relate appear if anything to be enhanced. It is important not to see dementia purely as a degeneration, but to realize that a core of the personality remains and relationships can become simplified and more immediate. (📖 Chapters 4, 16, 17, 19, and 21).

Place of care and death

- Dementia often precipitates institutional care (Table 1.1, and 📖 Chapter 20).
- In the USA, 67% of dementia-related deaths occur in nursing homes. This compares with 38% of cancer patients dying at home and 35% in hospital, and a national average of 55% hospital deaths for all causes.
- A review of place of death for those certified as having died of AD, dementia, or senility in England between 2007 and 2009 showed that 59% had died in care homes, 32% in hospital, and only 8% in their own homes.

Causes of death

Mavis died at home with dementia. She was cared for there with a full package through until death and with full equipment as well. There was ongoing specialist support to advise upon her needs and the minimization of her distress until death; death was peaceful at home with family present.

Joy died in a nursing home. She could not be managed at home but as a result of good advance discussions about illness, when she developed her final pneumonia, she stayed in the nursing home where she lived, and avoided dying in the emergency department. Her family and also the staff she knew were with her at the time of death. She had had an advanced dementia. Her death certificate gave pneumonia as the cause of death but did not mention dementia.

- Dementia is a terminal illness, associated with earlier death.
- In the UK, an estimated 60,000 deaths each year are attributable to dementia, which, however, contributes to a substantial number of other deaths. This is about half the number of deaths attributable to smoking, but occurs in a much older age group. An analysis of death certificates from 2001–2009 in England showed that AD, dementia, or frailty was a cause or contributory cause of death in 15% of all deaths.
- A 10-year population based cohort study conducted by the Medical Research Council (MRC) in the UK concluded that 1 in 3 people over 65 suffer from dementia at death.
- Death certificates give very inaccurate epidemiological data, as dementia is often not listed as a contributory factor. Most people who die with dementia are certified of dying as a result of intercurrent illnesses which occur much more commonly in dementia than in comparable cognitively non-demented elders.
- Deaths certified as being caused by dementia are said to be stable in males, but increasing in females.
- Women with dementia tend to survive longer than men.
- Vascular dementia (VaD), Lewy body dementia (DLB), and frontotemporal dementia have a shorter prognosis than AD.
- In AD, the more rapid the cognitive decline, the shorter the prognosis tends to be.
- Post-mortem series of people with AD and other dementias show bronchopneumonia and ischaemic heart disease to be the commonest immediate causes of death. Heart disease was slightly less frequent in AD than in VaD, and heart failure was a commoner cause of death in VaD.
- Pulmonary emboli were found in around 1 in 8 patients in one series, and unsuspected malignancies in between 4 and 8%.
- 60% of people with VaD die within 5 years of diagnosis, often of other cardiovascular conditions, e.g. myocardial infarction, stroke.
- A death-certificate analysis of nearly 900 deaths from advanced dementia in Holland suggested that 35% died of cachexia/dehydration, 20% of cardiovascular conditions, and another 20% of acute respiratory conditions. It is unclear to what extent cachexia/dehydration actually

contributed to death rather than being terminal events in people who were very ill. The clinical diagnosis of dehydration in people who are cachectic can be difficult; in this series it is not clear how this diagnosis was established other than through the clinical opinion of the certifying doctor.

- A recent study found that hospital deaths from concurrent conditions are significantly higher for men but not women with AD across a broad spectrum of concurrent conditions: myocardial infarction, heart failure, hip fracture, gastrointestinal haemorrhage; and men also have a higher risk of contracting pneumonia. The authors of this research suggest poorer care for male dementia patients might be responsible, but the reasons remain unclear.[2]

Laditka JN, Laditka SB, Cornman CB (2005) Evaluating hospital care for individuals with Alzheimer's disease using inpatient quality indicators. *Am J Alzheimers Dis Other Demen* **20**, 27–36.

Palliative care of people with dementia

Specialist palliative care of people with dementia has been slow to take off. Reasons for this include:

- An early concentration on cancer by specialist palliative care.
- A fear of being inundated by numbers, submerging other patient groups.
- A very different, much slower, disease trajectory requiring a different model of care.
- A different balance between medical and social needs from other illnesses seen by specialist palliative care.
- Difficulty in determining when palliative care should get involved.
- A dearth of information about the late stages of dementia, leading to a lack of clarity about the role of specialist palliative care.

There were some pioneering voices, most notably Ladislaus Volicer in the USA, who laid the groundwork for subsequent work with people with dementia. Another significant impetus was the number of patients with acquired immune deficiency syndrome (AIDS) dementia (ADC) being looked after by some palliative care units. However, even recently, involvement of specialist palliative care has been limited. Over the last few years a number of projects have been under way to explore the contribution palliative care could make to this field. For example, in the UK the National Council for Palliative Care, the Alzheimer's Society, and others have got together to plan the way ahead. It is clear that:

- Advanced dementia has a number of characteristics which make it amenable to palliative care.
- There is a great need for detailed information about end-stage dementia to allow the planning and delivery of appropriate services.
- The care of people with advanced dementia must equally focus on their carers, who often are under tremendous strain.
- The provision of care must follow people across the different care environments of home, residential care, or hospital.

Indira was a 75-year-old Indian lady with advanced dementia. She could not talk but cried out. She seemed to be especially upset by moving and also had a history of arthritis. Simple analgesics were of little use but she settled considerably with the use of opiate analgesia. Her family were pleased to see her distress settle.

David was a 64-year-old man with an advanced dementia. He had been psychotic during his illness but now could only shout and call out. No one could understand what he was saying any longer, but he looked afraid and fearful. His eyes stared and he would cry out for help. The physicians and his family agreed that he appeared distressed and various medicines were tried to alleviate this. Antidepressants and analgesics had little effect, but antipsychotics helped, and with them he seemed settled. It was agreed that despite their harm they were appropriately used to palliate his distress. He died a few weeks after admission but his family were pleased that he was much more peaceful in his last days.

Further reading

Blight A (ed) (2007) *Progress with dementia – moving forward: addressing palliative care for people with dementia*, pp. 1–24. National Council for Palliative Care, London.

Knapp M, Prince M (2007) *Dementia UK: a report into the prevalence and cost of dementia prepared by the Personal Social Services Research Unit (PSSRU) at the London School of Economics and the Institute of Psychiatry at King's College, for the Alzheimer's Society: the full report.* Alzheimer's Society, London.

Chapter 2

Dementia and its management

Introduction

Older people have always been known to lose faculties, and so-called 'senility' was thought to be a normal feature of aging. In the 1960s and 1970s, it became clear that the degree of cognitive decline was related to pathological lesions in the brain and the decrease in the brain chemical acetylcholine (ACh). AD was found to be the most common cause of dementia, and for many lay people the term is now synonymous with dementia. Originally AD was used to describe YOD, but it now refers to dementias in all ages where the major pathological features are neuro-fibrillary plaques and tangles (📖 Chapter 2, Types of dementia, pp. 20–26).

Partly because aging populations have more time to develop dementia, partly because of increased awareness and better case definition, and probably partly because of a change in the frequency of risk factors, estimates of numbers worldwide have increased from just 150 in 1945 to 35.6 million in 2010,[1] with 4.6 million new cases being diagnosed each year.

Other factors which have changed our appreciation of the problem of dementia and the public perception of it include:

- Better recognition through increased awareness and screening instruments.
- A decrease in the stigma of the disease, enabling more people to admit that they or their relatives have it.
- A greater understanding of the pathological processes and different types of dementia.
- The development of drugs to treat the condition, which has encouraged people to seek treatment and services to look for dementia.
- Advocacy and lobbying by and on behalf of people with dementia.
- More prominence in health planning with increasing numbers of older people.

This chapter provides an overview of the different dementias, but many of the themes will be dealt with in more detail in later chapters (see cross-references in the text).

1 Wimo A, Prince M (2010) *World Alzheimer report 2010: the global economic impact of dementia*, p. 53. Alzheimer's Disease International, Northbrook, IL.

What is dementia?

Dementia is a progressive and generally irreversible condition which is characterized by:

- Impairment of memory and at least one other global cognitive function (such as comprehension, learning, language, learnt behaviour, etc.), with an associated
  - decline in overall functioning,
  - change in personality (such as coarsening of social behaviour, loosening of emotional control or lack of motivation),
  - in a setting of clear consciousness.

The irreversibility criterion of dementia is not absolute. Some of the secondary causes of dementia may be treatable (e.g. deficiencies of vitamins such as B12) and the cognitive deficits may be partially or wholly reversible. With ongoing developments in the treatment of dementias its progress may eventually be alleviated, arrested, or even reversed in more people. This book focuses on the irreversible dementias.

Risk factors for getting dementia

Increasing age is the single most important risk factor (Table 2.1). YODs are much rarer (🕮 Chapter 3). Although genetic factors play a role in these cases, their overall contribution is relatively small and often related to environmental factors in complex ways; our current understanding of the genetics of dementia is still developing. The risk of dementia is associated with:

- Increasing age (the prevalence doubles every 5 years after the age of 65 years).
- Down's syndrome (high risk for people over 40 years of age) (🕮 Chapter 3).
- Having two copies of the apolipoprotein ε4 (ApOε4) gene.
- Heavy alcohol intake throughout life.
- Head trauma (any trauma causing loss of consciousness).
- Poor education—people with higher levels of education function better for the same level of pathological change.
- Vascular risk factors and heart disease (e.g. hypertension, obesity, high blood cholesterol levels, diabetes).
- Surgery (especially following heart surgery and fractures).

Table 2.1 Age-stratified prevalence of dementia

Age range	Prevalence rate (%)
65–69	1.4
70–74	2.8
75–79	5.6
80–84	10.5
85–89	20.8
90–95	38.6

Symptoms of dementia

For a more detailed discussion see 📖 Chapters 4 and 10.

As AD is the most common cause of dementia the main symptoms listed here apply principally to this illness. Where other dementias differ in their symptoms, this will be noted in their descriptions. There are four broad categories of symptoms of dementia:

- Cognitive symptoms.
- Behavioural and psychiatric symptoms.
- Functional impairment.
- Personality change.

Cognitive symptoms

The key to understanding how and when cognitive symptoms present is to consider two aspects:

- *Cognitive capacity* is the capacity of a person to acquire, recall, process, and utilize information. It is affected by brain disease, previous educational ability, personality factors, and learned coping skills. Cognitive capacity is also affected by social networks. Spouses or children may over time start to compensate for a lot of deficits so that the person affected may overtly or unconsciously rely on other people's cognitive powers to compensate for failing memory.
- *Cognitive challenge* describes demands upon cognitive skills. With frequently used cognitive tasks (e.g. the names of familiar people, words, objects, or activities) cognitive challenge is low. The highest challenges come from unfamiliar tasks (e.g. operating a new appliance), complex (e.g. income tax returns), or recent events.

Signs and symptoms of dementia will become manifest when cognitive challenges exceed cognitive capacity. For example, when maintaining a routine in a familiar environment one can cover up cognitive decline for a long time, but this becomes obvious when one has to learn new routines in an unfamiliar environment. Early on in dementia the most demanding tasks trigger minor difficulties or mistakes. Later, most everyday tasks suffer.

The main cognitive symptoms of dementia are:

- Rapid forgetting: new information is forgotten more quickly.
- Slower learning: new information is learnt more slowly.
- Repetitive speech and repetitive questioning.
- Confabulating: the manufacturing of often plausible memories to fill in gaps.
- Misplacing objects: sometimes in very odd places. This may lead to delusions of theft.
- Recent memory loss: more distant memories are more robust.

Orientation to time and place

- Difficulty in remembering appointments: initially people may use lists or diaries, but then must rely upon other people to remember. Others will simply deny they had any appointment.
- Disorientation to time: this is often one of the early signs of cognitive loss. Patients forget what day or month it is. Later they lose their sense of time of day. Of course in institutional care, even those who do not have dementia may become disorientated because there are few clues as to what day it is.

- Day–night disorientation: people who wake up at night start thinking it is day time (this is also partly due to a reversed sleep–wake cycle: see 📖 Chapter 2, Symptoms of dementia, pp. 15–19 and 📖 Chapter 10, Sleep disturbance, pp. 196–199).
- Disorientation to place: people with moderate dementia often do not know where they are and get lost in unfamiliar settings. Later on, they may get lost in familiar settings, even at home. Even in advanced disease, people will often remember their home addresses if they have lived there for a long time. At times, however, they may think they are living at a previous address.
- Disorientation to person: dementia affects recognition of other people, first those who are only slight acquaintances, then people who are far more familiar, e.g. spouse and other family members. See 📖 Chapter 2, Symptoms of dementia, pp. 15–19 and 📖 Chapters 10 and 11.

Speech difficulties

Speech difficulties occur early in AD but are usually overshadowed by the memory loss. In other types of dementia, e.g. frontotemporal dementia, these are more prominent and occur earlier. The main effects are word-finding difficulties, and producing and understanding speech (expressive and receptive dysphasias). Word-finding difficulties manifest as:

- Reduced range of/simpler words: people's vocabulary will diminish subtly and they tend to use simpler words (e.g. dog instead of terrier) or older words (e.g. wireless instead of radio).
- Pauses in speech/incomplete sentences: people may forget words and so sentences may be interrupted or become incomplete.
- Circumlocution: being unable to make the point, patients may talk around the point in an attempt to compensate.
- Incorrect words/names: people may use the wrong words or names for objects or people (e.g. saying 'bird' instead of 'bread'). If persistent this is known as a substitution. Some patients may be aware they are using the wrong words and get frustrated; others may be oblivious to what they are doing. Later, words might be made up (neologisms).
- Expressive and receptive dysphasias: in pure expressive dysphasia the syntax breaks down and sentences consist of apparently random but individually correct words. In pure receptive dysphasia sentences are syntactically correct but as the person cannot understand what is being said to them, their answers bear no resemblance to the conversation.

Apraxia

Apraxia is the inability to perform learned movements. Actions which are more practised are more resistant to decline. In dementia we often see:

- Inability to use devices: initially new or unfamiliar household devices are troublesome, but later these difficulties extend to familiar devices.
- Dressing apraxia: difficulty putting on clothes, e.g. buttoning shirts, putting pants on before trousers, along with other problems of activities of daily living (ADL)

Agnosia

- Agnosia is the non-recognition of objects, people, or sensations which is not caused by sensory deficit (e.g. poor eyesight), problems with attention (e.g. distractibility in delirium), or level of consciousness, but by central neurological damage. It is a failure to grasp the meaning and significance of the object perceived. Agnosias can be visual, auditory, or tactile, for example.

- Non-recognition of objects: the object perceived is not recognized despite previous familiarity. These agnosias may be specific to a particular sensory type. In visual agnosias, an object that is not recognized by sight might be quickly identified by its feel. Two-dimensional drawings of an object may be particularly difficult to interpret.
- Non-recognition of people, e.g. relatives may not be recognized because their faces are not recognized (*prosopagnosia*—this is different from not remembering their name). They can, however, still be identified by other means, e.g. their voice. A possibly related impairment may contribute to the Capgras delusion, where familiar people are misidentified as identical-looking impostors because the feeling of familiarity associated with recognition is lost.

Behavioural and psychological symptoms of dementia (BPSD)

These symptoms can be caused by the pathological process but also by people's personalities and other people's reaction to the person with dementia. Several symptoms can occur.

Delusions and other odd ideas

Delusions are bizarre beliefs which cannot be understood. Some delusions appear to have no precipitating cause (primary delusions); others (secondary delusions) arise from identifiable causes, e.g. forgetfulness. Common delusions are:

- Delusions of theft: things have been stolen (some are in fact misplaced).
- Phantom boarders: the idea that intruders are living in the house.
- Misidentifications: of people, of one's own image in the mirror, of pictures, or of images on television.

Hallucinations and illusions

Hallucinations are common in dementia and occur in any sensory modality (most commonly visual or auditory) in the absence of sensory stimuli and in clear consciousness. People with dementia may commonly hear voices or see intruders.

Vivid and repeated visual hallucinations suggest dementia with DLB. Hallucinations occur early in DLB but at a more advanced stage in AD.

An *illusion* is a distorted sensory perception (e.g. seeing a snake instead of a crack in the floor). Illusions are commoner when there is limited sensory input (e.g. dim light, deafness), when people are just waking up or going to sleep, or when delirium is present. When described to others, they can be hard to distinguish from the delusional beliefs that people with dementia may experience.

Distress

Distress has multiple causes (□ Chapter 6) and each individual requires a good attempt to identify the cause. Distress may be evidenced by disturbances of mood, anxiety, and behaviour.

Mood disturbances

Several types of mood disturbances may occur:

- Depression (📖 Chapter 10, Depression, pp. 178–184) is very common, especially in VaD. In the early stages it is very difficult to distinguish between depression and early dementia. Later, depression is more difficult to detect, though screening tests may help. People with depression and dementia may look sad, say they are low, be tearful, and struggle to enjoy themselves. Loss of appetite, weight loss, loss of energy and poor motivation, emotional flattening, and social withdrawal may be present. Tearfulness can be due to emotional lability (sometimes happening after a stroke) where crying is not accompanied by a persistent low mood. Some depressed people can laugh at times, but still respond to treatment with antidepressants.
- Elation is less common. It can be due to impairment of the frontal lobes of the brain, either as part of a generalized atrophy in AD or more focal damage as in VaD or frontotemporal dementia. People may be inappropriately cheerful

Anxiety (📖 Chapter 10, Anxiety, pp. 191–192)

Anxiety is common and often caused by a fear of not coping . Early in the illness, being lost in a new place might cause anxiety. Later on even being out of sight of a relative can cause panic. Co-existing depression can aggravate anxiety.

Changes in behaviour (📖 Chapter 10, Agitation and aggression, pp. 193–195)

- Agitation: can be manifest by inappropriate vocalizations (e.g. screaming or repetitive words or phrases), pacing, wandering, rummaging, repeatedly dressing and undressing, fiddling with objects, fidgeting.
- Apathy: others may be indifferent to events around them, less interested in interacting with people, or speak less spontaneously. Day-time dozing is common. Apathy may represent depression.
- Disinhibition: (e.g. making inappropriate comments to others), is commoner and people with dementia may make impulsive and reckless decisions. People may get very irritable with carers and attack them.
- Irritability and aggression: the person with dementia can become irritable, impatient, argumentative, or verbally or physically aggressive. Both internal and external factors cause this. While some may have always been short-tempered, others might be in pain, uncomfortable, frightened, psychotic, or depressed. Others are just poorly cared for (e.g. being spoken to in a patronizing way).
- Sleep–wake cycle disturbances: it is common for people with dementia to have disturbed sleep–wake cycles, e.g. they will sleep during the day and be wide awake at night. As a result some try to leave the house or do daytime chores even in the middle of the night.
- Change in eating habits: people with dementia usually lose their appetite (also seen in depression) and weight loss is common. Overeating is less common. Food preferences may change (e.g. wanting sweeter foods may signal frontal impairment). Hyperphagia (putting too much food into one's mouth) occurs in some people with severe frontal lobe damage.

Functional impairment

Daily living skills become impaired. This starts with the most complex and least often used skills (e.g. managing investments, cooking a complex meal) and slowly spreads to day-to-day tasks (e.g. managing household bills, shopping), and then basic skills (e.g. dressing, finding the toilet etc.).

Personality change

Relatives and spouses often note changes in personality. Changes in behaviour, habits, flattening of affect, and irritability at not being recognized are some of the most difficult symptoms for them to cope with.

Types of dementia

There are various ways of classifying dementias, each of varying utility depending on the context in which the term is being used.

Genetic

Most dementias are *sporadic* with no obvious inheritance patterns. Rarely, dementia is an inherited (and inheritable) genetic condition, e.g. Huntingdon's disease (autosomal dominant) and some pedigrees of young-onset AD. People with Down's syndrome usually develop AD in middle age because they have an extra copy of the gene that codes for the protein thought to cause dementia (🕮 Chapter 3). Most dementias have much more complex causes, with minor inheritable risk factors playing a small part (most commonly having two copies of the ApOε4 gene).

Primary and secondary dementias

If the mechanism by which an illness causes damage is neurodegeneration, e.g. in AD, the resultant dementia is a *primary* dementia. If the dementia is part of a broader illness where the neurodegeneration is a consequence of a broader disease process, the syndrome is a *secondary* dementia, e.g. vitamin deficiencies, brain tumour.

Late and early onset ('pre-senile') dementias

This is an arbitrary definition based on whether or not dementia has started before or after the age of 65 years (which is a rather outdated administrative threshold for 'old age' to start).

Differentiation by brain area

Dementias can also be characterized by the site of the main brain pathology.

Cortical dementias involve the cerebral cortex. Some areas of the cortex may be damaged earlier or more severely than others, e.g. AD, frontotemporal dementias. The symptoms produced are specific to the cortical areas affected.

Subcortical dementias involve the 'deep' structures underneath the cortex. These dementias involve only minor memory loss but instead have more pronounced slowing of thought processes, lowered mood, and movement disorders. Parkinson's dementia is an example.

Cortico-subcortical dementias are a mixture of both cortical and subcortical types; symptoms are a mixture of the two, e.g. DLB.

Multifocal dementias have multiple discrete areas of the brain involved, e.g. CJD. The symptoms depend on the area of the brain affected.

Differentiation by pathology

Different symptom clusters may suggest particular types of dementia, which can help predict progression, prognosis, and treatment. Some types overlap considerably (e.g. VaD and AD). Some types have important clinical consequences, e.g. neuroleptic drugs in DLB may be lethal.

AD (🕮 Chapters 4, 10, and 12)

AD causes 40–60% of dementia. It is rare before the age of 45 and is much commoner after age 75. A family history is found in up to 50% of those developing AD by age 90, but the interplay of genetics and environment is complex. Symptoms are seen earlier where Alzheimer's and vascular pathology co-exist.

Pathology

The main pathological features are *plaques* and *tangles*.
- Plaques are abnormal accumulations of a protein (β-amyloid) surrounded by inflammatory debris.
- Tangles are composed of tau protein resulting from the destruction of intracellular tubules.

Abnormal accumulation of β-amyloid appears to initiate brain cell death. Cell loss occurs most in areas associated with memory (initially the hippo-campus) and those which produce neurotransmitters linked to memory (ACh etc.). There is loss of cortical tissue, with a reduction in the brain tissue in the folds of the brain (gyri) and an enlargement of the gaps in the folds (sulci). Apart from the hippocampus, the frontal, temporal, and parietal lobes, and the nucleus of Meynert are most affected. These areas play important parts in memory, behaviour, and decision-making, association, language, and spatial orientation.

Risk factors (see 🕮 Chapter 2, What is dementia?, p. 14)

Clinical features and course (see 🕮 Chapter 2, Symptoms of dementia, pp. 15–19).
- Typically starts insidiously, progresses gradually. It is often difficult for relatives to remember a definite start to the symptoms.
- Functional stages of dementia (🕮 Chapter 4, Staging systems, pp. 58–62).
- Time course for dementia is 2.5–12 years from diagnosis, with an average of about 4.5 years.

Diagnosis
- Requires a careful history from the patient and a collateral history from a reliable informant, and at least a simple memory test.
- Tests (e.g. blood biochemistry, brain computed tomography (CT) scan) should be done to exclude other causes. Generally:
  - CT scan shows general shrinkage, enlarged ventricles, and prominent brain sulci.
  - Magnetic resonance imaging (MRI) scan shows similar findings. Can pick up shrinkage of the hippocampus and medial temporal lobe.
  - Single photon emission computed tomography (SPECT) scanning using 99mTc-HMPAO (Tc-hexamethylpropyleneamine oxime) shows a global decrease of perfusion that is more prominent in the fronto-parietal lobe.
  - New developments include detection of hyperphosporlyated τ-protein or β-amyloid protein in CSF and visualization of amyloid in the brain using a specific marker by PET scanning.

Treatment

Management is both pharmacological and non-pharmacological. There is growing awareness that the way we treat people with dementia has an enormous influence on symptomatology and behaviour, as well as the progression of impairment (🕮 Chapter 17). Rehabilitative approaches, the use of appropriate technology, informed care, and a number of other therapies are also important (🕮 Chapters 11, 20, and 23).

Current specific pharmacological treatments (see Box) aim to improve memory in two ways:
- Acetylcholinesterase inhibitors (AChEIs) stop the breakdown of ACh, the neurotransmitter associated with memory. These drugs only help memory in about 30–40% of cases. There are associated benefits in other non-cognitive areas which relatives and carers often value highly.
- Glutamate blockade: memantine blocks the action of low levels of glutamate (usually released by damaged and dying cells) at the hippocampus but allows larger physiological levels of glutamate to act. It also helps in other cognitive and non-cognitive areas.

Promising treatments for AD in development include attempts to stop amyloid protein aggregation or to remove it. Symptomatic treatments are crucial and are described elsewhere.

Drugs for AD

AChEIs—donepezil, galantamine, rivastigmine

AChEIs are indicated in early and moderate AD to slow down or reverse memory loss. Over 6 months of use, a third of patients show improvement, a third stay stable, and another third deteriorate despite the medication. The National Institute for Health and Clinical Excellence (NICE) has recently accepted that these drugs improve function and global condition but not behaviour, although the behavioural results for galantamine are mixed. There are some data suggestive of longer-term benefit but this remains to be confirmed. NICE also noted an Alzheimer's Society survey of users and carers who also felt that these drugs made patients 'happier, brighter, more aware and more active …calmer and less aggressive …more independent and taking care of personal needs'. This survey is of course unblinded and unrandomized, carried out in the face of NICE resistance to funding such drugs in early dementia at the time.

Adverse effects are mainly gastrointestinal (GI; nausea, diarrhoea, vomiting), insomnia, headache, dizziness and high blood pressure (b.p.). AChEIs are metabolized by cytochrome P450 (CYP450) enzymes and are prone to interactions through this (📖 Appendix 2).

Memantine

Indicated for moderate to severe cognitive impairment. NICE accepts that memantine produced global improvement at 6 months; a slowing down in functional loss (Functional Assessment Staging (FAST) Scale); some improvement in cognitive performance at 3 months, not maintained at 6 months; but no effect on behavioural difficulties.

The main adverse effects are dizziness, hypertension, and constipation. There is a theoretical potential for interactions with other N-methyl d-aspartate (NMDA) receptor antagonists (📖 Chapter 8, Adjuvant analgesics, pp. 126–131). More important is the possibility of interaction with other drugs that share the same renal tubular secretion mechanism, such as cimetidine, ranitidine, metformin, quinidine, and some diuretics.

VaD

This is the second commonest form of dementia, affecting 25–40% of people with dementia. VaD is most commonly multi-infarct.

Pathology
Brain cells die due to lack of oxygen (ischaemia). Cell death can be diffuse or focal, and progression can be acute (e.g. following an infarct) or chronic and slow. The commonest cause is multiple small thrombi or emboli.

Risk factors
Are those associated with cardiovascular disease, e.g. ischaemic heart disease, high blood cholesterol, diabetes, smoking, peripheral vascular disease, cardiac arrhythmias, hypertension, and increased blood viscosity.

Clinical features and course
VaD presents more variably than AD. Certain features may be commoner, though it really can be quite hard to differentiate VaD from AD clinically. Suggestive signs include:
• Sudden onset and periodic exacerbations.
• Step-wise deterioration, i.e. clinical plateaus followed by sudden declines which when put on a graph look like steps.
• Worsening confusion at night (called 'sundowning').
• Some preservation of cognitive areas.
• Slower thinking processes.
• Depression.
• Emotional lability (laughter or tearfulness without any apparent trigger and without concomitant prolonged alterations of mood).
• Focal neurological signs and symptoms.
• Cardiovascular risk factors.
• The prognosis is poorer and even harder to predict than in AD.
• Death from stroke or a heart attack is commoner.

Other types of vascular dementia
• Binswanger's disease (also known as lacunar dementia, progressive subcortical vascular encephalopathy) results from multiple infarcts of the subcortical areas (seen on MRI scan). There is a more subcortical picture with mild pyramidal signs (asymmetrical reflexes), hemiparesis, rigidity, limb and gait ataxia and pseudobulbar palsy (dysarthria, dysphagia, mood lability). Depression and other psychiatric symptoms may be found. Modern imaging techniques are picking up more cases.
• CADASIL (cerebral autosomal dominant arteriopathy with subcortical infarcts and leukoencephalopathy) is a rare familial form of pre-senile VaD.

Differentiation from AD
This is hard, especially where ischaemic damage is slow and diffuse, with insidious onset of symptoms. Brain imaging may show extensive ischaemia. VaD may still respond to cholinesterase inhibitors.

Severe cognitive deficits occasionally follow a single major stroke. However, many go on to have other strokes (even if not major) and may develop a progressive cognitive decline.

Diagnosis
Diagnosis is made from a careful history, physical examination, and brain imaging (CT or MRI). Carotid Doppler studies are occasionally useful, as are echocardiograms. There are no clear diagnostic criteria agreed for VaD because it has such varied pathology and subtypes have not been clearly defined.

Treatment
- Treatment is really secondary prevention, designed to prevent a recurrence of the strokes and minimize their effects.
- Improve circulation: treat arrhythmias, give aspirin and other antiplatelet drugs.
- Treat hypertension, high blood cholesterol, and optimize diabetic control.
- Maintain general health: avoid dehydration, balanced diet, sustainable levels of exercise.

Mixed dementia
Most dementias are probably a mixture of VaD and AD type dementias.

DLB
This form of dementia (10–20% of all cases) is fairly common and contains features of both Parkinson's disease (PD) and AD. Patients with DLB are at risk from worsening illness or death from the use of antipsychotic medication.

Pathology
- DLB is one of the synucleinopathies in which there is an accumulation of aggregates of the protein α-synuclein. These diseases include PD, multisystem atrophy (MSA), and pure autonomic failure.
- The key pathological feature is cortical Lewy bodies. Lewy bodies comprise α-synuclein and ubiquitin (a cell stress protein) in brainstem nuclei, substantia nigra, paralimbic, and cortical areas.
- The substantia nigra is depleted of cells and dopamine as in PD. There are plaques in similar numbers to AD but fewer tangles.
- Vascular pathology occurs in about 30% of cases.
- Shrinkage of the brain is particularly prominent in the temporal lobe, parietal lobe, and the cingulate gyrus.

Risk factors
No known risk factors; age of onset can be as early as 50.

Clinical features and course
- Memory: many patients initially complain of poor short-term memory but this is initially mild (unless complicated by depression or fluctuating consciousness). Depression may aggravate the severity of the memory problem, the bradykinesis (slow movement), and bradyphrenia.
- Bradyphrenia (slowness of thinking) may be a prominent feature of DLB. It may present as an ability to get there answer right, but taking a long time to get.
- Word-finding and visuospatial difficulties occur early.
- Executive dysfunction is more prominent and earlier in DLB than in AD, with mental inflexibility, indecisiveness, and lack of judgment. This can be tested easily using neuropsychological tests such as the trail-finding test.
- Fluctuations in consciousness: occur from minute to minute. Inattention and unresponsiveness for up to several minutes may mimic transient ischaemic attacks (TIAs). This is thought to occur because of a sudden loss of ACh production.

- Visual hallucinations are prominent and typically complex and detailed, e.g. animals, people. Patients often realize that they are not real, but more rarely the content is distressing. Care must be taken not to blame all hallucinations on DLB. Visual hallucinations can occur in AD and VaD where they are fragmentary. They can also be caused by dopaminergic drugs like levodopa in people with PD. These need to be distinguished from visual hallucinations and illusions found in delirium (e.g. caused by strokes or TIAs).
- Parkinsonian symptoms may develop after the first symptoms of dementia are present, or may precede the cognitive symptoms. People with DLB may have a flexed posture, shuffling gait, reduced arm swing when walking, bradykinesia (slow movement), and bradyphrenia (slowness of thinking). Tremor is rarer than in PD.
- Falls are increased due to both autonomic and cognitive dysfunction.
- Spontaneous muscle twitching (myoclonus) is common, mild, and widespread and can be mistaken for the myoclonus of CJD (📖 Chapter 3, Main types of YOD, pp. 40–46).
- Sensitivity to neuroleptic drugs: dopamine-blocking neuroleptic drugs have a disproportionately severe parkinsonism effect; cognitive decline and death may be accelerated. Due to concerns over the mortality of antipsychotics in DLB, NICE has recommended the use of memantine for those with severe behavioural and psychological symptoms of DLB.
- Progression is steady and fairly quick.

Diagnosis
The agreed diagnostic criteria require two of the following:
- fluctuating consciousness
- recurrent visual hallucinations and
- spontaneous Parkinsonian symptoms (i.e. not due to drug treatment).

Supportive features include falls, neuroleptic sensitivity, and non-visual hallucinations.
  DLB must be distinguished from AD, VaD, PD, psychotic depression, and rarer neurological illnesses like progressive supranuclear palsy (PSP) and MSA:
- CT and MRI scans show relative sparing of the medial temporal lobe and peri-ventricular white matter lesions (hyperintensities) may be prominent.
- SPECT scanning using 99mTc-HMPAO (binds to glucose) shows a global decrease of perfusion more prominent in the occipital lobe.
- Even more useful is SPECT scanning using FPCT [2β-carbomethoxy-3β-(4-chlorophenyl)-8-(-3-fluoropropyl) nortropane; binds to dopamine]—there is reduced uptake in the putamen and caudate nuclei (like PD).

Treatment
- There is substantial evidence that AChEIs, e.g. rivastigmine, are very effective in quite a few DLB cases, restoring the balance between ACh and dopamine so inattention, agitation, and hallucinations are decreased.
- As there is a need to avoid neuroleptics, antidepressants and benzodiazepines are more useful. The latter help in myoclonus (📖 Chapter 9, Neurological symptoms, pp. 163–166).

- Cautious use of antiparkinsonian dopamine-enhancing drugs (e.g. co-careldopa) will often help parkinsonian symptoms, and a higher dose can be used if combined with AChEIs.
- Dopamine agonists are very likely to worsen hallucinations and should be avoided.

Frontotemporal dementias (Pick's disease)
Fairly common in the elderly, but one of the commoner dementias in younger people (📖 Chapter 3, Main types of YOD, pp. 40–46).

HIV-associated dementia
Most commonly occurs in younger people (📖 Chapter 3, Main types of YOD, pp. 40–46).

Transmissible spongiform encephalopathies (prion diseases) and CJD
These are discussed with dementias in younger people (📖 Chapter 3, Main types of YOD, pp. 40–46).

PSP
PSP is an illness which, though related to PD, can be very difficult to differentiate from other neurodegenerative diseases as its early symptoms are non-specific and later progress is variable between individuals.

- Early symptoms include fatigue, headaches, dizziness, difficulty walking and balancing (including backwards falls), depression, mild personality changes, memory problems, and pseudobulbar symptoms (dysphagia, dysarthria, dysphonia, and labile affect). These symptoms may last years and are easily misdiagnosed.
- Later symptoms are numerous but still very variable and include:
  - Gaze palsy: the patient cannot look down on command but the eyes move down when the head is tilted. This is not always present.
  - Eye symptoms: difficulties in opening and closing eyelids, blurred vision, a slow rate of blink (leading to dry eyes), tunnel vision, light sensitivity.
  - Swallowing difficulties, leading to the risk of aspiration pneumonia.
  - Motor difficulties: muscle dystonias (including a mask-like facial expression), impaired handwriting, parkinsonian motor symptoms (bradykinesia).
  - Memory problems: memory loss is mild but aggravated by slow mental processes (bradyphrenia) and initiation, sequencing, and planning difficulties.
- The disease responds poorly to levodopa.
- People become immobile in the later stages and death is within 6 years of onset, usually from infections.

Cortico-basilar degeneration (CBD)
Similar to PSP, though rarer, but cognitive symptoms predominate. Limb rigidity is less symmetrical and control of limb movements may be so difficult that some patients feel as if they have no control (so-called 'alien limb').

Huntington's disease
Discussed in Chapter 3 (📖 Chapter 3, Main types of YOD, pp. 40–46).

What is *not* dementia?

Dementia could be confused with other conditions. However, some of these conditions can co-exist with dementia.

Delirium (📖 Chapter 10, Delirium, pp. 174–177)

- Delirium is a response of the brain to a stress which overwhelms its capacity to function well.
- It is more common in people with dementia and serious physical illnesses.
- It carries increased morbidity and mortality.
- Delirium commonly arises quickly (hours to days) and tends to fluctuate during the course of the day. Less commonly it can last longer.

Clinical features

- Impaired cognition (memory deficits, disorientation).
- Impaired consciousness (awareness of the environment).
- Impaired attention and concentration (the ability to focus on aspects of the environment and avoid distraction).
- Abnormal perceptions: the person experiences fragmentary and changeable
  - illusions
  - hallucinations
  - imagery—memories or dreams which cannot be distinguished from reality.
- Abnormal thinking (muddled thinking as manifested in speech).
- Abnormal behaviour (can be any mixture of *hyperactive* or *hypoactive* as described below).
- Disturbed sleep–wake cycle (daytime sleepiness and night agitation).

Disorientation to time, fluctuating consciousness, and distorted thinking and speech are key features. Delirium and dementia are hard to tell apart, and so it is important that medical causes of reversible confusion are always looked for in people with dementia who are unwell.

Types of delirium

Hyperactive delirium is manifest by agitation, over-alertness, irritability, agitation, easy distractibility, and tangential, rambling speech. Patients with *hypoactive delirium*, in contrast, are lethargic and unresponsive, with sparse slow speech. These patients are less often noticed, but are no less unwell. Hypoactive delirium is probably the more common form and is sometimes mistaken for depression.

Causes of delirium

The brain is susceptible to a number of physical stressors. If these exceed the brain's coping capacity, delirium can result. Older brains with more injury or disease are more vulnerable. Common stressors include:

- Infection: even minor infections, e.g. cellulitis, can cause a delirium if the person is susceptible. The commonest causes are urinary and respiratory tract infections and blood infections (septicaemia).
- Drug side-effects: commonest with drugs which interfere with cholinergic activity (such as antiparkinsonian drugs, atropine), antipsychotics, benzodiazepines (such as temazepam), opioid analgesics.

- Surgery: recovery from the surgery itself as well as the anaesthetic.
- Stroke and brain injury.
- Hypoxia: due to heart or lung failure or anaemia.
- Organ failure: such as kidney, liver, lung, heart.
- Metabolic disturbances: disturbances in electrolytes (such as sodium, potassium, calcium), malnutrition and dehydration as well as hypo- or hyperglycaemia.
- Endocrine disorders: disorders of thyroid, parathyroid, glucose metabolism.

The syndrome may be alleviated by helping the person to make sense of their environment, and it is useful to consider:

- Poor lighting.
- Unfamiliar environments.
- Sensory impairments.
- Pain, discomfort, immobility.
- Tiredness.

Note that given a severe enough brain stressor, even healthy brains become delirious. Conversely with a severely diseased brain, even minor stressors can cause delirium. People who have recovered from delirium have fragmentary memories of the event.

Prognosis

Recovery from delirium is slower than usually thought, and may take months. The prognosis is often poor with incomplete recovery frequently being seen[2].

Depression (📖 Chapter 10, Depression, pp. 178–184)

In clinical use the term depression denotes a severe and prolonged low mood and associated behavioural and cognitive features. It is important in the context of dementia and palliative care because:

- It is very common at any time during the course of a dementing illness (i.e. the two can co-exist, especially with VaD).
- It may mimic dementia and thus lead to misdiagnosis of dementia.
- It may be the first sign of a dementing illness or a serious physical illness such as cancer.
- It is treatable and distressing.
- It is common in dementia.

Table 2.2 compares depression and dementia.

If in doubt always check for any underlying physical illness and treat for depression as the symptoms of low mood can be helped and will make any underlying dementia clearer.

Vascular depression

Vascular lesions in the brain are associated with depression. It is thought that these lesions play a part in causing or aggravating depression. 'Vascular depression' has been postulated as the association between extensive subcortical ischaemic lesions and the first onset of depression after the age of 50. The causative link has not been proven. Many late-onset depressive illnesses progress to dementia.

---

2 Adamis D, Treloar A, Martin F, Macdonald A (2006) Recovery and outcome of delirium in elderly medical inpatients. Arch Gerontol Geriatr **43**, 289–98.

Table 2.2 Main differences between depression and dementia

Depression occurring without dementia	Dementia complicated by depression
Memory problems start *after* the onset of low mood	Memory problems start *before* the onset of low mood
Start of illness tends to be more precisely recognized	Onset of illness usually is more insidious and difficult to pinpoint except in retrospect
Short duration of illness (months)	Longer duration of illness (years)
Low mood sometimes worse in morning	Low mood usually constant
Anhedonia (loss of enjoyment)	Flat affect (unresponsive to events) may mimic this
During questioning testing subject does not make an effort, often saying 'I don't know'	During questioning makes an effort and confabulates or becomes very upset if fails to answer or remember
Tends to be self-critical	Can blame others
Orientation normal	Disorientation
Early morning wakening	Nocturnal exacerbation of confusion
Past history of depression throughout life	No or recent history of depression
Memory problems both for recent and distant memories and may selectively remember upsetting memories	Temporal gradient (recent memories lost first and worst) and no emotional filtering of memories
Delusions and hallucinations in severe illness with themes of worthlessness, derogatory towards person	Hallucinations more often bizarre and may not be derogatory towards person

Amnestic syndromes

These are syndromes of non-progressive memory impairment caused by specific medical conditions or substances. Memory impairment may be permanent and severe, so from the point of view of palliative care these can be managed as a dementia. Several syndromes are of relevance:

Alcohol-related dementia (📖 Chapter 10, Delirium, pp. 174–177)
Alcohol is neurotoxic, and chronic and heavy drinking will cause memory impairment both directly and because of other factors like poor nutrition and head injury. There is no clear syndrome with global cognitive impairment including memory, concentration, and executive functions. *Korsakoff's syndrome* is the result of brain damage to specific areas of the brain and presents as a fixed retrograde amnesia (i.e. memory loss up to a particular point in time) and anterograde amnesia (inability to lay down

new memories). If alcohol is stopped, progression may be arrested and some improvement may even be seen over years.

Cerebrovascular disease

Infarcts and haemorrhages in the brain can cause significant and extensive cognitive impairment depending on the size and location of the lesion.

Head injury

Cognitive impairment can be caused by brain damage due to direct traumatic injury, hypoxia, and toxins. The degree and pattern of impairment will depend on the insult, the location of the injury, and the volume of brain tissue affected.

Case study

Patsy, a 74-year-old woman with AD, was referred by her dementia care nursing home as she was refusing to eat and drink, losing weight rapidly, and had gone from fully mobile to bed bound within weeks. The general practitioner (GP) had recently stopped her regular diazepam as she was sleeping during the day. He could find no swallowing impairment.

On assessment Patsy appeared very frightened and anxious and was able to answer few questions. She said she felt something sticking in her throat, which hurt, but due to poor short-term memory could not remember for how long, or if this happened when swallowing. Her daughter-in-law reported that she often complained of abdominal pain. Patsy's nurse had not been aware of any pain or discomfort, but had not asked Patsy about this. There were no oral infections, ulcers, dental problems, or dysphagia.

Further questioning of the nurse and relative revealed that Patsy had a long-standing anxiety problem and had been on regular diazepam for several years. She was often anxious and tearful. She had become too frightened to sleep in her own room at night, often spent nights awake, sleeping on an off during the day to make up. Patsy appeared low in mood, with a flat affect and no eye contact.

The palliative care nurse specialist suggested that Patsy should have a psychiatric review. Meanwhile she was started on regular paracetamol for pain and fluconazole for pharyngeal thrush. A laxative was started for her undiagnosed constipation.

Psychiatric review next day diagnosed a paranoid, agitated depression with some degree of diazepam withdrawal. Diazepam was restarted once daily and p.r.n. (as needed), with an antidepressant. Mood, anxiety, appetite, sleep, and mobility improved after about 4 weeks; she put on weight and was again able to sleep in her own room.

Clearly Patsy's physical deterioration was not due to dementia progression, as first thought, but to undetected mental health problems.

Beyond the medical model

The 'medical model' of illness has been powerful in understanding illnesses and their treatment. It postulates that a characteristic set of physical changes to the body occur together and constitute an illness with a characteristic set of symptoms, signs, and course. By recognizing this pattern one can treat the illness. With more complex morbidity such as mental illness, chronic disease, and dementia, however, it has limitations. It is simplistic to attribute all the effects of dementia to brain disease. Society's management of people with dementia, to which the medical model has contributed significantly, greatly amplifies the impact of the illness on individuals (📖 Chapter 17). Some indeed describe dementia in these terms, eschewing the medical model altogether. The immense challenges for carers are described in 📖 Chapters 21 and 22.

Key components of the care process

Dementia is complex, changing, and its effects profound and far-reaching. The focus of care should be about improving the quality of life for the patient and their family, by treating the illness itself but also by helping the person and their family keep their voice and as much dignity, choices, and control over their lives as possible.

Treatment of the illness

- Diagnosis should be as early as possible, and communicated to the patient and their family, to allow for planning for the future.
- Assessment should be comprehensive, holistic, and continue throughout the illness.
- Treatment should be multimodal (i.e. not just with drugs) and aims to:
  - delay progression, e.g. by drugs , mental, and social activities
  - maximize function, e.g. work with personal strengths (📖 Chapter 17)
  - minimize impairment, e.g. provide aids and adaptations (📖 Chapter 11)
  - treat positive symptoms, e.g. depression, hallucinations (📖 Chapter 10).

Management of the person and the family

The key to managing the whole person is to provide

- Appropriate, timely, and relevant information about all aspects of dementia, services, benefits, etc. (📖 Chapters 16 and 24).
- Choices about current and future treatments (e.g. whether or not they want a particular drug or resuscitation) (📖 Chapter 18).
- Counselling to the patient and to their family to deal with the emotional trauma of the illness and its consequences (📖 Chapter 16).
- Provide breaks from caring for the family (respite) (📖 Chapter 22).
- Practical advice on day-to-day issues, e.g. benefits (📖 Chapter 24).
- Connection to a bigger support network, e.g. local day centres, groups.
- A connection to other services and agencies as and when needed.
- Advocacy for when the patient's or family's voice is not being heard.
- Provision of a physical environment that assists independence and selfhood (📖 Chapter 11).

The professionals

Many professional disciplines are involved in dementia care. Most operate within multidisciplinary teams. The composition of such teams varies, especially in different countries. Regardless of who delivers the care, cooperation with other professionals in a team is the best way to deliver good care.

The old-age psychiatrist

A doctor trained and specializing in the mental health of older people with particular expertise in:
- Psychiatric assessment, diagnosis, and treatment of psychiatric symptoms using drugs, and often psychological treatments.
- Behavioural and psychiatric symptoms of dementia and depression.
- Risk management, mental health legislation, and assessment of mental capacity.
- Clinical leadership to old-age psychiatry teams.

The geriatrician

A doctor trained in the medical care of older people with particular expertise in:
- Physical assessment, diagnosis, and treatment of physical illness, especially neurological disease.
- Treating delirium and dementia.
- Treating people with advanced or terminal physical disease.
- In some countries, e.g. in Australia and New Zealand, uncomplicated dementia is dealt with primarily by geriatricians.

The neurologist

A doctor trained in assessing and treating neurological illness with particular expertise in:
- Assessing and diagnosing dementia in younger people.
- Neurological assessment and treatment of neurological disease.

In some countries, such as Germany, a neurologist takes the lead in diagnosing and treating people with dementia.

The district nurse/long-term matron

District nurses (DNs) and long-term matrons have a central role to play in the ongoing care of those with dementia, and will be especially good at assessing physical need and solutions to physical and practical difficulties. Many will also be able to manage mental symptoms well, though they are also likely to need the support of others.

The psychiatric nurse

Specialist psychiatric nurses are key professionals in dementia care. Some nurses are specialized in dementia care and some can prescribe medication. They have training and experience in medicine and often psychological treatments but primarily try to improve or maintain optimal health and quality of life. They provide expertise in:
- Assessment and diagnosis of dementia.
- Monitoring and follow-up of patients and carers.

- Personal care and support to people with dementia.
- Some psychological treatments, e.g. cognitive behavioural therapies.
- Advocacy, outreach, and liaison.

The clinical psychologist

Psychologists are clinicians trained to study the human mind including cognition and behaviour. They do not have medical training but have other considerable expertise in dementia care including:

- Cognitive testing (if specialized in this they are called neuropsychologists) to help with the screening, assessment, and diagnosis of dementias.
- Advice on maximizing function and minimizing impairment in dementia.
- Behavioural assessment and management of behavioural disturbances in dementia.
- Psychological therapies to support patients and carers.

The occupational therapist

A clinician trained to maximize a person's abilities in daily living, work, or leisure. Independence and a sense of well-being are achieved through:

- The restoration, preservation, and promotion of skills and confidence.
- The opportunity to perform meaningful and creative activities.
- The modification of the environment or provision of tools or aids to compensate for any deficits.

They have expertise in and will advise upon

- Assessment of existing skills and abilities.
- Modifying environments to maximize functioning and minimize risk.
- Organizing and monitoring meaningful activities tailored to the person's individual needs and personality.
- The appropriate place of care (e.g. home/residential/nursing care).

Occupational therapists are taking a lead in developing intelligent sensors and networks which monitor the activities of people with dementia living at home by themselves. These sensors allow risky behaviour to be monitored and addressed as they happen and allow more people to live at home for longer (see 📖 Chapter 11, Physical disabilities, pp. 212–220).

The social worker

A specialist trained in social models of disability and deprivation. Social workers have been at the forefront in moving dementia care beyond the medical model and understanding dementia in a social context. Within the dementia team social workers take a leading role in:

- Assessing and reinforcing formal and informal social support networks.
- Assessing, advising, and advocating for patients and their families of their rights to financial help and benefits.
- Advising and guiding patients and families about options for residential care and home care.
- Devising and monitoring packages of home care services for individuals.
- Investigating suspected cases of abuse involving older people.

The speech and language therapist

A clinician trained in the assessment and treatment of disorders affecting speech and swallowing. They are essential in assessing speech and swallowing in later stages of dementia and help to minimize the risk of dysphagia and to enhance communication when speech is impaired.

The physiotherapist

A clinician specializing in the enhancement, restoration, and preservation of functioning and well-being through manipulation, mobilization techniques, and prescribing strengthening exercises. They have a role in the later stages of dementia when immobility and imbalance are starting to have an effect.

The GP or family doctor

A central component of good dementia care. Although not usually a member of a dementia care team, the GP will be the first port of call when worries about memory or behaviour emerge. GPs will screen and medically investigate people with failing memories before referring them to a specialist for diagnosis. They will often also start treatments for depression. Once a diagnosis is made, GPs work closely with dementia care teams to continue supporting patients and their families even when people move into residential care. A lot of palliative care in patient's and residential homes is provided by GPs.

The specialist palliative care physicians and nurses

These ought to be involved in the care of at least some people with advanced dementia, especially where there is ongoing distress and symptom control is challenging. Perhaps they also ought to be more often involved where distress appears to be due to physical pain more than mental distress.

Further reading

Baldwin C, Capstick A (eds) (2007) *Tom Kitwood on dementia: a reader and critical commentary*, annotated edn. Open University Press, Maidenhead.

UK Department of Health (2009) *Living well with dementia—a national dementia strategy*. Department of Health, London.

Various authors (2008) Clinical aspects of dementia. In Jacoby R, Openheimer C, Dening T, Thomas A (eds) *Oxford textbook of old age psychiatry*, pp. 417–504. Oxford University Press, Oxford.

Young-onset dementia (YOD)

Introduction

YOD refers to dementia with an onset before the age of 65. It is rare but presents major challenges. AD represents only 30% of all YODs, including some cases with a strong autosomal dominant inheritance. There is a broader range of conditions that cause dementia in the young, which may be difficult to diagnose. Clinical features, and other effects of the illness, may be different from the effects in older people, both in terms of the dementia itself and its effect on the person with dementia, family, and carers. A dementia affecting someone in their 40s or 50s will have a profound effect on their own and their spouse's employment and financial situation as well as on their family life. Furthermore, YOD often presents with more behavioural problems in fitter, healthier people, increasing the burden of caring. In 2002, the Alzheimer's Society estimated that there were about 18,500 younger people with dementia in the UK.

Epidemiology and implications for management

The epidemiology of YOD is summarized in Table 3.1.

Table 3.1 Epidemiology of YOD (onset 30–64 years)

YOD	Prevalence/100,000	Proportion of total (%)
AD	21.7	30
VaD	10.9	15
Frontotemporal lobar degenerations	9.3	13
Alcohol-related dementia	8.3	12
DLB	6	8
Huntington's disease	4.7	6
Dementia in multiple sclerosis	4.1	6
Dementia in Down's syndrome	1.6	3
CBD	1.0	2
Prion disease	1.0	
Dementia in PD	1.0	
Dementia due to carbon monoxide poisoning	0.5	
Other causes	4.1	

Reproduced from Sampson EL, Warren JD, Rossor MN (2004) Young Onset Dementia. *Postgrad Med J* **80**, 125–39, with permission from BMJ Publishing Group Ltd.

Characteristics which distinguish younger from older people with dementia

People with YODs
• Are more likely to have an unusual cause for their dementia.
• Are often aware that something is wrong and feel more powerless and frustrated.
• Are often initially misdiagnosed, most commonly with depression.
• Tend to decline at a faster rate.
• Are usually physically more fit and active.
• Are more often in employment and bearing financial responsibilities.
• Have dependant family members such as children.
• Have younger carers who are more often in employment.
• Do not fit easily into service configurations (adult, older mental health services, or neurology), presenting major management challenges.
• Will have to manage a wide range of responses from others to their diagnosis because their circumstances are so unusual.
• Are more likely to experience a lack of knowledge or understanding of YOD by the medical profession.
• May consequently find it difficult to access appropriate information and support, which can result in delay in diagnosis and reduced support.
• Often struggle at work, change jobs and fail again, ending up unemployed.
• May find that moving jobs will have jeopardized their sick pay and pension rights.
• Hopefully find that physicians are often more thorough and interventionist in diagnosis and treatment, as there is more potential for reversibility or improvement.

Special sensitivity and support is needed for people with YOD and their families. Teenagers may be faced with caring for a parent with dementia at a time when they expected to be forging their own lives. Carers, and young carers in particular, have a number of entitlements under the Carers' Act to a personal assessment of their own needs and support, but many professionals are not aware of these entitlements (□ Chapters 22 and 24).

Issues in diagnosis

In YOD potentially treatable conditions may be more common, including:
- Chronic subdural haematomas.
- Tumours.
- Inflammatory conditions.
- Infection.
- Normal pressure hydrocephalus.
- Encephalopathies.
- Autoimmune disorders, e.g. systemic lupus erythematosus (SLE), HIV.

However, a reversible cause of dementia is still found in only a small minority. Progressive forms of dementia are the norm. Some are familial including:
- Some cases of AD.
- Huntington's disease.
- Some cases of CJD.
- CADASIL.

These are detected more commonly, but remain very rare. These conditions can be particularly illuminating for research on the pathology of dementia.

Main types of YOD

AD

- Although still the commonest cause of dementia in this age group (see Table 3.1), only about 5–10% of all AD cases occur in younger people.
- Onset is often subtle, presenting with low mood, worry, and struggling to cope at work.
- Early treatment with antidepressants is common, but progression may be rapid and illness may have a relatively short course.
- Epilepsy is commoner in advanced stages than with older-onset AD (📖 Chapter 9, Neurological symptoms, pp. 163–166).
- Some affected people will have a strong family history. These account for less than 2% of all AD cases overall. Inheritance is autosomal dominant with strong penetrance, i.e. children of an affected parent will have a close to 50% risk of being affected. If an individual bears the abnormal gene, he or she will develop AD. The mutations responsible can be on
- Chromosome 21, causing abnormal amyloid precursor protein (APP) to be formed. This mutation may partly account for the increased risk of AD in people with Down's syndrome, who have trisomy of chromosome 21, where three chromosomes can produce amyloid.
- Chromosome 14, causing the abnormal protein presenilin 1 to be formed. Presenilin 1 is part of the enzymatic complex responsible for cleaving the β-amyloid peptide from APP. There are a large number of different mutations of the responsible gene; most have complete penetrance.
- Chromosome 1, causing the abnormal protein presenilin 2 to be formed. Again there are a number of possible mutations of the responsible gene, and again presenilin 2 is involved in APP metabolism, causing increased plaque deposition.

All three abnormalities will lead to abnormal excess formation of the 42-amino-acid form of β-amyloid peptide over the normal 40-peptide variety. This in turn is thought to set off biochemical cascades which result in neuronal damage and neurofibrillary tangles and senile plaque deposition.

Family members of some people affected by young-onset AD may be offered genetic testing. Predictive genetic testing for APP and presenilin abnormalities is available but should be coupled with appropriate counselling if contemplated. Family members have a right to know if they want to know, but equally their right to choose not to know must be respected.

Genetic testing is also possible for the ApOε4 gene, which can sometimes be a risk factor for AD. However, the association of this abnormality with the disease is much looser than the familial autosomal dominant AD, is not predictive, and testing is a much more ethically contentious matter. People with the abnormal gene might not develop AD, and people without it are still at risk of developing the illness.

AD in Down's syndrome

- AD is common in older people with Down's syndrome, 50% of whom now survive to age 60. The relationship between the two conditions is complex and has been the subject of much study.

- Down's syndrome is more common in families with a history of AD, and mothers who have children with Down's syndrome before the age of 35 (but not older mothers) run a five-fold risk of developing AD. It has also been suggested that mosaicism with trisomy 21 (where some cells in the body, but not all, have an extra chromosome 21, which is the defining feature of Down's syndrome) may account for some cases of Alzheimer's in later life.
- The neuropathological brain changes of AD are universal in all people with Down's syndrome by age 40. The clinical syndrome of AD occurs in 10–25% of people with Down's aged 40–49 years and in up to 75% of those aged over 60. Vascular disease, which is common in older people with Down's, also acts as a risk factor.
- The presence of AD shortens prognosis in Down's syndrome.
- The development of dementia may go unrecognized for some time as some of the deficits may be put down to the underlying learning disabilities (Table 3.2). A number of useful screening tools exist, such as the Dementia Scale for Downs Syndrome and the Dementia Questionnaire for Mentally Retarded Persons.
- Management of the dementia is along conventional lines. The need for environmental stability is even higher than with other people with dementia. If change is needed, as far as possible environmental changes should be gradual and frequent rather than sharp and infrequent.
- Remember that cataracts are common in older people with Down's syndrome, and impaired eyesight can compound the cognitive problems. Cataracts should be actively sought and serious thought given to whether correction is indicated. The same holds for other sensory deficits.

VaDs

VaDs (📖 Chapter 2, Types of dementia, pp. 20–26) are rarer. Some are caused by hypertension and hypercholesterolaemia with or without diabetes, others by vasculitides such as SLE and giant cell arteritis. If the cause of vasculopathy is treated, they may stabilize, allowing a longer course. Prevention of further vascular disease is important.

DLB (📖 Chapter 2, Types of dementia, pp. 20–26)
Frontotemporal dementias (Pick's disease)

This is a group of conditions with focal atrophy of the frontal and/or temporal lobes. Previously known as Pick's disease, this now refers to a pathological subtype of frontotemporal degeneration. There are three clinical syndromes:

- Frontotemporal lobar degeneration (FTLD), the most common type.
- Semantic dementia.
- Progressive non-fluent aphasia.

This description will focus on FTLD and the others will be discussed briefly.

Pathology

In FTLD there is bilateral shrinkage of the frontal and anterior temporal lobes. Most show spongiform degeneration of brain cells. A few cases show *Pick bodies* which are inclusions inside swollen brain cells. Pick bodies contain the protein tau (a component of tangles in AD). This variant is one of the tauopathies (which also includes PSP and CBD). Rarely, FTLD occurs as part of motor neuron disease (MND). A gene mutation on chromosome 17 causes some familial cases, but most cases seem sporadic.

Risk factors

There are no known risk factors except a positive family history.

Clinical features and course

- These often present without significant memory loss but have increasingly worsening organizational skills. In some, memory is well preserved until late in the illness, with the result that the diagnosis may be missed early on.
- A presentation of increasing personal chaos, untidiness at work, as well as personality change, irritability, and some depression ought to prompt consideration of this diagnosis.
- Affected individuals show a slow, insidious change in personality and behaviour:
  - Emotional blunting: emotions like embarrassment, fear, sadness, and pleasure are diminished.
  - Disinhibition: people react to any external event without any 'internal censorship' and there is little control over behaviour or speech. People are easily distracted, and may not see the effect they have on others.
  - Insight is impaired or absent.
  - Perseveration: thoughts, actions, and speech become 'stuck' and people cannot move on to other topics.
  - Dietary changes: a preference for sweet foods and in severe cases, hyperphagia to the point of stuffing food into their mouth and severe weight gain.
  - Dysexecutive changes: planning and sequencing (e.g. when cooking a meal or undertaking a journey) are impaired.
- Brain scans often (though not always) show frontal lobe atrophy.

Rare varieties of FTLD

Semantic dementia

This presents as breakdown in the knowledge base underlying language, so whilst the grammar and structure of words and sentences is intact, words become less specific and vague, e.g. 'the whatsit'. Orientation, visuospatial function, and memory are initially relatively well preserved. MRI scans show anterior temporal lobe atrophy worst on the left-hand side, and this is mirrored earlier by hypoperfusion in the same areas on SPECT 99mTc-HMPAO scanning.

Progressive non-fluent aphasia

This presents with selective language impairment where the structure of words and grammar break down and word production becomes difficult (e.g. stuttering, hesitant speech). People become mute in the middle stages. MRI scanning shows widening of the left sylvian fissures in the brain and SPECT HMPAO scanning shows poor perfusion around this area.

Treatment
- There is no specific treatment. AChEIs do not seem to help much and may increase agitation, but there may be some response to selective serotonin reuptake inhibitors (SSRIs) as they help with anxiety and compulsive behaviours. Higher doses may be tried.
- Sodium valproate and atypical neuroleptics may be needed for agitation and psychosis. These of course need to be coupled with behavioural approaches (📖 Chapter 10, Agitation and aggression, pp. 193–195)
- The marked behavioural and personality changes that occur early in FTLD may lead to earlier institutionalization than in those with late-onset disease.

Case study

Sally was 44 when her husband first noticed the change in her personality. Sally was a highly motivated businesswoman, who her husband describes as vivacious and funny. Initially, she seemed quite low in mood and less chatty. Her husband wondered if it was the pressure of her job and they talked about this but Sally did not think anything was wrong. Sally's manager also noticed her change in mood, motivation, and inability to complete her usual work. Her manager was worried about her and made an appointment for her to see the company doctor. An initial diagnosis of depression was made. The antidepressants seemed to help initially but her behaviour continued to change. She became quite rude to family and would make sexual advances to male friends. At work her manager noticed this behaviour and also that she could no longer plan her day and often missed appointments. This was very unusual for Sally and her manager made an appointment for her to see the doctor again. Following several reviews by the company doctor and changes in medication, a referral was made for her to see a neurologist. Following an MRI scan she was diagnosed with FTLD.

Transmissible spongiform encephalopathies (prion diseases) and CJD

- This group of illnesses is caused by prions, brain proteins whose role in normal brain functioning is as yet unclear.
- Normally soluble prion proteins can mutate into a folded insoluble form and in turn cause other prions to change into that folded form.
- Prion disease causes destruction of brain cells with the formation of the characteristic sponge cells.
- Prions can mutate spontaneously or be inherited (e.g. sporadic or familial CJD), or be transmitted by eating infected nervous tissue (kuru and new variant CJD).
- The prion disease that old-age psychiatrists and palliative care specialists are likely to meet is CJD. Other forms, such as fatal familial insomnia, are exceedingly rare.
- There are a number of forms of CJD:
  - Genetically inherited forms are very rare.
  - Sporadic CJD is uncommon, with 50–60 deaths every year in the UK.

- Variant CJD is probably linked to bovine spongiform encephalopathy (BSE) in cattle.
- Iatrogenic CJD is transmitted by medical or surgical procedures, most commonly in the UK via human growth hormone treatment, but also corneal transplants, neurosurgical procedures, etc.

Clinical features

- The illness progresses rapidly (death within 1 year, median 4 months) with loss of cortical signs and combinations of aphasia, visual impairment, behavioural and sleep disorders, autonomic problems, myoclonus, ataxia, and pyramidal signs.
- Clinical diagnosis can be supported by electroencephalogram (EEG), MRI and lumbar puncture which shows an elevated level of protein 14-3-3. However, this protein may also be raised in acute brain insults (e.g. herpes encephalitis, subarachnoid haemorrhage) or tumours (glioblastoma, paraneoplastic).
- A brain biopsy during life or at post-mortem is the only way to establish the diagnosis with certainty.
- Genetic testing is available to confirm the genetic variant (for families who want to know) but should be coupled with skilled counselling. The genetic form is very rare, and there is no means of prevention or treatment.
- Survival in variant CJD tends to be longer (often over a year compared with a few months in sporadic CJD).
- Variant CJD is more likely to present with psychobehavioural symptoms, while sporadic CJD tends to present with neurological features.
- AChIEs have not been shown to help and may increase agitation and extrapyramidal (rigidity, tremor, etc) and cerebellar signs (difficulty coordinating movement and balance).

HIV dementia

- Usually occurs in people who are symptomatic from HIV infection, although it may be the first AIDS-defining illness.
- The AIDS dementia complex (ADC) is not due to opportunistic infection but to an encephalopathy caused by the HIV virus itself. Infected monocytes and macrophages provoke damaging immunological reactions, e.g. via chemokines. HIV virus toxins cause further direct and indirect neuronal damage. This can be complicated by opportunistic infection, primary or metastatic brain tumours, vascular myelopathy, and adverse effects of some antiretrovirals.
- A lesser form, minor cognitive motor disorder (MCMD), with relatively little disturbance in ADL, is commoner than ADC since the advent of highly active antiretroviral therapy (HAART).
- Symptoms can be:
  - Mental (bradyphrenia or slow thought, apathy, poor concentration, memory loss, disorientation, anxiety and depression).
  - Motor (gait abnormalities, tremor, loss of balance and fine motor control, exaggerated reflexes and muscle tone).
  - Seizures.

- Cortical signs (apraxia, aphasia, and agnosia) are often absent, although dysphasias may sometimes occur and other cortical features may be found in the end stages.
- Progression is variable. In the terminal stages, profound dementia, aphasia, akinetic mutism, paraparesis, and double incontinence are common.
- Antiretroviral therapy can protect the patient from developing ADC and can in some cases partially or completely reduce the symptoms of ADC. Agents with high cerebrospinal fluid (CSF) penetration, e.g. lamivudine, nevirapine, and indinavir are preferred.
- Antidepressants and antipsychotics can be used to treat depression and psychotic symptoms, but sedation is fairly common.
- Psychostimulants such as methylphenidate (Ritalin) and dextroamphetamine (Dexedrine) have been used to improve attention, concentration, and psychomotor function. However, ADC is known to progress more rapidly in those with concurrent amphetamine abuse.

Huntington's disease

- This is a rare inherited disorder caused by an autosomal dominant gene encoding a protein called huntingtin. The resulting abnormal protein accumulates and destroys brain cells in the cortex and basal ganglia.
- The illness can start at any age and the larger the number of repeated gene sequences, the earlier the age of onset. The commonest age of onset is between the ages of 35 to 44 years.
- The illness lasts on average 20 years and death is commonly from pneumonia or cardiovascular disease. It presents with three main clusters of symptoms:
  - Movement symptoms: chorea (brief, non-repetitive, irregular muscle contractions which appear to flow from one muscle to the next). It starts with fidgeting and is sometimes disguised by the patient into pseudo-purposeful movements. It may be complicated by athetosis, which adds twisting and writhing movements. In later stages parkinsonian features (bradykinesia, rigidity, and postural instability) may emerge which develops into severe generalized spasticity.
  - Cognitive symptoms: there is a frontosubcortical syndrome. The frontal impairment presents as impaired verbal fluency, planning, and abstract thinking, and poor social functioning. The subcortical impairment presents as bradyphrenia and apathy. Memory and language are only mildly impaired at first.
  - Psychiatric symptoms: the main psychiatric complication is depression but this may be complicated by episodic mania (mimicking bipolar affective disorder). Other patients may become psychotic, or develop obsessive–compulsive disorders.
- Tetrabenazine may help the movement disorder and is indicated once the disorder is disabling or distressing. Side-effects include drowsiness, GI disturbances, depression, extrapyramidal dysfunction, and hypotension.

Table 3.2 Symptoms of dementia in Down's syndrome

Cognitive
- Forgetfulness of recent events (progressively long-term)
- Geographical disorientation
- Loss of previously learned skills
- Confusion

Affective
- Low mood
- Insomnia/hypersomnia
- Decreased concentration
- Aggression and irritability
- Anxiety and fearfulness
- Loss of interest and anergia

Behavioural
- Increased dependence
- Social isolation
- Excessive overactivity or restlessness
- Excessive uncooperativeness
- Personality change

Perceptual
- Hallucinations in any modality

Neurological
- Dysphasia leading to aphasia
- Agnosia
- Apraxia
- Gait disturbance
- Seizures
- Myoclonus
- Urinary incontinence
- Dystonias
- Loss of mobility

Reproduced from Stanton L, Coetzee RH (2004) Down's syndrome and dementia. *Adv Psychiatr Treat* **10**, 50–8, with permission.

Management of YOD

Medical

Thorough assessment of the dementia is essential. In view of the rather more medical and investigative approach, as well as the slightly higher possibility of finding reversible causes, YOD is more commonly seen by neurologists. Radiology and brain biopsies are utilized more frequently in diagnosis. Genetic advice and counselling may be required.

Best results will come from thorough assessment coupled with good counselling support and appropriate intervention. Management is, at its core, little different from that of later-onset dementia.

Social and legal implications

- The young age of people affected, often with young dependants and while holding down a job, has obvious financial and legal implications which need to be thought through carefully.
- Consider encouraging people with dementia to make a will.
- Those affected may also want to think about nominating a Lasting Power of Attorney (LPA), or put in place an advance statement of wishes. Be prepared to advise on the benefits and risks of advance refusals. Seek legal advice if required.
- Those in paid employment should consider the best time to give up work to maximize pension and entitlement to benefits. Changing work responsibilities may mean that they can stay in paid employment for longer.
- Driving may need to be given up early in the illness and will need to be handled sensitively. In the UK, Driver and Vehicle Licensing Agency (DVLA) guidance acknowledges that it is difficult to assess driving ability in those with dementia. The variable presentations and rates of progression are also acknowledged. In early dementia sufficient skills are retained and progression is slow, hence a licence may be issued subject to annual review. A formal driving assessment may be necessary. Poor short-term memory, disorientation, poor attention, and lack of insight and judgment are almost definite indications that the person is not fit to drive. Ideally it is the responsibility of the person affected by the illness to inform the DVLA who will then request medical reports and make a decision based on these. If the person refuses to inform the DVLA, then it may be necessary in the interests of public safety for the professional to do so.
- Carer burden is high and carers will need information, advice and support (📖 Chapter 22).
- Support for younger children requires a special approach and skill.
- Traditional ways of providing respite care which mainly cater for older people are often not suitable for the younger person with dementia.
- Ultimately placement in a nursing or residential home will be required for most, although many choose to keep their loved ones at home and this can be done through to death (📖 Chapter 20).

Palliative and end of life care

Palliative and end of life care for YODs reflect the norm for dementia—they are not categorically different from that for later-onset dementias. But the greater youth of the people affected may mean that they are more robust and more likely to reach a very late stage of dementia. So with dementias such as young-onset AD, the frequency with which contractures and intractable epilepsy occur will be somewhat greater. By contrast, death from intercurrent infection, stroke and heart disease at an earlier stage is less common. These patients and families must have timely and appropriate access to the palliative care approach and its specialist services when needed.

Further reading

Bayer A, Reban J (eds) (2004) Younger people with dementia. *Alzheimer's disease and related conditions, a dementologist's handbook*, pp. 270–5. MEDEA Press, Prague.

Advanced dementia

Progression of dementia

- Disease progression in dementia is often slow and gradual. Major sudden changes in severity are unusual, and even with the vascular dementias the stepwise progression often spoken of usually involves multiple tiny steps. A clear and sudden transition to palliative care is rarely seen.
- This differs from the model often seen with cancer and most organ failures of a progressive illness with a sharp transition towards palliative care. In cancer care there comes a point at which curative, very burdensome therapies no longer work. They are abandoned for palliative treatments and symptom management with the aim of maintaining function for as long as possible.
- In dementia the prognosis may be just as short, but it is much less predictable and a clear transition from curative, very burdensome therapies to a more palliative approach is less clear cut. The implication of this is that it may be more difficult to base a decision to move towards palliative care upon prognosis than it is upon needs.
- Beyond that, dementia is often associated with delirium and other concurrent medical illnesses. A patient who develops a pneumonia or a hip fracture may be hospitalized and become much more disabled. Such illnesses can often cause permanent step-wise deteriorations in function. This accounts for so many residential and nursing care admissions after being in hospital for a major illness.

When is dementia advanced?

The need for palliative care generally increases as dementia advances. Various criteria define advanced dementia.

Definitions of advanced dementia

Advanced dementia indicates disease progression leading to total dependence on others, requiring care equivalent to placement in a nursing home.

It can also be defined formally by the score achieved on a number of special staging schemes, which are discussed below (☐ Chapter 4, Staging systems, pp. 58–62):
- <10 on the Mini Mental State Examination (MMSE).
- Stage 3 (some would include Stage 2) on the Clinical Dementia Rating (CDR).
- Stages 6–7 on the FAST score of the Global Deterioration Scale (GDS).

Advanced dementia

- Patients with AD spend around twice as long in moderately severe to severe dementia as they do in the earlier stages of the illness. The advanced phases are the ones in which patients will benefit most from palliative care.
- Progression tends to be more rapid in younger patients, and quickens as the disease progresses.
- Psychobehavioural symptoms (e.g. depression, agitation, delusional behaviour, wandering) predominate in advanced dementia until the late severe stages, where the clinical picture tends to become a more purely biological one, e.g. progression to aphasia, inability to walk, sit up unaided, hold head up.
- Patients with advanced dementia lose their ability to communicate their needs and wishes unambiguously. This has important consequences for the assessment of signs of discomfort and general day-to-day care, as well as for their ability to participate in decision-making around their care.
- In advanced dementia, the impact on carers is often very pronounced. Patients with advanced dementia are no longer able to live independently, and depend on either the constant presence of carers or admission into an institution. The former may place a very heavy burden on carers, while the latter may lead to institutionalization and depersonalization.

Cognitive changes in advanced dementia

In advanced AD memory is not the only cognitive function to be impaired.

Memory

For most lay people, dementia represents a loss of memory. The ability to form, learn, and retrieve memories is profoundly affected in dementia. In order to understand what is lost and what is relatively preserved until late, and what the effect of this is on function and personality, it is useful to break memory down into its constituent components:

• Declarative (or explicit) memory deals with facts and events; one can consciously access these memories. This can be further broken down into:
  • Episodic memory: this refers to the ability to remember one's own experiences. Thus you remember your name, what you had for breakfast this morning, what Great Aunt Clara gave you for Christmas, or when you last had lunch. Episodic memory is impaired in early AD but becomes extremely impaired in advanced AD. Autobiographical memory (for events in one's life—for example about one's youth), a subset of episodic memory, is also lost in late AD.
  • Working (or immediate or short-term) memory, for example the ability to immediately repeat a number or a phrase, is preserved. Strangely, digit span (the longest sequence of random digits one can remember—normally seven plus or minus two for adults) is often reduced early on in the disease but may improve again in the late stages.
  • Semantic memory is memory for learned facts, i.e. knowledge—the date of the start of the Second World War, what one uses a screwdriver for, and the alphabet. Semantic memory is relatively well preserved in early AD, but becomes profoundly reduced in advanced AD.
• Non-declarative (or implicit) memory deals with memory which is expressed in behaviour, without the person being aware they are remembering something as they do it. This is often preserved until late in AD. It includes:
  • Procedural memory, such as opening a box of matches or using a key in a door, overlearned skills like driving a car or doing up shoelaces, habits and conditioned responses.
  • Perceptual priming is memory related to (often visual) cues. Thus a nursing home resident might quickly learn the shortest route out of the building, and may repeatedly go missing.

Attention

The ability to focus and to shift attention when required may both be impaired. Reaction times may be slowed. People with dementia may become unable to complete more than one simple task at a time. Thus, for example, talking while walking can for some increase the risk of falls, and listening while eating can worsen the chances of aspiration.

Simple attention span may not be so affected; it is possible to administer simple cognitive tests lasting up to 30 minutes to patients with advanced dementia, but not longer.

Other aspects of perception
- Visuospatial ability (the ability to perceive spatial relationships between objects) is significantly affected in AD, although the exact pattern differs greatly from person to person (📖 Chapter 11, Cognitive disabilities, pp. 209–211).
- Unilateral inattention is common, so that one side of the field of vision may be ignored.
- Visual sensitivity to contrast is often reduced.
- Recognition of objects is often severely impaired, as is pattern recognition, spatial judgment, and perceptual organization (the perception and organization of relationships between the various patterns perceived). This contributes to, for example, getting lost, wandering, and disorientation even in familiar settings.
- Visuospatial impairment becomes very severe in late-stage AD, and may contribute to a feeling of great insecurity in one's surroundings and a severe sense of unfamiliarity.

Thinking and reasoning
The ability to think is affected early on. Abstract reasoning is lost. Boundaries between concepts become less distinct, leading to vague and woolly thinking. Many patients with early or moderate AD talk of the fuzziness in their heads. Ultimately this leads to a loss of decision-making capacity.

Expressive functions
These include speaking, physical gestures, drawing, manipulating objects, and so on.

Language deteriorates fairly quickly after the onset of AD. Speech becomes less rich, e.g. a narrower vocabulary is used; speech flows less smoothly with gaps and interruptions; and the affected person speaks less and less. Spontaneous speech is replaced by speaking only when someone else initiates an exchange. Comprehension also diminishes fairly early on. The ability to name things is affected. In late AD speech can be affected in many ways:
- Comprehension is impaired; even simple one-step instructions are not followed. The ability to follow even simple logic is lost.
- Perseveration of speech (the uncontrollable repetition of a particular response) is common: 'Help me, help me, help me'. The same questions can also be repeated over and over. Groaning and other non-verbal expressions are also frequent.
- Echolalia (repetitions of others' vocalizations) and palilalia (repetition of one's own speech) are frequent; the latter may sound like stuttering.
- Naming objects is impaired, and this is further worsened by perceptual deficits.
- The basic syntax (using words to form sentences and phrases) of speech is preserved until relatively late, but is impossible to follow as general terms ('it') are used for description without any clue as to what they refer to.

- The ability to repeat words or even read text without understanding its meaning is at times preserved until late, although reading accuracy does suffer. Writing deteriorates at least as quickly as speech, often more so.
- Eventually speech becomes mumbling and impossible to follow.
- People with advanced AD may become severely aphasic or mute. Unlike patients suffering from other organic aphasias, they become unable to also make their meaning known by using non-verbal gestures or intonations—a useful distinguishing feature when in doubt.

Apraxias (loss of the ability to carry out learned purposeful movements) are common, and impairment is often severe in advanced AD. The ability to perform everyday activities (dressing up, toileting, feeding) is often lost in moderate dementia. Understanding and utilization of even simple tools disappears. Eventually the patient finds it very difficult to perform any intentional acts. The repeated fingering of certain objects, shredding of tissues or rummaging found in moderate dementia gradually disappears in very late illness.

Executive function

- Executive function describes the ability to assess a situation, plan, and act. It includes the ability to respond to novel situations, to override habit and to correct errors in performance. It is essential for independent goal-directed behaviour.
- Insight into the degree of impairment is common early on in the illness and worsens with time.
- Distractibility often interferes with the ability to carry out even a simple task.
- Perseveration in activity also interferes with purposive behaviour.
- Executive function is severely affected in advanced AD so that affected individuals do not initiate or carry out purposive activity independently.
- Eventually there is no responsiveness to changes in the environment.

Emotional behaviour

- Emotional behaviour may be relatively preserved until late.
- Patients with AD can become very clingy to caregivers, and insecure when they even leave the room; or on the other hand (and increasingly with disease progression), show apathy and lack of involvement.
- Similar behaviour can happen in institutions: patients can form greatly trusting or paranoid attitudes towards particular members of staff almost instantly on first meeting them, and the attitudes to that person will often persist.
- Eventually emotional responses become very blunted. Smiling disappears, often there is little response to being touched, although many still find repeated touching or stroking of objects or of and by other people comforting.

Practical abilities and skills

All of these debilities combine together to produce a wide range of practical disabilities that come with advanced dementia including impairments

of instrumental ADLs, and later of the more basic ADLs (📖 Chapter 11, Basic concepts, pp. 205–206; Physical disabilities, pp. 212–220), including:
- The ability to cook, wash, shop, organize.
- Self-care, washing, dressing.
- Continence and the ability to feed oneself, etc.
- Mobility, etc.

Behavioural and psychological features

These are defined as symptoms of disturbed perception, thought content, mood, behaviour, frequently occurring in patients with dementia. They include:

- Agitation.
- Anxiety.
- Apathy.
- Culturally inappropriate behaviours.
- Delusions.
- Depression/dysphoria.
- Disinhibition.
- Disorders of appetite.
- Euphoria/elation.
- Hallucinations.
- Irritability/lability.
- Screaming.
- Sleep disturbance.
- Wandering.

Depression is often commonest early on in dementia, with behavioural disturbance and psychosis commoner a bit later.

Towards the end, these difficulties may settle, though ongoing management of them is often required. BPSD are discussed in detail in 📖 Chapter 10.

Physical changes

A number of physical changes occur in severe dementia.

Weight loss

In women, weight loss can precede the appearance of AD by over 10 years, suggesting that the illness starts much earlier than hitherto believed. Weight loss remains a feature of AD throughout the illness. The issues of feeding and diet are discussed in 📖 Chapters 9 and 13. Severe inanition, with its accompanying increased risk of infection and complications such as pressure sores, is common in advanced AD and other dementias.

Falls and disorders of balance

Falls are common in people with dementia. A community survey in Sweden found that 10% of residents with dementia had fallen at least once in the previous week. There are several reasons behind this phenomenon. Slowness of movement and reaction, visuospatial deficits, distractibility, the presence of extrapyramidal symptoms in some patients, and drug effects such as postural hypotension and slowed reaction times all contribute. In later dementia, increasing stiffness and joint contractures may supervene, and most patients become bedbound. See 📖 Chapters 11 and 12.

Epilepsy

Epilepsy of the grand mal type or partial seizures is relatively common in advanced dementia and may require treatment with anticonvulsants (📖 Chapter 9, Neurological symptoms, pp. 163–166).

Staging systems

It is useful to try and work out when dementia is reaching an advanced stage, to enable better care, better planning, and to allow communication around prognosis.

Many use scores such as the Folstein MMSE. A score of <10 here implies advanced dementia. However, such scales are often dependent on socio-economic background, level of intelligence, visual and hearing ability, as well as cultural factors. Moreover, they often register change better in the mild to moderate phase of dementia than at the more severe end.

Scales which use observation of function are better. Most depend on information furnished by observers. Staging systems can be useful in:
• Identifying the care needs of an individual.
• Working out the needs of populations with advanced dementia.
• Identifying which groups will benefit from a particular intervention in a research study or in clinical practice.
• Monitoring disease progression in an individual, with an eye to prognostication along broad lines.

However, formal staging must supplement and never substitute for a personalized assessment of needs and capabilities.
• Global staging systems look at cognition, behaviour and function. Three global systems are discussed here: CDR, the GDS, and the FAST scale of the GDS.
• These staging systems were developed for AD, but also appear valid for other tautopathies [supranuclear palsy, CBD, frontotemporal dementias (Pick's disease), Down's syndrome dementia] and perhaps for other dementias.
• Other indicators exist, but some do not allow a detailed assessment of the severity and impact of dementia, and others are not in widespread use. They are not discussed further.

CDR[1]
• The CDR scores dementia sufferers on each of six domains (see Table 4.1) and rates each finding as normal, questionable, mild, moderate, or severe.
• Changes in CDR score are slow and may be difficult to see from year to year, so clinically its usefulness in this context is limited.
• Although Stage 2 is described as moderate dementia, it expresses a level of dependency on others that for many would imply moderately severe dementia.
• The CDR was initially developed for a prospective study of mild AD, and is less able to discriminate differences in late dementia.

The GDS
• The GDS was originally developed for AD.
• It classifies patients into one of seven categories ranging from normal to very severe dementia.

1 Hughes CP et al. (1982) A new clinical scale for the staging of dementia. Br J Psychiat **140**, 566–72.

Table 4.1 The CDR scale

Stage	0	0.5	1	2	3
Impairment	None	Questionable	Mild	Moderate	Severe
Memory	No memory loss or slight inconstant forgetfulness	Consistent slight forgetfulness, partial recollection of events, 'benign' forgetfulness	Moderate memory loss, more marked for recent events; defect interferes with everyday activities	Severe memory loss; only highly learned material retained; new material rapidly lost	Severe memory loss; only fragments remain
Orientation	Fully oriented	Fully oriented except for slight difficulty with time relationships	Moderate difficulty with time relationships; oriented for place at examination; may have geographic disorientation elsewhere	Severe difficulty with time relationships; usually disoriented to time, often to place	Oriented to person only
Judgment and problem solving	Solves everyday problems and handles business and financial affairs well; judgment good in relation to past performance	Slight impairment in solving problems, similarities and differences	Moderate difficulty in problems, similarities and differences; social judgment usually maintained	Severely impaired in handling problems, similarities and differences; social judgment usually impaired	Unable to make judgments or solve problems

(continued)

Table 4.1 Continued

Stage	0	0.5	1	2	3
Community affairs	Independent function at usual level in job, shopping, volunteer, and social groups	Slight impairment in these activities	Unable to function independently at these activities although may still be engaged in some; appears normal to casual inspection	No pretence of independent function outside home. Appears well enough to be taken to functions outside a family home	No pretence of independent function outside home. Appears too ill to be taken to functions outside a family home
Home and hobbies	Life at home, hobbies, and intellectual interests well maintained	Life at home, hobbies, and intellectual interests slightly impaired	Mild but definite impairment of function at home; more difficult chores abandoned; more complicated hobbies and interests abandoned	Only simple chores preserved; very restricted interests, poorly maintained	No significant function in home
Personal care	Fully capable of self-care	Needs prompting	Requires assistance in dressing, hygiene, keeping of personal effects	Requires much help with personal care; frequent incontinence	

Score only as decline from previous usual level due to cognitive loss, not impairment due to other factors.

Reproduced from Hughes CP et al. (1982) A new clinical scale for the staging of dementia. *Br J Psychiat* **140**, 566–72, with permission.

- Stage 6 describes moderately severe dementia, and Stage 7 very severe dementia (see Table 4.2). Once more, changes in GDS may be quite slow, especially in the earlier stages.

FAST

- FAST (Table 4.3) is a subsystem of the GDS, and concentrates on functional ability.

Table 4.2 The GDS (only Stages 6 and 7 are shown)

Stage 6	• May occasionally forget the name of the spouse upon whom they are entirely dependent for survival • Will be largely unaware of all recent events and experiences in their lives • Retain some knowledge of their surroundings, the year, the season etc. • May have difficulty counting by ones from 10, both backward and sometimes forward • Will require some assistance with ADLs. • May become incontinent • Will require travel assistance but occasionally will be able to travel to familiar locations • Diurnal rhythm frequently disturbed • Almost always recall their own name • Frequently continue to be able to distinguish familiar from unfamiliar persons in their environment • Personality and emotional changes occur. These are quite variable and include: delusional behaviour, e.g. patients may accuse their spouse of being an impostor, may talk to imaginary figures in the environment, or to their own reflection in the mirror • Obsessive symptoms, e.g. person may continually repeat simple cleaning activities • Anxiety symptoms, agitation, and even previously non-existent violent behaviour may occur • Cognitive abulia, e.g. loss of willpower because an individual cannot carry a thought long enough to determine a purposeful course of action
Stage 7	• All verbal abilities are lost over the course of this stage • Early in this stage words and phrases are spoken but speech is very circumscribed • Later there is no speech at all—only grunting • Incontinent: requires assistance toileting and feeding • Basic psychomotor skills (e.g. ability to walk) are lost with the progression of this stage • The brain appears to be no longer able to tell the body what to do • Generalized and cortical neurological signs and symptoms are frequently present

Table 4.3 FAST staging and time course of functional loss in AD (note: only Stages 6 and 7, i.e. severe dementia, are shown)

FAST stage	Clinical characteristics	Clinical diagnosis	Estimated duration in AD	Mean MMSE
6a	Requires assistance in dressing	Moderately severe AD	5 months	9
6b	Requires assistance in bathing properly		5 months	8
6c	Requires assistance with mechanics of toileting (such as flushing, wiping)		5 months	5
6d	Urinary incontinence		4 months	3
6e	Faecal incontinence		10 months	1
7a	Speech ability limited to about half a dozen words	Severe AD	12 months	0
7b	Intelligible vocabulary limited to a single word		12 months	0
7c	Ambulatory ability lost		12 months	0
7d	Ability to sit up lost		12 months	0
7e	Ability to smile lost		18 months	0
7f	Ability to hold head up lost		12 months or longer	0

Adapted from Table 2, p. 88 in Reisberg B et al. Clinical features of severe dementia: staging. In: Burns A, Winblad B (2006) Severe dementia. Wiley, Chichester. Copyright © 1984 by Barry Reisberg, M.D. Reproduced with permission.

• It is particularly suited to the study of advanced dementia in that it breaks down the advanced stages into a number of substages, when function is lost rapidly.
• Interestingly, FAST correlates closely with a number of anatomical changes (e.g. hippocampal volume) in AD.
• Stages 6 and 7 (which break down into 11 substages) describe moderately advanced and advanced dementia.

Identifying the need for palliative care

In dementia, an analogy with cancer is misleading: there are no 'curative' and 'palliative' phases. No treatment currently arrests or cures dementia except in very narrow situations due, e.g. to infection or vitamin deficiency. All treatment is palliative, aimed at best at slowing down progression; but no current treatment has a dramatic impact on this. Therefore all dementia management needs to be infused with a palliative approach (Chapter 5), which should also play a large part in specialist training:

- Are there any severe or persistent physical symptoms present?
- Is the combination of problems complex and ongoing?
- Is the patient persistently distressed without a clear psychiatric cause?
- Are there complex family needs in the context of advanced illness?
- Are there concurrent illnesses which limit prognosis?

The diagnosis of dementia and the likelihood of dying soon

Some people with advanced dementia will be happy, calm, and enjoy being with family or in their care setting. Discussion may enable better care planning and is often valued by families as an opportunity to think through the challenges they face.

Many people with advanced dementia, with good care, may be stable for years and do not die as quickly as expected, but it is important to try and work out when care should move to a more palliative approach: as an example, one of the authors looked after a patient who died 8 years after she became mute and 7 years after her discharge home from a dementia nursing home with total immobility and the need for full nursing care.

A number of criteria have been put forward to allow generalists and specialists to identify who should receive palliative care for dementia.

The surprise question

The 'surprise question' works well and is intuitive, with face validity. However, as the progress of dementia is often slow and subtle, clinicians may struggle to spot the likelihood of death within a year, particularly if their experience of end-stage dementia or care of the dying is limited.

The surprise question

A 'no' answer to the question 'Would you be surprised if this patient were to die in the next 6–12 months?'

Prognostic indicators guidance within the Gold Standards Framework (GSF)

The GSF (http://www.goldstandardsframework.nhs.uk/), whose implementation across primary health care is supported by the Department of Health in the UK, accepts a number of criteria for patients with dementia to be considered as needing palliative care. The current definition (issued September 2008) comprises disease-related criteria along with another criterion involving patient choice for palliative or comfort care. The criteria have yet to be validated formally in the advanced dementia setting.

Indicators for palliative care under the GSF

Prognostic indicators
- Co-morbidities or other general predictors of end-stage illness:
  - General physical decline
  - Reducing performance status/ECOG/Karnofsky score (KPS) <50%
  - Dependence in most ADLs

Specific indicators for dementia
- Unable to walk without assistance AND
- Urinary and faecal incontinence AND
- No consistently meaningful verbal communication AND
- Unable to dress without assistance
- Barthel score <3
- Reduced ability to perform ADLs
- PLUS any one of the following: weight loss >10% in the last 6 months without other causes; pyelonephritis or urinary tract infection (UTI); serum albumin <25g/L; severe pressure sores, e.g. grade III or IV; recurrent fevers; reduced oral intake/weight loss; aspiration pneumonia.

Patient choice for comfort care

A needs-based criterion
The National Council for Palliative Care (NCPC) has suggested that, given the problems of prognosis, a needs-based criterion may be simpler.

Needs-based criteria for a more palliative approach[2]

- (1) Does the patient have moderately severe or severe dementia?
- (2) Does the patient also have severe distress (mental or physical) which is not easily amenable to treatment?
  - OR severe physical frailty which is not easily amenable to treatment?
  - OR another condition (e.g. comorbid cancer) which merits palliative care services in its own right?

If criteria 1 and 2 co-exist, then the patient ought to have a full assessment of need and a focused analysis of why they are in distress and how best their symptoms can be improved and distress reduced.

Concurrent conditions needing palliative care

- Certain concurrent conditions, such as cancer, require palliative care in their own right.
- Often dementia will complicate and limit the treatment of the other illness due to reduced physical tolerance to treatment because the individual is unable to understand why he or she is being made to suffer often uncomfortable treatment, such as chemotherapy.
- It is often right in such circumstances to limit curative treatment and to palliate more. Equally, however, a nihilistic attitude to treatment

2 Gibson L, Hughes J, Jordan A, Matthews D, Regnard C, Sutton L, Treloar A (2009) *The power of partnership. Palliative care in dementia*. National Council for Palliative Care, London.

because of the presence of dementia is to be condemned. Decisions must be individualized, and cost and benefit weighed up for that patient considering all their physical, emotional, and social circumstances (📖 Chapter 13).

Diagnosing the last days of life
See 📖 Chapter 14.

Entitlement to discussion and detailed reassessment
Patients have a right to expect, if they want it, a discussion of prognosis, likely problems, and what can be done to reduce distress and suffering (see 📖 Chapters 16 and 18).

Conclusion
The need for palliative care is identified by a combination of prognosis and the current clinical state and needs of the patient. Having identified that need, a good quality holistic reassessment is required and then care provided by combinations of dementia services, general medical services and specialist palliative care services. Partnership working and mutual understanding and education are required.

Chapter 5

An overview of palliative care

Fundamentals

Definition

Palliative care has been defined by the WHO as: 'an approach that improves the quality of life of patients and their families facing the problem associated with life-threatening illness, through the prevention and relief of suffering by means of early identification and impeccable assessment and treatment of pain and other problems, physical, psychosocial and spiritual'. Palliative care:

- Provides relief from pain and other distressing symptoms.
- Affirms life and regards dying as a normal process.
- Intends neither to hasten nor to postpone death.
- Integrates the psychological and spiritual aspects of patient care.
- Offers a support system to help patients live as actively as possible until death.
- Offers a support system to help the family cope during the patient's illness and in their own bereavement.
- Uses a team approach to address the needs of patients and their families, including bereavement counselling, if indicated.
- Will enhance quality of life, and may also positively influence the course of illness.
- Is applicable early in the course of illness, in conjunction with other therapies that are intended to prolong life, such as chemotherapy or radiation therapy, and includes those investigations needed to better understand and manage distressing clinical complications.

A bit of history

Cicely Saunders, founder of the modern hospice movement, developed her ideas first at St Joseph's Hospice in Hackney and later at St Christopher's Hospice in Sydenham, London, which she set up in 1967. She brought together a group of professionals who made significant contributions to pain and symptom control, to understanding the psychological impact of terminal illness and adaptation to it, to social work with families facing loss, and to the study of bereavement. Two years after the foundation of St Christopher's inpatient unit, the hospice launched the world's first specialist palliative care home care team. Cicely Saunders' ideals fundamentally influenced the setting up of the first UK hospital palliative support team at St Thomas' Hospital in London in 1971. Since then palliative care has spread worldwide. Over 8000 palliative care units are now found in over 100 countries—a drop in the ocean compared to the size of the problem, but the rate of growth over 40 years has been phenomenal. In some countries and regions, such as the UK or Catalonia in Spain, palliative care units cover the whole geographical area, although for many others coverage is still sparse and haphazard. Palliative medicine has become a recognized specialty in many countries with specialist training programmes and accreditation.

See http://www.helpthehospices.org.uk/hospiceinformation/ for details of palliative care in the UK and around the world.

Foundations of palliative care

Cicely Saunders based her work on a number of essential principles:

• The patient is a whole person, an interplay of physical, psychological, social, and spiritual dimensions. These are not separate, but rather terms of convenience expressing a very complex unitary reality. Patient assessment and management must always keep this cardinal principle in mind. Care must therefore be delivered by a multidisciplinary team uniting different specialists who can together address this complex reality. Open communication within the caring team is crucial. Boundaries between the different professional skill sets are blurred, as each professional has to be able to relate to the patient as a whole person, while retaining the integrity of their own profession. For example all health care professionals have to be able to recognize and respond to psychosocial and spiritual distress, and not just see the patient as a physically diseased body.

• The family, rather than the individual, is the unit of care. They all suffer from the illness that in a narrow, pathological sense is the patient's, but in a richer sense is an illness of the group of people centred around that person. It affects each individual in a personal and different way, but the 'family' (however it is defined for that particular patient) also has its own illness. Relationships are the stuff of person-centred care. This also implies that care does not finish when the patient dies; the care of the bereaved has always been considered an integral part of palliative care.

• Symptoms and the process of adaptation to life-threatening illness can be analysed scientifically in the same way that any other illness can, to suggest effective ways of management.

This view of palliative care as an interplay of two ecologies, one internal to the patient and the other comprising their relationships, is expressed for example in the concept of 'total pain'. Pain is not merely physical pain, but encompasses mental pain as well as existential or spiritual pain.

Cicely Saunders insisted that pain in advanced disease is the product of an interaction of physical, psychosocial, and spiritual factors, and could only be adequately addressed if all these factors were understood and attended to. Interestingly, functional imaging is now starting to reveal the mechanisms by which emotion and state of mind influence pain.

Perhaps even more than other terminal illnesses, dementia combines mental and physical disability. Dementia is a condition where pain is often physical, but distress is also very often mental. Issues of carer burden, impact, and meaning strongly validate Cicely Saunders' concept of total pain.

Who delivers palliative care?

A useful distinction has been made between the following types of care:

- General palliative care: a palliative care approach can be used to advantage by anyone caring for people who are ill. Basic palliative care skills can be easily learned and are useful not just in dealing with patients with terminal illness but also with anyone with chronic disease, and are also applicable to many acute illness situations. An emphasis on symptom control, an awareness that one is dealing with a whole person and with family as well as patient, a respect for patient autonomy, and a policy of open and sensitive communication are the hallmarks of this approach.
- Supportive care: in illnesses such as cancer, where aggressive treatment at an early stage can be curative, the well-being of the patient can be ignored in the concentration on cure. 'Best supportive care' has come to denote the same principles already enunciated, in the awareness that people facing potentially life-changing illnesses and treatment face difficult symptoms and major physical, psychological, and social adjustments. Information and efforts at rehabilitation are key.
- Specialist palliative care: this is provided by multidisciplinary teams, key members of which will have had specialist training. Specialist palliative care teams look after patients with more complex problems and provide advice and education to other services.

The multidisciplinary team

Specialist palliative care is delivered by a multidisciplinary team. The precise composition of the team varies according to the population served, but in general the core members are:

- Specialist doctors.
- Specialist home care nurses.
- Inpatient unit nurses.
- Social workers and/or psychologists.
- Chaplain/spiritual care .
- Physiotherapists.
- Other therapists, e.g. occupational therapists, art and music therapists, complementary therapists.

Teams also often include psychiatrists, speech and language therapists, and dieticians. Teams with more specialist interests will have other relevant members as necessary.

Why refer for specialist palliative care?

Patients are usually referred to specialist palliative care for one of several reasons:
- Symptom control.
- Psychosocial support for the patient, including respite admissions.
- Psychosocial support for the family, including respite admissions.
- Terminal care.
- Rehabilitation.
- Staff support in particularly difficult situations.

In most services, patients are under specialist palliative home care for the last few months before their death. In the UK, the average length of stay in inpatient palliative care is around 13 days, as patients are treated for acute problems and then discharged back into the community, or into nursing homes, usually with specialist palliative home care.

The concept of appropriate care

One of the distinguishing features of palliative care is the attention which is given to ensure that decisions will benefit patients in the round. All treatments are assessed in terms of whether or not they are appropriate. Key factors feeding into the determination of appropriate care are:
- Burdensomeness.
- Likely benefit/futility of proposed treatment.
- Balancing benefit with possible side-effects.

The outcome of treatment must be looked at in conjunction with the social and psychological implications before a choice is made to follow one particular option. A good sense of judgment, born of examined experience and knowledge of the individual, is fundamental to good palliative care practice. This is discussed in more detail in Chapter 13.

Where is palliative care delivered?

People who are terminally ill require care that follows them in whichever environment they live. Much care is delivered by generalists. However, specialist palliative care input is often involved. A comprehensive specialist palliative care service will comprise care at home, in hospital, in nursing or residential care homes, and in specialist palliative care inpatient units or hospices. The following discussion addresses generalist and specialist palliative care delivery in a general context (i.e. not relating to dementia), because this background is useful for understanding service delivery to people with dementia. For a discussion of issues of care delivery specifically to people with dementia see 📖 Chapter 20.

At home

- Studies consistently confirm that most people, when asked, would like to be cared for and die in their own homes rather than in an institution.
- GPs and DNs provide much of the end of life care in the community. A GP in the UK with a list of 1700 patients would have about 17 dying patients each year. An old study by the Audit Commission in the UK[1] showed that palliative and terminal care took up 40% of a DN's time.
- In the UK, care outside working hours is provided by GP deputizing services. These may lack information about the patient, may not know they are also under specialist palliative care, and, under pressure from other visits they may have to do, may at times refer people for emergency hospital admission who could be cared for properly at home. Greater sharing of information between deputizing services and specialist palliative care home care teams, and the easy availability of specialist advice 24 hours a day, may improve this situation.
- Many patients at home are under specialist palliative care home care teams. The average length of stay under the care of such a team is several months. Some people whose condition stabilizes will be discharged, only to be re-referred when their care needs change again.
- Patients will also sometimes avail themselves of day-care facilities. Specialist palliative care day care varies enormously, from the purely social to the heavily medicalized. Day care allows people who are otherwise housebound and who become very isolated a chance to get out of their home, to socialize, to meet other people in the same situation, and to discover and enjoy new activities and a new side of themselves. This counters the feeling of diminishment that people who are dying feel, and transmits the feeling that there is still life to be had much more effectively than talking about it would.
- Determinants of home death vary from country to country.
- A recent systematic review found the following factors were strongly associated with death at home for cancer patients:
  - low functional status
  - expressed preference for dying at home
  - the presence of home care, particularly when this is more intensive
  - living with relatives
  - extended family support.
- In the UK the number of home cancer deaths has fallen over the last decade.

- Few empirical data exist regarding determinants of home death in people with dementia.
- But is now clear that supporting people to live at home until they die with dementia is feasible and can have excellent outcomes (see 📖 Chapter 20).

Specialist palliative care home care teams usually consist of specialist nurses with doctor and social worker or psychologist support. They visit patients at home to provide advice on symptom control and to give emotional support to the patient and family. A number of services provide 24 hour visiting or telephone support; this is encouraged by the National End of Life Care Strategy.

Hospitals

- In the UK, after a fall in the number of hospital deaths from 1985 to 1994, these have again increased. In England, in 2006, 58% of all deaths occurred in hospital (including deaths from acute illness). In Canada the trend goes the opposite way, with increasing numbers of hospital deaths through the 20th century being reversed in the last 5 years of the millennium. In the USA hospital deaths have also diminished.
- Hospital is rarely the ideal place to care for the terminally ill. The attention to detail, time, and space their care requires is rarely available in what can be a busy and impersonal place.
- The National Audit Office (NAO) in the UK surveyed where people died in Sheffield in northern England. They showed that many people who died in hospital could have instead been managed at home or in care homes at the end of life. Of the 40% of care home residents who died in hospital, just under half could have been looked after in the care home to the end.
- A few hospitals have dedicated palliative care beds.
- Most care is carried out by hospital specialist palliative care teams (SPCTs), which often comprise a consultant, specialist nurses and, increasingly, a specialist social worker. Some teams have other members, e.g. a psychologist. SPCTs usually have a consultative and a training role.
- In England and Wales, since the Calman–Hine report into cancer care in 1995, hospitals are only accredited to treat cancer if they have a consultant-led SPCT. The resultant rise in SPCT numbers has produced a greater appreciation of their usefulness and better integration with other hospital services.
- SPCTs often see a broader range of patients than inpatient or home care units. They are also often called upon to advise in certain situations, e.g. where issues of withdrawing or withholding treatment, or particularly complex symptom control situations arise, even outside the palliative care context, e.g. in intensive care units.
- Patients with dementia present particular problems (📖 Chapter 20). Hospital palliative care teams have a role in conjunction with old-age psychiatry in advocating for these patients with their carers.

Hospices

- In people with cancer, the proportion who want to die at home decreases from 90% to 50% as death approaches, the difference being made up mostly by a wish to die in a hospice.

- The number of hospice units in the UK is larger than in most countries, but still small. In 2008, there were 223 inpatient units in the UK, with 3226 beds. Four-fifths of the beds are provided by the voluntary sector, mostly with a minority of their costs funded by the government, while the other fifth are NHS beds.

- Voluntary hospices receive an average of 38% of their funding from the NHS—some receive 100%, others no funding at all. The difference has to be made up by fundraising.

- A comparatively small proportion of deaths (5%) occur in specialist palliative care inpatient units, or hospices. In England, 17% of cancer deaths occur in hospices. Non-cancer admissions still form a very small percentage of overall hospice admissions (6% nationally in the UK in 2005–2006, though 25% for some individual units), so the impact on non-cancer place of death is very small overall.

- Hospices are relatively short-stay units, the average length of stay in the UK being about 2 weeks. This includes both patients who die within a day or two of admission and those who have a much longer stay because of complex needs.

- Patients can be admitted for symptom control, psychosocial need, or terminal care; some units also admit for respite and rehabilitation.

- About 50% of admissions to hospices in the UK end with the patient dying as an inpatient; in the other 50% the patient is discharged home or to a nursing home.

- The number of patients with dementia as their primary diagnosis who die in hospices in the UK is very small, though figures are higher for some countries, e.g. the USA. However, perhaps as many as a third of patients in palliative care inpatient units may have some degree of cognitive impairment.

Care homes

- 16% of all deaths in the UK occur in care homes. The NAO in the UK carried out a survey of deaths in Sheffield and found that 29% of the frail patients in their sample died in care homes along with 7% of cancer deaths and small numbers of unexpected and chronic illness deaths.

- There is a growing recognition that residents of care homes have rarely received the kind of service they deserve. Even when care in the home itself is excellent, few other community resources address the needs of older people in residential care.

- A comparison of 10 countries published in 1997 showed that Iceland and Denmark have a high rate of institutionalization of older people (>10%) while for most other developed countries the figure lies closer to 5–8%. Thus the proportion of older people who still live at home is still surprisingly high in most developed countries. However, the proportion of older people in institutions increases as they become frailer or when they are more isolated.

- In the UK, the number of residents in nursing homes is falling significantly year on year. It has decreased by 14% since 2004 (NHS Information Centre). The number of people in general beds fell more sharply than the number in mental health nursing homes, though this too is decreasing.

- A number of studies in various countries, including the UK, suggest that 50–70% of people admitted to nursing homes die in the first 2 years. Mortality is highest in the first 6 months, and then levels off slowly.
- Up to 75% of nursing home residents in the UK have dementia, often undiagnosed. Many people with dementia end up in nursing homes, the proportion increasing with age (Chapters 1 and 20).

Trends

A study published in 2008 by Gomes and Higginson[2] showed that home deaths could reduce by 42% by 2030 if current trends continue. The number will be taken up by institutional deaths. Given the diminishing number of care homes over the past years, what makes this figure particularly worrying (implying as it does that only 1 in 10 will die at home in 20 years' time), is the implication that much of the slack will have to be taken up by acute hospitals. It is clear that new models of care need to be put in place quickly to stop this potential catastrophe both in terms of care provided and economics.

References

1 Audit Commission (1999) *First assessment: a review of district nursing services in England and Wales.* Audit Commission, London.
2 Gomes B, Higginson IJ (2008) Where people die (1974–2030): past trends, future projections and implications for care. *Palliat Med* **22**, 33–41.
3 Ruth K, Pring A, Verne J (2010) Variations in place of death in England: Inequalities or appropriate consequences of age, gender and cause of death? National End of Life Care Intelligence Network, Bristol, 82.

Implications for the palliative care of people with dementia

Affected individuals die of or with advanced dementia, and a palliative care approach, with its detailed management of symptoms, its awareness of impending death, and its care for patients and families in the round, would greatly benefit people with dementia and their relatives. It is crucial that this approach is taught and practised in dementia units, in care homes and by primary health care teams.

People with dementia and cognitive impairment can come under specialist palliative care for two reasons. Most are currently referred for concurrent illnesses—they may have cancer or heart failure, for example, and happen to also have dementia. A growing number of units will also now accept patients for whom end-stage dementia is the primary diagnosis. The current set-up of specialist palliative care described above should work well for people with conditions such as cancer and organ failure who also have dementia, as they tend to have a relatively short illness with many acutely symptomatic episodes. However, end-stage dementia often follows a much longer time course. Symptoms are rarely as acute, and social problems are often even more dominant than in the rest of specialist palliative care. A different model of care is therefore needed to sustain the care of those in whom dementia is the primary illness, less medicalized, though with an excellent medical safety net. This model has to be more geared to cope with slowly progressive illness, and more able to work with and through existing services, for example community mental health teams for older adults. This enables the palliative care team to both improve their collaborators' skills and to reach more affected individuals in a more sustainable manner. Joint working also brings new knowledge and expertise to specialist palliative care, which can then use this in the care of those whose dementia is a secondary illness. Everyone gains through collaborative working, but effective communication is key.

Further reading

Department of Health (2008) *End of life care strategy – promoting high quality care for all adults at the end of life*. Department of Health, London.

Gibson L, Hughes J, Jordan A, Matthews D, Regnard C, Sutton L, Treloar A (2009) *The power of partnership. Palliative care in dementia*. National Council for Palliative Care, London.

Chapter 6

Distress in dementia

Severe distress in dementia: physical and mental pain

Not all those who have dementia suffer. Some are happy and comfortable and some even become more serene as a result of being 'let off' the worries of responsibility, etc. But dementia can be very distressing for both patient and family. Distress can be caused by:

- Physical pain.
- Depression.
- Psychosis.
- Fear and anxiety (e.g. poor understanding of what is happening).
- Insomnia.
- Hunger and diet.
- Boredom, isolation.
- Spiritual or existential upheaval.
- Poor environment or inappropriate environmental interventions.

Each one of these causes will have its own appropriate treatment (📖 Chapters 8, 9, 10, and 19).

In late dementia, patients become unable to verbalize the cause of their distress; it also becomes much harder to tell if someone is having psychotic symptoms. Even in those who were deluded or hallucinated (psychotic) earlier in the course of their illness, it may be impossible to tell if they remain so. But the distress may persist and remain treatable using the same treatments that were indicated earlier Beyond this, existential pain requires assessment and treatment.

Mental and existential pain

- Mental pain frequently presents as agitation, distress, or BPSD. The causes of the behaviour problems and challenging behaviour for that patient at that time need to be understood and explored in terms of treatability and preventability.
- Existential pain remains important in dementia. It requires proper exploration, understanding, and discussion. The distress and the reality of parting are important and bring needs and challenges of their own which must be assessed and addressed.
- All forms of distress need addressing and treating, whatever their origin.

Identifying distress, understanding the cause

In advanced dementia the symptoms and signs of physical, mental, or existential pain may be indistinguishable. Scales designed to measure pain in uncommunicative patients with dementia will be positive for either physical or mental pain. GPs and psychiatrists are often quite adept at identifying distress in people with dementia, but the full range of options for the skilled management of some forms of mental pain in dementia requires the expertise of old-age psychiatry.

Sometimes it is important not to treat distress aggressively if it can be tolerated for some periods of time. Distress in dementia often fluctuates. It may sometimes be better to allow distress, wandering, and challenging behaviour for part of the day, so that the better parts of the day are of greater quality without the effects of medication. Just like the rest of us, people with dementia have moments of unhappiness, which need to be allowed to occur.

But where distress is severe, the clinician must:
• Analyse and address the underlying cause.
• Alleviate the distress itself if the cause is irreversible.
• Ensure the burden of treatment does not outweigh the benefit.
• See the patient as a whole and balance treatments against their effect upon that whole, rather than a single disease measure (📖 Chapter 13).

This resonates with the description of 'total pain' set out by Cicely Saunders (📖 Chapter 5, Fundamentals, pp. 67–68).

Antipsychotics and balancing good and harm

The example of balancing the risks and benefits of antipsychotics in BPSD, and the effect of Omnibus Budget Reconciliation Act of 1987 (OBRA) in the USA, is discussed later (📖 Chapter 10, BPSD, pp. 171–173). As a result of directives to stop such medicines some patients returned to chronic distress and a resurgence of hallucinations, fear, and behaviour that challenges. Others were switched to medicines that may well be more harmful. There is no doubt that antipsychotic drugs are overused when behavioural measures, antidepressants, or analgesics, should be utilized instead. But dementia may be severely distressing for some patients, and there are cases where the use of antipsychotics for BPSD is justified. The excess mortality and morbidity from these drugs may sometimes have to be accepted if it is the only effective way of controlling severe distress.

Further reading

Treloar A et al. (2010) Ethical dilemmas: should antipsychotics ever be prescribed for people with dementia? *Br J Psychiat* **197**, 88–90.

Providing comfort and care

Beyond the specific medical treatments, distress is most powerfully reduced by the provision of good comfort and care. Being cold, poorly dressed, and sitting on a sore bottom in urine and faeces causes great distress. Separation from home, and isolation in settings (which may include home) where there is almost nothing going on and no social interaction, is a major cause of distress (📖 Chapters 17 and 20).

Living well with dementia can reduce distress

Living well with dementia also effectively reduces distress. Those working with dementia often see people in the very late stages, bedbound patients who can barely talk but who still give to those who care for them. Just recently one of us saw a patient, bedbound and dying, who had been in conflict with her daughter for years. Whenever the daughter provided care she would resist and insult her. But the day before she died, she looked up at her and said she loved her. Others continue to be Granny or Granddad and are still valued and enjoyed by those around them right to the end. Palliative care is about allowing those who are dying to live well while they die, and this is no less so in dementia.

Case history (missed pain)

Bob has a severe dementia and has been calling out day and night. When nurses come to him he pushes them away and he is often tearful and also eating poorly. He becomes very angry with carers when they provide care. He sleeps poorly and is often up and wandering at night. He has already been given antipsychotic medication but there has been little benefit. Enquiry reveals a past history of depression.

He is treated with an antidepressant, and improves. His family report that he is more able to smile now and interact.

Case history (antipsychotics indicated)

Bert has a severe dementia and has been calling out day and night. When nurses come to him he pushes them away and he is most violent at times of toileting and personal care. He seems fearful and also is thought to be seeing things and people who are not there. He seems to believe that he is being poisoned. A trial of low-dose antipsychotic is successful, but then these are stopped by a visiting GP responding to the concern about their use. His distress recurs and after discussion and explanation of risks with his daughter, she asks for them to be restarted.

Chapter 7

Principles of physical symptom assessment in dementia

Key issues in symptom assessment

Good, detailed assessment is the key to palliative care, as it is to all health care. In palliative care, this involves a number of important considerations:

- Symptoms are problems in their own right, not just signposts to an underlying diagnosis.
- Successful symptom management requires a thorough assessment of the severity, pattern, and impact of each symptom.
- The impact on function and day-to-day life must be looked into meticulously.
- Diagnostic tests should be used sparingly in people who are frail, and only after working out the expected burden and benefits.
- A good history plus a detailed physical examination will usually determine the likely cause for a symptom and hence its management.
- In BPSD (📖 Chapter 10), the underlying cause MUST be understood.
- In frail individuals, symptoms are very often multifactorial. Treatment may need to reflect this.
- Signs must be carefully observed and interpreted with an understanding of the broad range of causation, especially in people with limited or no verbal capacity.
- In advanced illness there is often multisystem disease and a number of other illnesses present. The clinician has to consider the effect of any proposed intervention across all these different conditions, so assessment will have to include the status of concurrent conditions. During assessment, an idea must be formed of how potential treatments are likely to be tolerated by that individual.
- At times one remains uncertain as to the origin of a symptom and has to treat it empirically. However, even in these cases there is usually a logical way to proceed.
- Blunderbuss approaches to symptom management often do more harm than good, especially in frail individuals.

In order to appreciate the limitations of symptom assessment in people with dementia, one needs first to understand the principles of symptom assessment in the general population and how it is different in older people and in people with learning disabilities.

Symptom assessment in the general population

Because symptoms are by definition what the person experiences, the gold standard for symptom assessment is the affected person's own evaluation of them. Subjectivity is not a problem: symptom assessment could not be anything but subjective.

For any symptom it is important to delineate:
- How severe it is—on average and at its most intense.
- How frequently it occurs.
- How long it lasts. Does it come on suddenly at great intensity or build up gradually to a peak? Does it diminish suddenly or gradually peter out?
- Whether there is a pattern to its occurrence, e.g. time of day, position.
- Whether the symptom has changed since it first occurred, e.g. is it more or less intense, more or less frequent?
- The quality of the symptom, e.g. pain, may be burning, pricking, or dull.
- Whether there are precipitating or relieving factors.
- Whether any other associated symptoms or signs occur in association with that symptom. For example, is dizziness associated with nausea, palpitations, or vertigo?
- What effect it has on day-to-day function. Does it impede sleep, getting to the shops, climbing stairs? Do some activities feel less safe since its onset? Has it affected relationships at home? Has it made the person more dependent, snappier, or more depressed? The effect on function is of the utmost importance, yet is rarely delineated in enough detail.
- What meaning having the symptom carries for the person. For example, pain can represent tumour progression to patients with cancer, even if the pain is not due to tumour in the first place, and unless this is dealt with, symptom control can be very fraught.
- This also implies an awareness of the cultural resonances of that symptom. For example, pain may be seen as God's will and to be accepted, which can sometimes create a tension between well-meaning clinician and patient or family. Equally, some high achievers find the possibility of limitation intolerable, and this impacts on their interpretation of and response to their symptoms. Some symptoms may be inexpressible in some cultures—for example conditions interpreted in the West as depression or psychosis may have a different explanation attached to them in some cultures. Without an understanding of these nuances, attempts at symptom control are likely to fail.

Most clinical symptom assessment is not formalized. The symptom is explored in a systematic but individualized and flexible manner. A detailed history often allows one to diagnose a symptom or shortlist to a very narrow field. Even if one lacks the knowledge of symptom assessment to fully integrate the mass of detail, a full history is well worth taking. It makes consultation with colleagues more fruitful, improves one's understanding of the impact of that symptom on that individual, and often suggests fruitful pharmacological, physical (use a walking stick; get up to walk slowly, in stages), or behavioural interventions.

Common formal symptom intensity measurement scales

Formalized assessment methods are essential in research and may be very helpful in clinical practice (Table 7.1). Well-validated tools measure what they are meant to measure; they give consistent results; and they give similar results if administered by different individuals. They are also likely to cover most of the important areas of enquiry.

However, formalized assessments also have limitations. They may not cover the problem faced by the patient. The absence of questions about a particular symptom in screening questionnaires may lead the casual observer to think that symptom is far less common than it really is. The person being assessed may misunderstand questions or statements on questionnaires— detailed cognitive testing of the questionnaire before launch may reduce the frequency of this happening. At times, although a person may appear to have filled in a rating scale appropriately, this may be based on an erroneous understanding of the questions. In particular, people with dementia should be helped by appropriately trained professionals when completing symptom assessment tools to avoid such pitfalls. In this situation, assessment scales completed by professionals are more common than in other areas of health care.

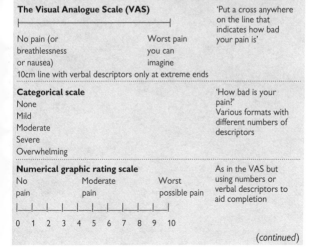

Table 7.1 Commonly used symptom assessment scales, using pain as the example

The Visual Analogue Scale (VAS)		'Put a cross anywhere on the line that indicates how bad your pain is'
No pain (or breathlessness or nausea)	Worst pain you can imagine	
10cm line with verbal descriptors only at extreme ends		
Categorical scale None Mild Moderate Severe Overwhelming		'How bad is your pain?' Various formats with different numbers of descriptors
Numerical graphic rating scale		As in the VAS but using numbers or verbal descriptors to aid completion
No pain	Moderate pain	Worst possible pain
0 1 2 3 4 5 6 7 8 9 10		

(continued)

Table 7.1 Continued

Graphical methods The Wong–Baker Faces Scale for pain[1] **Wong-Baker FACES™ Pain Rating Scale** 0 — No Hurt 2 — Hurts Little Bit 4 — Hurts Little More 6 — Hurts Even More 8 — Hurts Whole Lot 10 — Hurts Worst © 1983 Wong-Baker FACES™ Foundation. Used with permission.	Originally designed for children, the patient has to pick the face which most reflects the intensity of their pain. Many variations, with 6, 7 or even 11 faces.
Complex questionnaires The McGill Pain Questionnaire The Brief Pain Inventory	Time-consuming, but able to explore various dimensions of a symptom (e.g. sensory, affective, and evaluative dimensions for pain in the McGill Pain Questionnaire), and able to cross-check answers through different questions

1 Pautex S, Herrmann F, Le Lous P, Fabjan M, Michel JP, Gold G (2005) Feasibility and reliability of four pain self-assessment scales and correlation with an observational rating scale in hospitalized elderly demented patients. *J Gerontol A Biol Sci Med Sci* **60**, 524–9.

Symptom assessment in older people

Most people with dementia are older. In this age group there are additional issues to be aware of:

- Older people are often more stoical, although this may vary across cultures, and may be less likely to report discomfort, pain, or other troublesome symptoms.
- Particularly in institutions, older people may be afraid that complaining of symptoms could label them as difficult, and they may fear they are putting an extra burden on care staff. Similarly, at home, they may not want to worry relatives and therefore will underreport or underplay symptoms.
- Professionals (including care home staff) may not give much attention to assessing symptoms in older people. In younger people symptoms will usually only occur if there is some underlying acute pathology. In older people, symptoms are often present chronically, and may be mistakenly accepted as the inevitable cost of being old. This may lead to a nihilistic attitude to symptoms in older people, so that detailed assessment and active management may be mistakenly dispensed with.
- Older people may use euphemisms to describe unpleasant experiences and symptoms. For example, they may say something does not feel right, it bothers them, they may insist on calling a pain a discomfort, or they may even describe it as feeling sick. If one does not grasp their true meaning one can end up ignoring what they are saying or seriously underestimating the severity of a pain. Older patients with chronic pain use more descriptors for their pain than acute pain patients.
- Older people may not be able to use some assessment instruments as effectively. As many as 30% of cognitively intact older people may find the VAS confusing and may fill it in incorrectly (see Table 7.1).

Symptom assessment in people with learning disabilities

- People with learning disabilities often have an impaired ability to communicate verbally or through other means. Their capacity to form abstract concepts may also be reduced. Both of these can impact greatly on their ability to communicate and explain discomfort or other subjective symptoms. They may not be able to understand, or they may misunderstand, certain questions or questionnaires, and give misleading answers.
- The behavioural responses to pain appear to be similar to those of the normal population, although in autistic children they tend to be more exaggerated.
- There is a risk that unsettled behaviour due to discomfort may be automatically attributed to the learning disability or presented as a behavioural problem so that its true significance as, say, a sign of pain, is lost. This is termed 'diagnostic overshadowing', where all problems are attributed to the underlying condition without making a real effort to explore them. A meta-analysis of this phenomenon in 1995 found a small to moderate effect of diagnostic overshadowing.
- Surveys of professionals involved in the care of people with learning disabilities have repeatedly revealed that identifying symptoms correctly was one of their greatest anxieties.

Symptom assessment in people with dementia

In dementia, many of the issues are shared with learning difficulty, with some key differences. In dementia the impairment is by definition progressive, often following a lifetime of intellectual normality, whereas learning disabilities are usually stable over many years if not throughout life. In both, additional neurological or sensory impairments may complicate the problem (📖 Chapters 4, 9, and 11).

- People with mild to moderate dementia are likely to be able to follow pain assessment scales practically as well as people without dementia. In a study comparing four self-assessment scales in people with dementia, Pautex et al.[1] showed that only 12% of 160 participants were unable to understand any of the scales on offer. 97% and 90% of people with mild or moderate dementia, respectively, understood at least one scale. Thus although one may have to try different methods of pain assessment until one settles on the most appropriate one for the individual, assessment should not be vastly different from that of people with no intellectual impairment. There are no data in the literature relating to assessment of other physical symptoms, but it is likely that similar considerations hold.

- In advanced dementia the situation is somewhat different. Even here, Pautex et al.[2] found that 40% of patients were able to use at least one self-assessment scale correctly. In a later study she was able to elicit comprehension from 61% of study participants. It is worth bearing in mind that at this point tolerance to extensive investigation or long questionnaires is poor. Often, verbal utterances by the person affected can give strong indications that they are in pain. A patient may complain, for example, that their arm feels heavy, or that their foot is on fire. However, in late advanced dementia, communication problems become severe, verbalization eventually becomes non-existent, and observation by relatives or professional carers becomes the key to symptom assessment.

Approaches to the observational assessment of symptoms

In dementia, symptoms are caused by both physical pain and mental pain/distress, and the signs of distress have multiple causes. Never consider only a single cause of distress.

Most people with very advanced dementia become verbally uncommunicative. They still convey a lot through their behaviour, but the precision and subtlety of verbal communication is lost. Eventually, neurological changes may also limit the range of behavioural expressions of distress, although one can detect distress in anyone who is not deeply comatose—who would not feel distress in any case.

The intensity and frequency of some symptoms remain easy to evaluate and measure. Breathlessness, for example can be seen and graded:

- At rest.
- On exertion: how much exertion, e.g. how far one has to walk before becoming obviously short of breath?
- Length of recovery time.

This misses out the all-important affective component of breathlessness, but apart from eliciting the presence of distress it is difficult to investigate this further without speech, even more so as concept formation is also impaired. Similarly, one can count the number of episodes of vomiting, measure the volume of vomit, and look at what has been brought up. Constipation can be assessed through stool frequency and consistency.

Volicer, the pioneer of palliative care in dementia, recorded symptom frequency rather than intensity in his Symptom Management at End of Life in Dementia (SM-EOLD) scale, presumably because intensity is so difficult to judge without verbal communication. Such a scale is certainly helpful in assessing the effectiveness of one's care in a group of patients over time, or in a single patient over time. Its usefulness in evaluating an acute symptom in the here and now is clearly more limited.

Attempts to measure symptom intensity based on the effect on day-to-day life become extremely difficult. How does one judge which symptom of many is having what impact? How does one differentiate the impact of a symptom on activity or mood from frailty, depression, or other factors in someone who is unable to verbalize? And how does one quantify impact on activity in someone whom far advanced dementia has rendered practically immobile and uncommunicative?

The problem with assessing more objective symptoms as detailed above is more an administrative one: information is likely to be lost across staff handover between shifts, and unless one has robust systems and training in place to record such symptoms faithfully, the results can be very misleading.

What is lost irretrievably is the ability to delineate the subjective symptoms, such as nausea, or indeed pain, with any precision, as well as the affective component of any symptom and the meaning of that symptom for that person. There are ways around this to some extent, although the methods are often different for clinical management and research. These complementary approaches should, however, cross-fertilize by what has been learnt in each context.

Clinical approach to observational symptom assessment

The verbally uncommunicative patient cannot give a history, but a history can be elicited from family members, carers, or professionals who know the person. One should:

- Obtain as clear a description as possible of any objectively observable symptoms (such as breathlessness or vomiting): frequency, time pattern, intensity, precipitating or relieving factors. The level of detail serves two purposes
  - the diagnosis rests in the detail; a good history will usually point to one or perhaps two or three possible causes for a symptom, which can then be worked through
  - in eliciting a more detailed account one can go some way to judging the credibility of witness reports.
- Note any behavioural expression of discomfort or altered function (Table 7.2). Discomfort is often associated with pain behaviour, although it may be due to other sources of distress. Not all pain behaviour is the same. A recent study hypothesized that some behaviour is meant to protect against further injury or pain (guarding,

touching, rubbing); such behaviour is consistently related to the physical pain being experienced. Other pain behaviour (especially facial expression such as grimacing, moaning, and groaning) communicates the presence of pain to others; this type of pain behaviour appears to be more responsive to the social situation. Both are of course important in assessing clinical pain, but they fill in slightly different parts of the picture.

- Look at how the behaviour has changed from when the person was well. The person may become withdrawn, avoid company, or they may show unaccustomed agitation or even aggression without a clear cause.
- Look in particular for situations that the patient is avoiding, or that elicit the abnormal or changed behaviour.
- Cross-check the accounts of as many people as possible, paying particular attention to those who know and care for the person most.
- Put it all in the context of the patient's past history and known illnesses.
- Examine the patient in detail with an eye for any suggestive signs, cross-checking any suspicions derived from the history, and ruling out alternative explanations.

Table 7.2 Behaviour suggesting discomfort even in severe cognitive impairment

Agitation, fidgeting	Repetitive verbalizations
Repetitive movements	Decreased cognition
Tense muscles	Decreased function
Body bracing	Withdrawal
Increased calling out	Changes in sleep pattern
Tears or crying	Panic

Formal symptom assessment

There are many situations in which symptom assessment needs to be done formally, using structured validated assessment tools. These include research, sometimes to establish a formal diagnosis or quantify a problem or a deficit, but often in clinical situations. In research conditions, formal assessments protect clarity and exclude extraneous confounders which might muddy the results. On the other hand, in clinical situations formal assessments must always be coupled with other approaches, as one wants to collect as much evidence as possible to clarify the context of a situation, which can have a determining effect on interventions and outcomes.

Pain assessment
- For most people with dementia, a number of pain assessment tools which are available for use in non-demented patients can still be used,

and it is often a question of finding out which one suits that particular person best (📖 Chapter 7, Symptom assessment in the general population, pp. 82–84).

- The use of self-reports has long been considered the gold standard for pain assessment. However, this has been questioned recently in a number of papers. Some studies have hypothesized that people with dementia are simply less likely to express pain verbally, but concurrent behavioural and physiological indicators of pain have suggested they do have pain they are not reporting.[1] Functional MRI (fMRI) studies also suggest that pain perception may be increased but verbalization may be reduced. This is not to reduce emphasis on self-report, but to point out that self-report needs to be triangulated with other behavioural evidence, which is emerging as very robust in the pain literature.

In those who are verbally uncommunicative, diagnosis will often have to be made from the observations of others, and specialist assessment tools are needed. This inevitably leads to a number of issues:

- As already pointed out, casual observations can be very misleading. If someone is seen during the brief moment they are in pain and the assumption is made that they are in pain most of the time, the resulting prescribing can be dangerous. Equally, if a person is seen only rarely and happens not to be in pain when seen, one can assume they are not in pain the rest of the time, when they well may be. A systematic attempt at observation, and at utilizing the best available evidence (e.g. asking those who know the person most intimately), has to be made.
- Observers may need training in order to be reliable.
- Health care assistants (HCAs) will often be around the person in an institution longer than perhaps anyone else, and know them better than other staff members. Therefore some pain scales are aimed at HCAs to complete. However, some have questioned the ability of some HCAs to undertake such a complex task as evaluating pain in an uncommunicative patient. There is no empirical evidence to either back up or reject this claim, but until such evidence is available, a combination of training and cross-checking with other staff seems advisable. Many clinicians, however, greatly value the observations of HCAs and other untrained staff who can often provide evidence which clarifies a situation which can be otherwise read in more than one way. As always this evidence will have to be probed and assessed.
- Observation will reveal distress, but may not reveal the cause of distress, which could be pain or hunger or frustration or any of a large number of other potential causes (📖 Chapter 6).
- Pain should be checked both at rest and on movement (obviously related to the movements the patient would usually be exposed to in real life) to build up a useful picture.
- There are several factors to be weighed up when choosing a formal pain assessment tool for a particular situation:
  - Has the measure been properly validated? Has it been tested to show it measures what it says it measures, that it does so

---

1 Kunz M, Mylius V, Scharmann S, Schepelman K, Lautenbacher S (2009) Influence of dementia on multiple components of pain. *Eur J Pain* **13**, 317–25.

consistently, that different individuals using it will come to similar conclusions, that it correlates well with other validated measures of the same phenomenon, and that it is applicable to the situation at hand? Many pain instruments for dementia have only been validated in very limited settings, and one must be aware of these limitations when using them. They may still be useful in other settings, but only if the limitations are understood.

- Is the measure practical, within the grasp of the people applying it, and is it likely to be used properly and persistently? An approximate measure is better than no measure at all. Thus, a long and involved pain tool will probably soon fall into disuse in most hospitals or nursing homes, and it may be better to be pragmatic and adopt a shorter, less perfect measure which staff will actually use on an ongoing basis. On the other hand, simpler tools may miss less common types of pain which are more likely to be picked up on more nuanced and detailed instruments. One needs to choose the best tool for the task in hand.

- Some tools are more dependent on a shared cultural understanding of certain norms or behaviours than others. In some cities, nursing home and hospital staff can be highly multicultural, and there is often a high proportion of staff who have recently arrived from other countries, whose grasp of the language is limited, and who have had their nurse training in a very different cultural context with different norms. The situation is even more difficult when a large proportion of transient agency staff are employed, who cannot be trained into a shared understanding of particular tools. Here again, it may be better to use a simpler tool that is more robust across cultures than a complex, more nuanced one, as using the wrong tool can leave it open to misinterpretation of language or of descriptors. An example of a tool which appears to be relatively culturally robust is PAINAD (Pain Assessment in Advanced Dementia), as it relies mostly on simple objective observation of behaviour. Recent studies showed a high sensitivity but a high false positive rate (unsurprising for a scale based on observation), and a floor effect, i.e. it was not good at picking up low levels of pain.

Pain assessment tools

- A systematic review of pain tools used in severe dementia[2] recently concluded that no instrument for use in people with dementia achieves a high level of validation. It indicated that two instruments are currently the best validated.

- The first is Doloplus-2 (an online version of which can be found at http://www.doloplus.com/), which has been tested more widely and comprehensively than any other instrument. Developed in French, Doloplus-2 has been validated in a number of other languages (Norwegian, Chinese); validation of the English version

2 Zwakhalen SM *et al.* (2006) Pain in elderly people with severe dementia: a systematic review of behavioural pain assessment tools. *BMC Geriatr* **6**, 3.

is ongoing. Doloplus-2 assesses responses (sleep, verbal reaction, and problems of behaviour) in 10 situations which would be expected to evoke pain. It does not measure instantaneous pain but is more of an ongoing pain assessment instrument. In some respects it appears to help those who may forget about the physical component of distress in dementia, to spot distress that is caused by physical pain. Some authors have emphasized the need for training in the administration of Doloplus-2 as untrained staff may find it difficult to use.

- The second is PACSLAC (Pain Assessment Checklist for Seniors with Limited Ability to Communicate; this pain scale can be seen online at http://www.rgpc.ca/best/PAIN%20Best%20Practices%20%20ML%20Vanderhorst%20(June%2007)/PACSLAC.pdf), which is one of the few instruments where the items were specifically generated for pain in people with dementia, and is the only scale which focuses primarily on subtle changes in behaviour. PACSLAC is long, having 60 questions in four domains, but it is quickly filled in as the answers to the questions are of tick-box type. A shorter version has been produced.
- Other scales which rated equally highly in the systematic review are PAINAD and the French ECPA.
- Some other instruments are of recent origin and have not yet been widely validated.
- Different people may express distress differently. This has been acknowledged in the design of one tool for assessment of distress in people with severe communication difficulties. This is DisDAT (the Disability Distress Assessment Tool; not to be confused with the much earlier DS-DAT, or Discomfort Scale – Dementia of Alzheimer's Type), developed in Newcastle, UK, originally for people with learning disabilities. It relies on getting carers to record in detail the person's appearance, vocal signs, habits, mannerisms, and posture, when content and when distressed. This enables staff noting the observations to crystallize what they pick up almost intuitively, and it allows patterns of response to be passed on to others less familiar with the person, so they too can observe responses meaningfully. It also permits teams to establish and record baseline behaviours and appearance for new patients for comparison later. Its other great strength is that it deepens an understanding of pain presentation as it is used; not only does it allow pain to be assessed, but simultaneously develops staff attitudes and confidence in their own observations. It is easy for pain assessment tools to reduce the patient into an impersonal subject to be observed; DisDAT if properly used, can have the opposite effect, making the carer more aware of the subject as a person. The richest information comes from the whole team and family working together, as the documentation points out (see http://www.disdat.co.uk/). Figure 7.1 shows the first page of the DiSDAT tool.
- For research purposes, the analysis of facial expressions by detailed coding carried out by specially trained assessors has been well validated in people with AD. There is good evidence that facial expression of pain is consistent across different levels of cognitive attainment, and is a highly reliable tool for assessing pain.

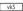 **Disability**
Distress Assessment Tool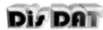

Client's name:	
DoB:	Gender:
Unit/ward:	NHS no.:
Your name:	Date completed:

Names of others who helped complete this form:

DisDATis

Intended to help identify distress cues in people who because of cognitive impairment or physical illness have severely limited communication.

Designed to describe a person's usual content cues, thus enabling distress cues to be identified more clearly.

NOT a scoring tool. It documents what many staff have done instinctively for many years thus providing a record against which subtle changes can be compared. This information can be transferred with the client or patient to any environment.

Only the first step. Once distress has been identified the usual clinical dicisions have to be made by professionals.

Meant to help you and your client or patient. It gives you more confidence in the observation skills you already have which in turn will help you improve the care of your client or patient.

INSTRUCTIONS FOR USING DisDAT ARE ON THE BACK PAGE

SUMMARY OF SIGNS AND BEHAVIOURS

Appearance when CONTENT		Appearance when DISTRESSED	
Face	Eyes	Face	Eyes
Tongue/jaw		Tongue/jaw	
Skin		Skin	

Vocal signs when CONTENT	Vocal signs when DISTRESSED
Sounds	Sounds
Speech	Speech

Habits and mannerisms when CONTENT	Habits and mannerisms when DISTRESSED
Habits	Habits
Mannerisms	Mannerisms
Comfortable distance	Comfortable distance

Posture & observations when CONTENT	Posture & observations when DISTRESSED
Posture	Posture
Observations	Observations

Known triggers of distress (write here any actions for situations that usually cause or worsen distress)

Fig. 7.1 The first page of DisDAT
DisDAT ©2006 Northumberland Type & Wear NHG Trust and St. Oswalds Hospice. Reproduced with permission.

Assessment of symptoms of mental/pain or distress

This is discussed in 📖 Chapter 10.

Assessment of non-pain physical symptoms

While the assessment of pain in people with dementia is problematic, the formal assessment of other physical symptoms is as yet rather undeveloped. Only two scales have been found to have some degree of limited validation in this context:

- The SM-EOLD scale was developed by Volicer to assess symptoms at the end of life. The scale looks at the frequency rather than the severity or subjective impact of symptoms (which in people with advanced dementia will often be impossible to ascertain except by educated guess, especially without highly trained staff). It assesses pain, shortness of breath, skin breakdown, calm, depression, fear, anxiety, agitation, and resistiveness to care.
- The Palliative Care Outcome Scale (POS) has been validated in a sample of terminally ill Dutch demented and non-demented patients. The authors feel there is some validity for POS in GDS groups 5 and 6 (📖 Chapter 4, Staging systems, pp. 58–62) but doubt it has validity in GDS 7 patients. This is unsurprising; some questions appear to lack face validity in this context, as they ask about the subjective effects of symptoms which can only be guessed at in people with this much impairment. It is difficult to quantify impact on day-to-day life, as well as to attribute it to a particular precise cause without a certain amount of corroborative evidence, when someone is extremely physically impaired anyway.

There is therefore an urgent need to develop and validate instruments to measure non-pain symptoms in these patients. In the meantime, certainly for those with far advanced dementia, clearly observable symptoms can be assessed in a limited fashion, as noted above.

On the other hand, the assessment of the more subjective symptoms such as nausea, or the impact of 'objective' symptoms on the patient is currently undeveloped.

Limitations of observation

There are a number of major limitations of observation which need emphasizing further:

- Observation is a blunt instrument, and can never reveal the subtleties that can be explored by close questioning.
- Some symptoms which have no external manifestations, such as nausea, can only be guessed at by inference (for example, has the person developed a *new* food aversion?). Whenever possible, direct questioning of the person affected is very useful, although cross-checking against other sources of information, such as observations by others, is always invaluable.
- Many more symptoms are far less reliably assessed in those who cannot easily express themselves (advanced dementia).
- Proxy reports need to be interpreted very carefully. Several studies (though not all) have shown that relatives systematically underestimate patients' physical status and overestimate their symptoms compared with patients' (and professionals') own accounts.
- Observation of facial expression and behaviour are snapshots in time.
- Many people, especially in institutions, are observed only for a very small part of the full day. It is all too easy to generalize from a transient problem which happened to be observed to the rest of the time when the person lies unobserved. The more major the intervention resulting from an observation, the more desirable it is to have multiple points to confirm a consistent pattern.

- Perhaps the greatest limitation of observation is the polyvalence of many of the signs. Distress representing pain, psychosis, depression, hunger, annoyance, frustration, or any of a large set of other feelings may show up in exactly the same behaviour.
- In particular, the presence of BPSD can confound and invalidate the use of observational symptom assessment systems. The relation between BPSD and pain or other symptoms has still been little explored. But it has been clearly argued that many of the BPSD are merely an expression of distress with its polyvalent causes. Mental symptom are discussed more fully later (📖 Chapter 10).

Some tentative conclusions may be drawn:

- In mild to moderate dementia, self-assessment of symptoms is reliable, although one may have to try various tools to find the most suitable for that patient.
- Even in severe dementia, self-assessment is likely to be possible in around half of patients. It should therefore be attempted first, before observation by others is used as the main source of evidence.
- Corroboration with the observations of relatives or staff is very useful. This helps to confirm or cast doubt on self-assessment. It also helps practitioners sharpen their skills at using third-party observations for occasions when this is the sole evidence available. And it gives the clinician invaluable insight into the outlook of the carer.
- Different people may present symptoms differently—hence individualize.
- There is a need to cross-check information with other observers, over time, and factor in examination, known medical and other problems, and response to management.
- Symptoms must be understood in terms of their cause, rather than merely because they exist.
- Treatment is often guided by that understanding of cause.

References

1 Pautex S, Herrmann F, Le Lous P, Fabjan M, Michel JP, Gold G (2005) Feasibility and reliability of four pain self-assessment scales and correlation with an observational rating scale in hospitalized elderly demented patients. *J Gerontol A Biol Sci Med Sci* **60**, 524–9.

2 Pautex S, Michon A, Guedira M, Emond H, Le Lous P, Samaras D et al. (2006) Pain in severe dementia: self-assessment or observational scales? *J Am Geriatr Soc* **54**, 1040–5.

Chapter 8

Pain and pain control in advanced dementia

Introduction

We all have a deeply ingrained fear of severe pain, which can set off primeval reactions of panic and distress. We express our pain by verbalizing (telling others, moaning), by our expression, and by our behaviour. People with advanced dementia suffer from pain just like anyone else, but their capacity to conceptualize their experience, to respond constructively to it themselves, and to express it so that others can empathize and assist them is severely limited. In this chapter we will review what is known about pain, and about pain in dementia, and how this impacts on its assessment and management.

What is pain?

The IASP defines pain as: 'An unpleasant sensory and emotional experience associated with actual or potential tissue damage, or described in terms of such damage'.

The single most important concept to grasp about pain is that it is *subjective*: only the person feeling the pain knows what their pain is like, how intense it is, where it is located, and what quality the pain has. Pain assessment too has to depend on the sufferer's subjective narrative, as an objective view of a pain is an oxymoron; but this becomes very difficult when the person in pain has limited ability to express it, as in advanced dementia.

Another vital point that the IASP definition makes is that the sensory physiological event of pain is inseparable from the accompanying emotional experience. We now think that our experience of pain is produced by the interplay of three components (Fig. 8.1). Dementia can affect each of these.

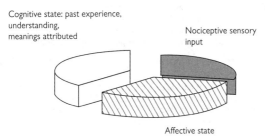

Fig. 8.1 Components of the pain experience

The biological wiring

For us to feel pain, the brain must perceive certain stimuli as painful. The neural circuitry of pain is complex; it requires:

- A receptor to detect pain.
- Pathways that transmit this sensation to the central nervous system (CNS).
- The CNS to integrate all pain-related inputs and fashion a response.
- Pathways back to the relevant parts of the body to effect a response.

Pain receptors (nociceptors)

- Painful stimuli are sensed by nociceptors, which are located in most organs, and can be stimulated by a number of changes in the tissue:
  - mechanical, e.g. strong pressure
  - thermal—significantly high or low temperatures
  - chemical, e.g. tissue acidosis from hypoxia, inflammatory mediators, e.g. bradykinin, nerve growth factor, interleukins, substance P.
- Receptors alter or transduce this response into electrical stimuli, which are transmitted along the axon of nerve pathway neurons to the cell body, which is located in the dorsal root ganglion (DRG) in the spinal cord (or, for the head, in the trigeminal nucleus for the trigeminal nerve).
- There are two basic types of pain receptor: Aδ-fibres and C-fibres.
- Aδ-fibres are myelinated; therefore they conduct pain rapidly, and are responsible for early pain from a painful stimulus (mostly heat and mechanical). They evoke sharp, pricking pain. Some Aδ-fibres are involved in hyperalgesia see below.
- C-fibres, by contrast, are non-myelinated, so conduct pain more slowly. They are polymodal, responding to mechanical, thermal, and chemical stimuli, and evoke a slow, burning pain.
- The pain threshold is the least experience of pain a subject will describe as painful (IASP definition). It is dependent on the nociceptive/discriminative component of pain. In other words, the point at which we start to feel pain is determined by the pain-transmitting circuitry.

Working out the origin of a pain

There are important differences between nociception from somatic structures (skin, joints, muscle) and visceral structures (internal organs), which influence how pain sensation is evoked, how it is felt, and how it can be treated. Failure to recognize these differences may lead to ineffective treatment and sometimes analgesic toxicity.

Superficial somatic pain

- Arises from the skin.
- Sharp, often burning in character.
- Focal to the site of injury, occurs in a well-defined area.
- Occurs immediately after the painful stimulus and is often of short duration.
- Responds to opioids, non-steroidal anti-inflammatory drugs (NSAIDs), somatic nerve blocks.

Deep somatic pain

- Arises from joints, muscle, tendons, bone.
- Pain is diffuse, over a much wider area than the precipitating stimulus.
- Distribution tends to be in the dermatome affected by the painful stimulus (see 📖 Appendix 4), but is at times remote from the site of origin. For example hip pain is often referred to the knee, diaphragmatic pain to the shoulder tip.
- Deep somatic pain is often associated with nausea and a sickening feeling, and if severe, with autonomic signs (tachycardia, pallor, sweating, b.p. changes, etc.).
- Can cause overlying skeletal muscle spasm, which may itself produce pain.
- Can take time to develop after the painful stimulus is applied, and is often slow to resolve.
- Responds to opioids, NSAIDs, somatic nerve blocks.
- Skeletal muscle spasm may need separate treatment by baclofen, diazepam, tizanidine, or other muscle relaxants.

Visceral pain

- Arises from the internal organs.
- Presents in two different ways:
  - Pain that is purely visceral is poorly localized, felt 'deep inside', and referred over a wide area across the midline of the body (hence the central chest pain of myocardial infarction).
  - When the inflamed organ is more superficial, as inflammation proceeds, it impinges on body wall structures, and pain develops many properties of deep somatic pain: felt over a large area in the same dermatome/s, often referred far from the point of origin, with overlying muscle spasm. For example with acute appendicitis, the inflamed appendix first produces midline peri-umbilical (visceral) pain, but when it impinges on the parietal peritoneum (abdominal wall—somatic), pain shifts to the right iliac fossa, and local tenderness and skeletal muscle spasm (guarding) develops.
- Visceral pain tends to feel very unpleasant and sickening and to be associated with autonomic changes.
- Visceral pain from solid organs (heart, pancreas) often responds to opioids and NSAIDs.
- Visceral pain from acute distension of a solid organ, stretching its organ capsule, is well localized and sharp. Pain from acute liver distension may respond to corticosteroids as well as NSAIDs.
- Hollow organs give rise to a particular pattern of visceral pain called colic.
- Colic comes on in waves, rising and falling to a cyclical pattern over a short time. It is due to distension of a hollow organ.
- Hollow organs have rings of smooth muscle in their wall to enable contraction and aid peristalsis. When smooth muscle is stretched, it contracts.
- Hollow organs can be cut, crushed or even burnt without evoking pain, but if they are distended, pain results as the smooth muscle contracts, presumably in an attempt to move the cause of distension along. Colicky pain occurs, for example, in renal colic, gastroenteritis, or bowel obstruction.

- Consider smooth muscle characteristics in managing colic (Table 8.1).
- Colic responds to antispasmodics, e.g. anticholinergic drugs, but less well to opioids.
- The vomiting that accompanies severe colic will usually disappear if the colic is controlled, without the need to give anti-emetics.
- Nerve blocks for visceral pain need to block local autonomic nerve plexuses. Alternatively, high epidural or spinal blocks may be needed, as the autonomic nerves supplying viscera originate high up in the spinal cord.

Table 8.1 Key differences between pain from skeletal and smooth muscle

Property	Skeletal muscle	Smooth muscle
Control	Voluntary	Involuntary
Properties	Contracts voluntarily	Contracts when stretched
Innervation	Somatic. Sensory (including for pain) and motor nerves	Autonomic: sympathetic and parasympathetic, for sensation (including pain) and activity
Pain	Deep somatic	Colic
Analgesia	Muscle relaxants, e.g. baclofen, diazepam	Anticholinergics, e.g. hyoscine butylbromide
Nerve blocks for resistant pain	Somatic blocks, e.g. epidural/spinal, peripheral nerve block, e.g. brachial block	Autonomic block, e.g. superior hypogastric plexus block, or high epidural

Pain pathways

There is a fast pathway which allows the brain to localize and characterize the nature of the pain—it serves the discriminative aspects of pain. Pain fibres travel to the DRG in the spinal cord where they synapse with second-order neurons. These ascend through the spinothalamic tract, together with temperature, touch, and visceral sensation, cross over to the other side of the cord, and go directly up to the thalamus and thence to the cortex.

Other, slower, more primitive, pathways subserve the affective and emotional feel of a pain: the palaeospinothalamic and spinoreticulothalamic tracts only reach the thalamus after making connections with brainstem regions.

The brain can also inhibit or modulate the intensity of pain traffic through descending inhibitory pathways (serotonergic and noradrenergic), which originate in the cortex, thalamus, and brainstem and synapse in the substantia gelatinosa of the DRG in the spinal cord.

The integrative role of the CNS

The CNS localizes pain and works out its characteristics, integrates it with other sensory inputs (e.g. visual and sound cues to danger), links it to past experience, and fashions emotional and behavioural responses, which are relayed back through appropriate pathways.

Acute and chronic pain: clinical differences (Table 8.2)

Acute pain is quite distinct from chronic pain in a number of ways. Affectively chronic pain has a totally different impact from acute pain, and often leads to prolonged disability and ongoing problems with employment and social role. However, there are also fundamental physiological differences, which explain why acute pain measures do not resolve chronic pain in the same way.

- Tissue injury causes local inflammation; inflammation in turn recruits adjacent nociceptors which become sensitized to pain, producing *hyperalgesia* (painful stimuli cause greater pain than normal) and *allodynia* (pain caused by normally non-painful stimuli, for example an inflamed joint can be very tender to light touch). *Peripheral sensitization* is the mechanism by which the pain receptors become more responsive to painful and non-painful stimuli.
- Ongoing painful stimuli also make the spinal cord, brainstem, and thalamocortical systems more excitable and amplify their response (*central sensitization*). This happens as a result of a cascade of changes in the neurotransmitters of the CNS. The CNS is a *plastic* system, changing in response to the traffic going on inside it.
- The altered chemical environment makes nerve cells behave differently, and sprout new connections to other areas in the CNS. The changes can maintain an ongoing pain state even though the underlying injury has healed. Responsiveness to medication can also be different from responsiveness in the acute state.

Table 8.2 Acute and chronic pain

Acute pain	Chronic pain
Has a clear cause	Causative injury often forgotten/unclear
Has a clear time course	Unknown time course, ongoing
Protective function—adaptive	Serves no protective function—maladaptive
Responds to conventional analgesics	Response to analgesics less predictable
Effect on affective state influenced by clear cause and time course	Effect on affective state influenced by uncertain cause and time course

Nociceptive, psychogenic, and neuropathic pain

Most pain we experience is nociceptive, i.e. it is produced by the action of a painful stimulus on a pain receptor. However, some pains do not result from painful stimuli.

- *Psychogenic pain* is pain produced mainly by emotional and psychological processes rather than tissue damage. Pure psychogenic pain is rare, but emotions influence pain perception and expression hugely (Chapter 8, State of mind and pain, p. 104)

- *Neuropathic pain* is pain produced by a lesion in the nervous system
rather than by a painful stimulus. The lesion can be compressive
(e.g. a disc prolapse in the spine, producing sciatica), infiltrative
(Pancoast tumour invading the brachial plexus) or due to damage to
the nerve itself by an intrinsic process (e.g. painful diabetic neuropathy).

The distinction between nociceptive and neuropathic pain is perhaps best
understood by an analogy. Nociceptive pain is akin to a well-functioning
car alarm. The stimulus (movement inside the car) is detected by sensors
and conveyed to a sound emitter which produces the characteristic
sound. In nociceptive pain the painful stimulus stimulates a pain receptor
and the impulse is transmitted up the CNS. Neuropathic pain is like a
faulty car alarm which goes off by itself, without provocation, day or night,
because the system short circuits. In the same manner nerve damage can
set up abnormal activity within the nerve which produces the painful sensation, and pain can come on spontaneously, without provocation or with
minimal cause.

Gladys was an inpatient in a nursing home. The nurses noticed she had
recently had a rash on one side of her chest wall, but thought nothing
of it as it started to fade a few days later. However, within weeks she
started to sleep less well, become agitated in bed, and uncharacteristically
preferred to be left alone. Even clothes or bedsheets rubbing against the
area of her by now almost faded rash would make her scream and hit out.
She had developed post-herpetic neuralgia, a type of neuropathic pain
which follows herpes zoster (shingles) in as many as 75% of the elderly.
She was started on gabapentin and the pain and changed behaviour eventually improved.

Recognizing neuropathic pain
- Neuropathic pain occurs in the known distribution of a peripheral
nerve or nerve root. In the case of central pain, neuropathic pain
occurs in a pattern subserved by a central structure. For example, post-
stroke pain can affect half the body, like weakness can.
- Fundamentally, however, neuropathic pain is recognized by the fact
that it is associated with nerve damage. This is usually a sensory deficit,
such as a numb area of skin, or an area of altered, unpleasant sensation
(dysaesthesiae), which may be subjective without being elicited as
numb on examination. Rarely, the damage can be very subtle, for
example changes in the skin temperature of different areas of the face
(due to vasomotor changes) in trigeminal neuralgia.
- Certain pain descriptors are often used in neuropathic pain, which may
be described as burning, shooting, pricking, ice-cold, like a tight band,
etc. These are suggestive but not diagnostic.
- There is often altered muscle power due to the nerve damage, and
some knowledge of anatomy will clarify the relation between pain and
weakness.
- Neuropathic pain is often episodic, and episodes are often spontaneous
(occur without a painful stimulus); hyperalgesia and allodynia also
occur, as does hyperpathia (painful stimuli are perceived to be

abnormally painful). These characteristics are shared with inflammatory pain, e.g. from an abscess or injury.
- Screening instruments exist to check whether a pain is neuropathic, for example the Leeds Assessment for Neuropathic Symptoms and Signs (LANSS) and PainDETECT.

State of mind and pain

The groundbreaking change in our conception of pain nowadays is our knowledge that how we feel pain is vastly affected by our emotional state and understanding (Table 8.3). The modern study of pain was born when Beecher noted that soldiers in World War II battles sometimes felt no pain despite horrendous injury until they were in a place of safety: fear and anxiety overrode the nociceptive input. Clearly psychological factors modulate the pain sensation. Numerous clinical and functional radiological studies confirm that emotional factors can totally override the physical sensory input. At the other extreme, pain can totally disable without an underlying physical lesion, purely due to psychological events.

- Pain is commoner in people who are depressed, and people with pain are more likely to suffer from major depression.
- Depressed cancer patients more often use affective terms to describe pain.
- The mechanism of this connection is unclear, although pain, depression, and anxiety share some neurophysiology and neurochemistry.
- Uncontrolled pain is a strong predictor of a desire for death.
- When both pain and depression are present both must be treated aggressively or neither may be dealt with successfully.
- Pain tolerance, i.e. the greatest level of pain which a subject is prepared to tolerate (IASP definition), reflects the affective/motivational element of pain.

Table 8.3 Factors affecting pain perception

Factors increasing pain	Factors reducing pain
Discomfort	Relief of other symptoms
Insomnia	Sleep
Fatigue	Sympathy
Anxiety	Understanding
Fear	Companionship
Anger	Creative activity
Sadness	Relaxation
Depression	Reduction in anxiety
Boredom	Elevation of mood
Mental isolation	Analgesics
Social abandonment	Anxiolytics, antidepressants

Reproduced with permission from Twycross R, Wilock A (1997) *Symptom management in advanced cancer*, 2nd edn. Radcliffe Publishing, Abingdon.

What we believe about the pain

The other essential component of pain is one's cognition of the pain. This comprises a number of interrelated elements:

- Memory of previous pain.
- Understanding of the cause and time course of the pain.
- Beliefs about consequences and meaning of the pain.
- Beliefs about treatment and treatability of the pain.
- Being able to fit the pain in the context of other things happening in one's life.

Mistaken cognitions can lead to pain-perpetuating behaviour: poor participation in treatment, problems taking medication, and activities that prolong or worsen pain. But cognitions also lead to anxiety about pain, which some consider to be as significant in worsening pain perception as depression. Working with cognitions through techniques such as cognitive behaviour therapy, or simply providing accurate information, can be a crucial step to good pain control.

Maisie was an 85-year-old woman with moderately advanced dementia who developed ovarian cancer. She had a distended, painful abdomen due to a combination of ascites and partial bowel obstruction from her tumour. She became very frightened and anxious every time she had colic. On talking to her it became clear she was afraid her abdomen would continue to grow until it burst. She had to be repeatedly reassured, but only really found some measure of peace when the symptoms of her obstruction were controlled with a syringe driver containing morphine and octreotide, and her ascites was partially drained under ultrasound guidance.

Further reading

Bennett MI, Attal N, Backonja MM, Baron R, Bouhassira D, Freynhagen R et al. (2007) Using screening tools to identify neuropathic pain. Pain **127**, 199–203.

Laird BJ et al. (2009) Are cancer pain and depression interdependent? A systematic review. Psychooncology **18**, 459–64.

Ochsner KN et al. (2006) Neural correlates of individual differences in pain-related fear and anxiety. Pain **120**, 69–77.

Pain in the elderly

- Pain is very common in the elderly. In a UK survey, 1/3 of women and 1/5 of men aged >75 had had pain for at least a week in the previous month in three or more body areas. Chronic pain is said to affect 50–80% of the elderly.
- Some pains are age-independent; others, both occupation-related and not (such as non-cardiac chest pain, abdominal pain, and orofacial pain), become rarer in old age; but pains mostly due to degenerative illnesses such as osteoarthritis become commoner with age.
- The elderly complain less of pain. There is evidence that the pain threshold is higher in the elderly, i.e. they need a higher pain intensity or duration to start to feel pain.
- Once the threshold is exceeded, the elderly are less able to tolerate severe pain than younger subjects.
- However, they are stoical and complain less.
- Frail men who have comorbid conditions suffer more intrusive pain.
- Pain can lead to social withdrawal and less utilization of services.

Pain in dementia

Effects of dementia on pain experience

Pain in dementia is common but often missed. This is partly because of communication difficulties and partly because of the difficulty people with advanced dementia have in conceptualizing pain. Dementia has a large impact on a person's experience of pain, which makes both the assessment and the management of pain more difficult. This happens because it alters all three components of the pain experience:

- Nociception.
- Cognition.
- Emotive component.

Effects on nociception

- The damage caused to the nervous system by dementias may impinge directly on pain pathways. This may reduce, intensify, or alter the sensation of pain.
- AD has little effect on the somatosensory cortex or on the thalamic nuclei, and therefore on the sensation of pain. Parietal disorders may have some effect on sensation.
- In VaD, the effect on pain sensation depends on the location of infarcts in the brain. Some infarcts, e.g. in the somatosensory cortex, may reduce pain sensitivity, whereas others can worsen or provoke pain. Thalamic infarcts may produce deafferentation pain, a type of neuropathic pain resulting from the loss of sensory input into the pain-carrying spinothalamic pathways; this can be very painful and difficult to treat.

Effects on cognition of pain

- In AD there is severe atrophy of structures key to the cognitive component of pain such as the amygdala, the anterior cingulate cortex, and the secondary somatosensory cortex. Damage to the insula affects the memory of past significant pains.
- In VaD lesions can be widespread and the effect on cognition and memory of pain can be varied and less predictable.
- Cognitive/evaluative components of the pain experience are severely and progressively disrupted in frontotemporal dementia. For example, patients may experience severe scalds because they do not anticipate that hot water can be damaging.

Effects on emotional response to pain

- AD damages the prefrontal cortex and the limbic system, altering the emotional response to pain.
- The actual effects vary from pain indifference to disinhibition.
- In VaD, again the effect depends on the location of infarcts. Prefrontal infarcts affect the emotional and motivational responses to pain.

Effect of dementia on pain expression

- People with mild to moderate dementia, and many people with severe dementia, can describe their pain usefully.
- As dementia progresses, there is less verbalization of pain.
- Behavioural responses to pain remain reliable.

- Facial expressions of discomfort are increased in demented patients compared with healthy controls. Detailed coding of facial expression is accurate and valid in dementia and remains a valuable research instrument. It is not practical in clinical assessment, but development of assessment methods based on facial expression may provide alternative means of assessment in non-verbal patients.
- See ☐ Chapter 7 for more information.

Epidemiology of pain in dementia

Prevalence of pain in dementia

- Estimates of the prevalence of pain in dementia vary from 28–83%. The variability can be accounted for by methodological differences, including different groups being studied and different assessment methods.
- A recent survey using PACSLAC (☐ Chapter 7, Symptom assessment in people with dementia, pp. 87–95), one of the best validated observational pain assessment tools in non-verbally communicative patients with dementia, arrived at a prevalence of 47%. Overall pain intensities were, however, mild.
- The literature is contradictory as to whether the prevalence of pain varies with the severity of dementia. Some work, including an important paper by Parmalee, suggested that pain is less common as dementia becomes more severe. Other studies disagree and show that the prevalence of pain does not change with the severity of dementia.
- A similar disagreement occurs in experimental studies of pain. Studies exist which suggest that patients with dementia have a higher, normal, or diminished pain tolerance compared with control groups. The prevailing view is that pain tolerance is increased in AD, and that the more advanced the disease the greater the increase in pain tolerance. The classic study underpinning this point of view is that by Benedetti, which showed that while pain threshold is unaffected by the presence of dementia, pain tolerance increases as dementia progresses. Other studies by Benedetti, Scherder and others suggest that the difference in pain tolerance is not due to a change in the sensory/discriminative mechanism ('biological wiring') of pain but in the cognitive and emotional dimensions detailed above.
- There are almost no comparable studies in VaD, but a study by Scherder (4) suggests that people suffering from VaD become less able to tolerate pain.
- Indeed, in any condition producing white matter lesions (more likely with a subtype of VaD but also AD, frontotemporal dementia, and PD), additional central pain may occur.
- The dominant view that pain tolerance increases with severity of AD has been challenged in a recent work by Kunz and colleagues which combined findings on subjective rating scales, facial expression, autonomic changes, and motor reflex responses to electrical pain stimuli. They found that while verbal expression and autonomic changes to pain decreased with progressive dementia, facial expressions to painful stimuli were significantly increased. The authors suggested that, rather than being increased, pain tolerance is reduced in people with dementia and therefore patients with

dementia suffer more pain even though in some ways they express it less. They also suggest that pain assessment in people with dementia should look at combining various measures, as subjective assessments alone tend to underreport pain.

- Clearly, even something as basic as whether people with dementia are more or less prone to pain than other individuals is as yet not settled .

Common causes of pain in dementia

Patients with dementia are elderly and tend to suffer from pains of degenerative origin. Common causes in advanced dementia include:

- Arthritis: osteoarthritis and less commonly rheumatoid or psoriatic arthritis.
- Back pain (from whatever cause).
- Pressure sores.
- Joint contractures.
- Constipation.
- Muscle spasticity.
- Local joint problems, e.g. tendinitis.

Incident pain (Chapter 8, Strong opioids, pp. 116–125), for example related to movement or weight bearing in the presence of joint problems, or to pressure sore dressing changes, is frequent.

How well is pain in dementia commonly managed?

Pain in people with dementia is rarely severe or particularly complex; however, it is often poorly managed for three main reasons:

- Failure to recognize the presence of pain, especially in people who are verbally uncommunicative.
- A fear that people with dementia may be abnormally sensitive to analgesics.
- The psychiatric training of many professional carers of people with dementia may make them tend to treat agitation with psychotropic medication without adequately assessing whether it is the result of pain and requires analgesia or a change in physical management.

There is a wealth of literature that shows that pain in dementia is often missed or inadequately treated. In a classic paper, Morrison and Siu compared daily analgesia in 59 cognitively intact patients and 38 patients with advanced dementia with hip fractures. Patients with advanced dementia received 1/3 of the opioid dose of patients with no cognitive impairment; but of the cognitively unimpaired patients, despite their much greater dose of opioid, as many as 40% still reported severe pain postoperatively. In another study, only just over 15% of cognitively intact and 24% of demented patients had a standing order for an opioid with their post-operative analgesia. This situation can be exacerbated by incidental factors such as overcrowding in the A&E department, which leads to less adequately documented pain assessment and analgesia for elderly people with hip fractures. Patients with dementia have also been shown to receive fewer NSAIDs, opiates, and paracetamol than cognitively intact controls with comparable pain. Inadequate analgesia is more likely in community patients with dementia if they are older, have advanced dementia (MMSE score < 10), or are more impaired in their ADLs. Less than half of a series of patients with AD and osteoarthritis were given analgesia, but osteoarthritis patients with dementia were more likely to be on benzodiazepines than other AD patients, presumably because the behavioural disturbance was misinterpreted and mistreated.

Control of pain in dementia follows the same principles of pain control in other situations, as described below. However a number of points need to be made.

• In a remarkable paper, Benedetti showed that the presence of prefrontal impairment in a subgroup of patients with AD led to the loss of a placebo response from their analgesia. The surprising effect of this was that the analgesia, shorn of its placebo component, was reduced so much that an increase in analgesic dose was needed to obtain good pain control. This finding applies only to a particular subgroup of people with AD; titrating the analgesic dose to comfort as outlined below should solve this becoming a practical issue.

• The undertreatment of pain in patients with dementia on psychogeriatric wards is borne out by a Dutch study which showed that, even after adjusting for the presence and severity of pain, patients on psychogeriatric wards were given less analgesia than patients on somatic wards. This points to the need for a greater cross-specialty expertise in the care of these patients.

• A recent review of pain in dementia by Scherder et al., some of the leading researchers in the field, pointed out that experimental pain tolerance 'does not represent the suffering from chronic pain, which is characterized by lack of control, and its impact on function and mood'.

Further reading

Benedetti F et al. (1999) Pain threshold and tolerance in Alzheimer's disease. Pain **80**, 377–82.

Benedetti F et al. (2006) Loss of expectation-related mechanisms in Alzheimer's disease makes analgesic therapies less effective. Pain **121**, 133–44.

Farrell MJ, Katz B, Helme RD (1996) The impact of dementia on the pain experience. Pain **67**, 7–15.

Gibson SJ, Weiner DK (2005) Pain in older persons. Progress in pain research and management, vol. 35. IASP Press, Seattle, WA.

Kunz M et al. (2007)The facial expression of pain in patients with dementia. Pain **133**, 221–8.

Kunz M et al. (2009) Influence of dementia on multiple components of pain. Eur J Pain **13**, 317–25.

Morrison RS, Siu A (2000) A comparison of pain and its treatment in advanced dementia and cognitively intact patients with hip fracture. J Pain Symptom Manage **19**, 240–8.

Parmelee PA, Smith B, Katz IR (1993) Pain complaints and cognitive status among elderly institution residents. J Am Geriatr Soc **41**, 517–22.

Scherder EJ et al. (2003) Pain assessment in patients with possible vascular dementia. Psychiatry **66**, 133–45.

Scherder E et al. (2009) Pain in dementia. Pain **145**, 276–8.

Principles of pain control

- Pain needs to be controlled if it disrupts day-to-day life.
- Occasional pain can be controlled with analgesics given p.r.n. Frequent or constant pain requires regular ('by the clock') pre-emptive analgesia.
- When possible, analgesia should be given by mouth. This allows the person in pain or the carer to give analgesia without waiting for a professional to attend, and restores some measure of control to the sufferer.
- Analgesia is guided by the WHO analgesic ladder (Fig. 8.2):
  - Step 1: mild pains should be treated with regular paracetamol or aspirin.
  - Step 2: if a full regular dose of these drugs does not control pain, switch to or add a weak opioid, e.g. dihydrocodeine, co-codamol.
  - Step 3: if a full regular dose of weak opioids does not control pain, switch up to a strong opioid, e.g. morphine, oxycodone.

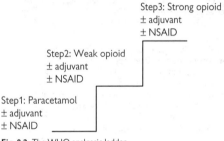

Step3: Strong opioid
± adjuvant
± NSAID

Step2: Weak opioid
± adjuvant
± NSAID

Step1: Paracetamol
± adjuvant
± NSAID

Fig. 8.2 The WHO analgesic ladder

Using the WHO analgesic ladder:
- At each step, give analgesia at the full dose and regularly.
- If this does not control pain, move up to an analgesic on the next step, not to another analgesic on the same step.
- Add NSAIDs and adjuvant analgesics at any step as necessary.
- Remember non-pharmacological means of pain control in conjunction with (or sometimes instead of) drug use.

Common analgesics

Drug interactions and metabolism (📖 Appendix 2)

Many drug interactions involve the cytochrome system of hepatic metabolism. A few preliminary notes may reduce confusion:

- Drugs may be active, i.e. have an analgesic action themselves, or only become active when metabolized to a daughter molecule. Similarly, metabolites can have intrinsic analgesic activity or they can be inactive.
- Enzyme inducers make the liver break down drugs more rapidly. They will therefore inactivate active drugs that have no active metabolites more quickly, but may well potentiate drugs with active metabolites as they increase the metabolism of the parent substance into its metabolites.
- Hepatic enzyme inhibitors slow down drug metabolism and hence prolong and potentiate the effect of active drugs, but they can reduce the effect of active metabolites.

Paracetamol

- Commonly used analgesic, antipyretic available over the counter.
- Lacks anti-inflammatory and antiplatelet properties.
- Dosage up to 1g q.d.s., although recently the Food and Drug Administration (FDA) in the USA has considered lower dosages.
- Mechanism of action not fully clear, but appears to be central and complex. May act on peroxidase site of cyclooxygenase, but also inhibits descending serotonergic pathways, appears to inhibit l-arginine nitric oxide pathways, and metabolites may have activity at cannabinoid receptors.
- Possible (though doubtful) association with GI bleeding.
- May increase the International Normalized Ratio (INR) in patients on warfarin if taken regularly.

Weak opioids

This includes drugs such as codeine, dihydrocodeine, co-codamol, and tramadol.

Codeine

- Produces its analgesic effect mainly through conversion to morphine, although other metabolites are also formed.
- Genetic variations in metabolism produce a spectrum of effectiveness, from slow metabolizers who get little analgesic effect to ultra-rapid metabolizers who can develop dangerous morphine toxicity from taking codeine.
- Its metabolism is also inhibited by CYP2D6 inhibitors (📖 Appendix 2) rendering its analgesia much weaker.
- It is a component of a number of compound analgesics, such as co-codamol (codeine + paracetamol). Co-codamol comes in three different strengths, 8/500, 15/500, and 30/500, the difference being in

the dose of codeine. It is important to know which dose of co-codamol one is dealing with.
- The variability of its effects and the great potential for interaction make some choose other weak opioids in preference to codeine.

Dihydrocodeine
- An active drug, not a prodrug, unlike codeine. Therefore despite similar genetic variations in metabolism and drug interactions to codeine, its analgesic effect is more consistent across individuals.
- Dihydrocodeine is a component (with paracetamol) of co-dydramol, which comes in strengths of 10/500, 20/500, and 30/500. Make sure you are aware of the dose you are prescribing, and do not use co-dydramol or co-codamol with paracetamol, as this can lead to inadvertent, and potentially fatal, liver toxicity.

Tramadol
- An opioid but also a weak inhibitor of norepinephrine and serotonin reuptake.
- Tramadol shows low affinity for the opioid μ-receptor, but its active M-1 metabolite has higher affinity and is a more potent analgesic.
- Tramadol is metabolized by the CYP2D6 cytochrome system, which makes it prone to genetic variability in metabolism and drug interactions. This is important if converting from or to other opioids (📖 Appendix 5, pp. 413–415)
- It can lower seizure threshold sufficiently to cause seizures at clinical doses, particularly when used with other opioids, neuroleptics, monoamine oxidase inhibitors (MAOIs), tricyclic antidepressants, or SSRIs. A history of seizures or other risk factors for seizures also increases the risk.
- Combined use with SSRIs carries a risk of serotonin syndrome (📖 Appendix 3, pp. 408–410).
- In renal failure, reduce the maximal daily dose and increase dose intervals.
- Dose adjustment is also recommended in liver failure and in the elderly.

NSAIDs
- NSAIDs are analgesic, anti-inflammatory (this is a separate function from their analgesia), and antipyretic.
- They inhibit cyclooxygenase (COX), thus blocking prostaglandin production at sites of inflammation. NSAIDs also play a number of central roles and individual NSAIDs will often have non-prostaglandin-mediated effects.
- There is genetic variability in the response to different NSAIDs and in their metabolism.
- There are two isoforms of COX, COX-1 and COX-2. Broadly speaking, COX-1 has a greater role in the housekeeping activities of the healthy body and COX-2 in inflammatory responses. However, this is a vast oversimplification as both isoforms take part in both processes, to a different degree in different tissues.

- NSAIDs can be classified into non-selective NSAIDs (block both COX-1 and COX-2 at clinical doses, e.g. ibuprofen, naproxen, diclofenac); selective NSAIDs (block COX-2 preferentially, but COX-1 inhibition becomes significant at the upper clinical range of dosage, e.g. etodolac, meloxicam), and COX-2 inhibitors (block COX-2 practically exclusively at clinical doses, e.g. celecoxib, etoricoxib).
- Although meta-analyses have not shown NSAIDs to be more effective than paracetamol in arthritis, patient preference does consistently favour NSAIDs. However, NSAIDs have a number of important adverse effects noted below.

Peptic ulceration

Gastric ulcers are 5–6 times commoner in people on NSAIDs; duodenal ulcers only 1.1 times more common. The risk is highest in the first month after starting the drugs but continues at a low level in the long term.

Risk factors for peptic ulceration on NSAIDs include:
- Age >60, with a linear increase in risk with increasing age.
- History of ulcer/GI bleed.
- Concurrent steroids, aspirin, anticoagulants, or SSRIs.
- High dose of NSAID/multiple simultaneous NSAIDs.
- Serious systemic disorders.
- Possibly, *Helicobacter pylori* infection.

The risk of ulceration, and of its serious complications (perforation, GI bleeding, gastric outlet obstruction) can be significantly reduced (📖 see box 'Using an NSAID').

Small bowel damage

NSAIDs can produce ulceration, bleeding, perforation, obstruction, and changes in bowel wall permeability, accounting for example for some examples of unexplained anaemia. Some think this problem equals peptic ulceration in scale.
- Currently there is no proven way of reducing this risk, except to use NSAIDs sparingly and at the smallest effective dose.
- NSAIDs affect the large bowel similarly: they also cause exacerbations of inflammatory bowel disease (Crohn's or ulcerative colitis).

Renal failure

Chronic NSAID use increases the risk of chronic renal failure. In infirm patients in particular they also can cause acute renal failure. Risk is highest in conditions of low effective circulating volume, such as bleeding, heart failure, diuretic use, and diarrhoea and vomiting. NSAIDs should therefore be avoided in such circumstances.

Thrombosis

Both non-selective NSAIDs and COX-2 inhibitors increase thrombotic risk (both myocardial infarction and stroke). The American Heart Association advises using other analgesics in preference to NSAIDs in patients with known, or at high risk of, heart disease They recommend using COX-2 inhibitors in this context only as a last resort. However, recent evidence suggests that celecoxib is actually safer than most non-selective NSAIDs.

Using an NSAID

- If there are major GI risk factors (📖 Chapter 8, Common analgesics, pp. 112–115), use nabumetone, celecoxib, or ibuprofen, which are the NSAIDs least likely to cause GI complications.
- Add a proton pump inhibitor (PPI; e.g. lansoprazole 30mg daily) or misoprostol 400mcg twice a day (b.d.), or if these are not tolerated, a *double-dose* H2 blocker (e.g. famotidine).
- Keep to the smallest dose that gives good pain relief and use a NSAID for the shortest time possible.
- If there are major cardiovascular risk factors, choose naproxen or celecoxib. Avoid ibuprofen or diclofenac.
- NSAIDs increase the risk of GI bleeding from low-dose aspirin to the extent that COX-2 inhibitors lose their GI safety advantage. Using aspirin with a NSAID also removes the protective effect of aspirin against thrombosis. Do not use aspirin and NSAIDs concurrently.

Further reading

Pace V (2008) Clinical pharmacology and therapeutics: nonopioids. In: *Cancer pain* (ed. N Sykes, MI Bennett, C-S Yuan), pp. 123–50. Hodder Arnold, London.

Strong opioids

Strong opioids are unique in that they have no ceiling effect: increasing the dose always increases the degree of analgesia. However, for any particular patient in any particular set of circumstances, there is a maximum dose that they can safely tolerate, although this can change as circumstances change.

Morphine

Pharmacology

- Morphine, the most commonly used strong opioid, is a μ-receptor agonist.
- It is metabolized mainly in the liver by glucuronidation.
- The main metabolite, morphine-3-glucuronide (M3G), has no activity at opioid receptors.
- Morphine-6-glucuronide (M6G) is an active metabolite, significantly more potent as an analgesic than morphine. Several other metabolites are produced, probably of lesser importance.
- Morphine metabolism also occurs in other tissues, especially the CNS.
- Morphine oral bioavailability varies hugely, from 15–64%, though it averages around 35%. This has major implications for conversions to and from other opioids, as conversion using morphine equivalent doses from tables can lead to overdosage of some and underdosage of other patients (🕮 Appendix 5, pp. 413–415).

Cautions

- *Morphine should be avoided in renal impairment.*
- While it is a remarkably safe drug if properly used in most settings, in renal failure metabolites accumulate and morphine toxicity can rapidly result, which can be fatal or extremely uncomfortable for the patient (🕮 Chapter 8, Strong opioids, pp. 116–125)
- As there are now many safe alternatives, there is no justification for using morphine in this situation (🕮 Chapter 8, Strong opioids, pp. 116–125)
- Morphine is surprisingly well tolerated in liver failure until this becomes severe and glucuronidation is finally affected.

> Opioids other than morphine are used increasingly, especially in situations of organ failure or intolerance to morphine. Some of these are complex to handle, and sometimes problems arise because of the circumstances in which a changeover from morphine is instituted, e.g. renal failure, where the risk of drug-associated problems is often marked. Some detail is given in the following account as non-specialists may find themselves looking after patients on unfamiliar opioids. In cases of doubt or unfamiliarity with the drugs in questions, palliative care or pain specialist advice should be sought.

Using morphine

1. It is usually easiest to start with immediate release (IR) morphine.
2. As a rough rule of thumb:
   - 1g paracetamol 4-hourly gives less analgesia than 2.5mg oral morphine 4-hourly.
   - 60mg dihydrocodeine or codeine 4-hourly is equivalent to 5mg oral morphine 4-hourly

   Hence when starting oral morphine because analgesia with other drugs is inadequate, convert the dose you are already giving to a morphine equivalent dose using the above (or 📖 Appendix 5), and then work out the new, stronger dose by increasing this by between 30% and 100%, depending on pain severity.

   For example, a patient with uncontrolled pain on paracetamol 1g q.d.s. can be converted either to dihydrocodeine 30–60mg 4-hourly or to morphine 2.5–5mg 4-hourly.

3. Dose increments if pain is uncontrolled should be as follows: 2.5mg| 5mg|10mg|15mg|20mg|30mg|40mg|60mg|90mg. Subsequently doses are best increased in 30–50% steps.
4. Once the dose of morphine needed has been established, for convenience and better adherence one can total the daily dose of morphine required and divide by 2 to give 12-hourly doses of modified release (MR) morphine.

   For example, a patient on morphine IR 10mg 4-hourly is taking 10 × 6 = 60mg daily, which can be switched to morphine MR 30mg b.d.

5. As a rough rule of thumb, p.r.n. doses for breakthrough pain should be roughly equivalent to the 50–100% of the 4-hourly dose the patient is on.

   For example a patient on 10mg 4-hourly (or 30mg morphine MR b.d.) should have morphine IR 5–10mg p.r.n. for breakthrough pain while a patient on 100mg 4-hourly (or 300mg morphine MR b.d.) should be given morphine IR 50–100mg p.r.n. for breakthrough pain.

   However, this is a rough rule of thumb, as breakthrough pain may vary widely (📖 Chapter 8, Strong opioids, pp. 116–125).

6. Always start an anti-emetic with morphine for the first week: good choices would be haloperidol 0.5–1.5mg nocte, or, in haloperidol-intolerant patients, cyclizine 50mg t.d.s. The anti-emetic can almost always be stopped within a week.
7. Opioids constipate, therefore laxatives should also be started at the same time and titrated according to response. Laxatives should be combinations of bowel stimulants and stool softeners, e.g. senna or bisacodyl (stimulants) plus liquid paraffin and magnesium hydroxide oral emulsion BP (e.g. Milpar) or lactulose or macrogol (softeners/osmotic laxatives) (Table 9.7).
8. Explain to patients or carers beforehand that while there may be some initial drowsiness, this is very likely to lift within a week.
9. Learn to recognize the signs of opioid toxicity (📖 Chapter 8, Strong opioids, pp. 116–125).
10. If in doubt, consult a palliative care colleague.

Diamorphine

- Diamorphine is broken down into morphine almost immediately in the body.
- Its one advantage is its very great solubility, which means that high doses can be given as stat injections or in syringe drivers in very small volumes.

Oxycodone

Pharmacology

- Oxycodone is a μ- and κ-opioid receptor agonist. The clinical implications of this are unclear.
- It has at least two active metabolites, although it is uncertain how much these usually contribute to analgesia. One of these, oxymorphone, is produced by cytochrome-based metabolism; in CYP2D6 ultra-metabolizers it may produce opioid toxicity even with low oxycodone doses

Clinical use

- Often a substitute for morphine in intolerant patients.
- To convert from oral morphine to oral oxycodone, give half the morphine dose as oxycodone, e.g. morphine 10mg by mouth (p.o.) = oxycodone 5mg p.o.
- To convert from subcutaneous (s.c.) morphine to s.c. oxycodone, divide the morphine dose by 2, e.g. 10mg morphine s.c. = 5mg oxycodone s.c.

Cautions

- Hepatic failure: more likely to cause toxicity than morphine.
- Moderate to severe renal failure: though slightly safer than morphine. Avoid if renal failure is at all severe.
- Elderly: bioavailability is increased by 15%. However, if doses are titrated to pain this should not present problems.

Fentanyl

In the UK fentanyl is used either as an injectable drug, mainly in anaesthesia, or as a transdermal patch for the control of cancer pain and chronic pain.

Pharmacology

- Fentanyl is a synthetic opioid with high affinity for the μ-receptor.
- It is unsuitable for oral use due to high first-pass metabolism.
- Its high lipophilicity makes transdermal and transmucosal routes possible.
- It has a high volume of distribution.
- Elimination half-life increases from around 15 minutes with single injections to 7–12 hours in steady-state conditions.
- Metabolism is predominantly in the liver. CYP3A4 inhibitors increase fentanyl concentrations (📖 Appendix 2).
- Conversion ratios from morphine vary in different individuals from 70:1 to 150:1. Variability similarly holds for conversion from other opioids. This has implications when switching from other opioids to a fentanyl patch.

- It takes much longer to wean the elderly off patches, because the elimination half-life of fentanyl after the removal of the patch increases from 20 hours in younger patients to 43 hours in the elderly.

Clinical use
- Fentanyl is less constipating than morphine, though laxatives are still usually required.
- It can be given via various routes:
  - Transdermal fentanyl ('fentanyl patch').
  - Transmucosal fentanyl: a number of proprietary preparations are available for treatment of breakthrough pain by buccal or sublingual transmucosal routes. **These are only to be used in patients already on strong opioids as fatalities have otherwise been reported,** and are licensed for use in cancer pain. They should be used under the guidance of a palliative care or pain specialist.
  - Fentanyl can also be used spinally or via a continuous s.c. or i.v. infusion; its use in these settings is outside the scope of this book.

Using transdermal fentanyl ('fentanyl patches')

Fentanyl's high lipophilicity, potency, and small molecular size make it ideal for transdermal (TD) use. It builds a skin and s.c. tissue depot from which it diffuses systemically. Steady state for transdermal fentanyl is reached after 17–48 hours.

In reservoir patches a membrane holds the drug in the patch; in matrix patches it is contained in a slow-releasing adhesive matrix. For any patient, use the same type consistently, as properties differ.

How to use
- Apply to hairless skin. Clip but do not shave hair. Avoid soap, oils, or cream (these alter skin permeability). Press firmly in place for at least 30 seconds.
- When converting from another opioid, cover the period until the fentanyl patch kicks in with the usual analgesia:
  - e.g. give oral morphine IR at 0, 4, 8, and 12 hours after applying the patch, then p.r.n.
  - e.g. give the last dose of 12-hourly morphine MR (modified release) at the same time as the patch is put on, then use morphine IR for breakthrough pain as normal.
  - e.g. continue analgesia through a syringe driver for 12 hours after applying the patch.
- Use p.r.n. medication liberally for the first 48 hours, as serum levels build up.
- If after the first 48 hours more than two p.r.n. doses are needed daily, increase the patch dosage by one step.

Some patients develop withdrawal symptoms when switched over to fentanyl due to variability in dose conversion ratios. Symptoms include yawning, sweating, lacrimation, rhinorrhoea, anxiety, restlessness, insomnia, dilated pupils, piloerection ('cold turkey'), chills, tachycardia, hypertension, nausea and vomiting, colic, diarrhoea, and muscle aches and pains. In these

(continued)

patients give p.r.n. doses of IR opioid, e.g. morphine, to cover the few days until the symptoms subside.

Patches need changing every 72 hours, rotating through four different body sites before returning to the original site again. Occasional patients need them changed every 48 hours.

In fever or with skin warming, increased absorption can cause toxicity. Absorption of transdermal fentanyl can be impaired in cachexia.

Opioid-naive patients must only be started on transdermal fentanyl by someone experienced in its use, as the dose they require would still be unknown, and the patches take a long time to wear off. This could lead to fatal fentanyl toxicity, which has been reported on many occasions due to incorrect use. In the USA the FDA warns against using fentanyl in opioid-naive patients.

Similarly, fentanyl patches should not be used for rapid titration of analgesia, but only where opioid requirements are stable.

Source: Twycross R, Wilcock A, Charlesworth S, Dickman A (2009) *Palliative care formulary*, 3rd edn. Radcliffe Publishing, Oxford.

Hydromorphone

- Hydromorphone is a μ-agonist that can be given p.o., p.r., or by s.c., i.m., i.v., or spinal injection. It is well absorbed from all routes.
- Its great solubility makes it attractive for patients on high opioid doses.
- It undergoes extensive first-pass metabolism to hydromorphone-3-glucuronide (HM3G), which accumulates in renal failure and may contribute to rare neurotoxicity (📖 Chapter 8, Strong opioids, pp. 116–125).
- The manufacturer suggests a conversion ratio of 7.5:1 from morphine, i.e. 7.5mg of morphine = 1mg of hydromorphone, whether p.o., s.c., or i.m. Others suggest that when switching from morphine to hydromorphone, 5mg of morphine = 1mg hydromorphone, but when switching from hydromorphone to morphine, a 1:4 ratio should be used.
- It should be used with caution in liver failure, and in severe renal failure due to the risk of neuroexcitation.

Methadone

- Methadone is a μ- and δ-agonist; unlike many opioids is not an alkaloid.
- It has NMDA-antagonist activity similar to ketamine (📖 Chapter 8, Adjuvant analgesics, pp. 126–131), which in theory makes it particularly useful for neuropathic pain, but no clinical study has examined whether this is so.
- It is highly lipophilic, so is rapidly absorbed.
- Oral bioavailability varies between 41 and 97% (usually 80%). This variability is one factor that makes conversion from other opioids difficult.
- It is distributed rapidly but then eliminated slowly (30–60 hours).
- Its half-life increases very significantly in the elderly, reportedly to 130 hours and sometimes longer.
- It has a high volume of distribution.
- Methadone has no active metabolites.

- It interacts extensively with enzyme inducers and inhibitors (📖 Appendix 2).
- The half-life of methadone increases significantly with increasing urine pH.
- It can prolong the cardiac QT interval and precipitate torsades de pointes, a cardiac arrhythmia which can lead into ventricular fibrillation and cardiac arrest. Use with other QT-interval-prolonging drugs (📖 Appendix 2) is not recommended.
- All these and other factors make methadone a difficult drug to use, and it should be reserved for palliative care and pain specialists.

Buprenorphine

- Buprenorphine is a partial μ-agonist and κ and δ-antagonist.
- Consequently it has a ceiling effect for respiratory depression, and higher doses will not make this worse. Psychotomimetic symptoms (hallucinations confusion, sedation) are said to be less common than with opioid agonists.
- Buprenorphine has a high first-pass metabolism, and is converted to a metabolite which crosses the blood–brain barrier (BBB) with difficulty and therefore produces little analgesia. It is therefore not a good oral opioid.
- Metabolism is intra-hepatic, and partly CYP3A4 dependent (📖 Appendix 2).
- It can be given by injection but in palliative care is more likely to be used s.l. (sublingual) or especially TD.
- s.l. buprenorphine is readily absorbed but reaches a plasma peak concentration at 90 minutes, and its duration of action is 6–8 hours.
- There are different TD preparations and it is important to be aware of which one is dealing with. Some are applied for up to 4 days, the manufacturers recommending changing twice a week on the same days of the week to facilitate remembering. They also suggest covering with the patient's usual short-acting analgesic for 12 hours after the first application, if moving from another opioid. Other, lower-concentration, preparations are applied every 7th day. The manufacturers recommend covering pain with p.r.n. immediate release analgesia when first applying the patch.
- In both types of patches, regular opioids must not be restarted until at least 24 hours after discontinuing a patch.
- Patch dose must not be increased until it has been up for at least 3 days.
- Patches should not be put on the same site within a week.
- For practical details about applying the patches see 📖 Chapter 8, Strong opiods, pp. 116–125.
- Buprenorphine is safe in renal failure but must be used with caution and at reduced dose in severe liver failure.
- It was feared in the past that concurrent use of opioid agonists for breakthrough pain or switching to buprenorphine from opioid agonists could reduce analgesia. This only happens at very high buprenorphine doses.

Recognizing and managing opioid toxicity

The right dose of an opioid is the dose that relieves pain without producing toxicity. The skill lies in choosing analgesic and regime to control pain without unacceptable adverse effects.

Just as one is not allowed to drive a car unless one can stop it safely, so *one cannot use opioids safely if one is unable to recognize opioid toxicity.*

Signs of opioid toxicity

- Sedation
- Nausea and vomiting
- Respiratory depression
- Sweating
- Pruritus
- Hallucinations
- Delirium
- Neuroxecitatory effects: myoclonus, allodynia, hyperalgesia, seizures

Sedation

- Sedation from opioids in cognitively intact patients tends to disappear after a week of continued use. There are no data around use in the cognitively impaired.
- Continuing sedation with opioids is rare if the pain is opioid-responsive (📖 Chapter 8, Strong opiods, pp. 116–125) and the right dose is used. The degree of sedation does NOT depend on the dose of opioid: some patients with minor pain can be heavily sedated on very small doses of opioid, and others with severe pain may not be sedated at all on a thousand times the same dose.
- A number of studies using neuropsychological testing have shown that on balance long-term opioids do not impair performance in people with cancer or those without cancer. In some cases, by taking away pain, they actually improve attention and performance. However, almost all these studies have been done on people with relatively high performance status, and none in people with cognitive impairment.
- If a patient on opioids appears sedated, exclude other causes (e.g. infection, hypercalcaemia, hyponatraemia, poor sleep). Unless sedation is severe, if the opioid has just been commenced, persist for a few days.
- If sedation is severe or persistent see 📖 Chapter 8, Strong opioids, pp. 116–125.

Nausea and vomiting

- Common in the first week of opioid use, then usually settle.
- Add haloperidol or cyclizine for a week to control.
- Persistent nausea and vomiting may require continued anti-emetic use or opioid switching.

Respiratory depression

- Although common in acute pain, e.g. post-operative pain and with i.v. opioids, it is very unusual in chronic opioid dosing, especially by mouth.
- Normal adult respiratory rates vary between 12 and 20 breaths/minute.
- This is the one symptom for which the use of naloxone should be considered. Naloxone can precipitate severe pain in people on

opioids, and is rarely needed as most problems will improve over a few hours anyway. However, severe respiratory depression can be fatal and justifies naloxone use (see box 'Using naloxone to reverse opioid induced respiratory depression').

Neuroexcitatory effects
- Myoclonus is common in opioid toxicity, although it can also be due to renal or hepatic failure, PD, AD, or CJD.
- Remove the cause if possible.
- First-line treatment is with clonazepam. Alternatives are sodium valproate, phenytoin, and barbiturates.
- Patients may also develop allodynia and hyperalgesia (📖 Chapter 8, The biological wiring, pp. 98–103) especially on high opioid doses.

Opioid responsive and opioid non-responsive pain

One of the commonest causes of opioid toxicity is the failure to recognize that the pain is not opioid responsive. The opioid is then increased repeatedly without effect until the patient becomes toxic but is still in pain. Opioid poorly-responsive pains include:
- Colic: responds better to anticholinergic drugs.
- Tenesmus: painful spasm of the anal sphincter with an urgent but mostly ineffectual urge to defecate, e.g. in rectal tumours or distension by hard faecal masses. Evacuate the rectum if possible. If there is no other treatment, a lumbar sympathetic block, a rectal stent if appropriate, or use of some calcium channel blockers are the treatments of choice.
- Bladder spasm: responds to antimuscarinics, e.g. oxybutinin, tolterodine, or trospium.
- Pressure sore pain: systemic opioids are often only marginally helpful in pressure sore pain. Pressure-relieving measures are very helpful. In cases of severe pain, topical opioids, e.g. diamorphine, are highly effective.

Using naloxone to reverse opioid induced respiratory depression

Indications
- Respiratory rate < 8/minute AND patient unconscious and/or cyanosed.
- Clinical signs are more likely to detect respiratory depression than pulse oximetry.[1]

Management
- Make up 400mcg naloxone to 10ml with 0.9% saline.
- Give 0.5ml (20mcg) every 2 minutes until the respiratory rate is satisfactory.
- Titrate doses to respiratory function, not level of consciousness, as pain from opioid withdrawal may cause severe agitation.
- Further doses may be needed as naloxone is short acting.

Based partly on Twycross R, Wilcock A, Charlesworth S, Dickman A (2009) *Palliative care formulary*, 3rd edn. Radcliffe Publishing, Oxford.

---

1 American Society of Anesthesiologists Task Force on Neuraxial Opioids (2009) Practice guidelines for the prevention, detection and management of respiratory depression associated with neuraxial opioid administration. *Anesthesiology* **110**, 218–30.

Incident pain and breakthrough pain

- Incident pain is pain precipitated by an action that is anticipated to cause pain. For example walking on a leg with an inflamed joint can cause a rapid flare-up of severe pain that subsides as soon as the weight is taken off the leg. Again, changing dressings on pressure sores can cause incident pain.

- Most incident pain has a very rapid onset and offset. This makes it impossible to treat properly pharmacologically if the difference between pain at rest and pain on provocation is at all marked. One would need two very different doses of analgesia: a low dose for the constant background pain and a much higher dose for the brief flare-ups. Using a high dose when the patient is not in severe pain will make them very drowsy.

- Incident pains can sometimes be treated by anticipatory analgesia, e.g. a small dose of oral or s.c. opioid 15–20 minutes before a painful dressing change.

- Explore non-pharmacological means, e.g. walking stick, nerve block.

- Incident pain is one type of *breakthrough* pain. Breakthrough pain is 'an abrupt, short lived and intense pain that "breaks through" the round-the-clock analgesia that controls persistent pain'[2].

- End-of dose pain is often confused with breakthrough pain. It occurs soon before the next regular dose of medication, e.g. 4-hourly morphine, is due. It is treated simply by increasing the baseline opioid dose by say 30% to make it last until the next dose takes effect.

- Breakthrough pain often lasts less than 30 minutes per episode, and often peaks at 3–5 minutes after onset. Giving say 4-hourly morphine for a pain with this profile risks the medication only starting to have an effect once the pain has worn off, and then staying in the system after the need for it has subsided, for long enough to make the patient drowsy for some time.

- A number of medications designed specially for breakthrough pain, such as mucosal fentanyl citrate lozenges or s.l. tablets, have been developed. The-se start to act within 15 minutes and still have an effect 2 hours later. Their pharmacological profile thus fits the breakthrough pain profile better. *They should not be used in opioid naïve patients and it is recommended that specialist advice be sought for their use.*

Anne was reported by care home staff to have become withdrawn, had gone off her food, and often screamed or cried when her dressings were changed. Examination revealed a frail old lady with a necrotic area on her foot, with thick pus issuing from underneath, and totally exposed tendons to the toes on the dorsum of the foot. The GP, fearful of adverse effects, would only prescribe p.r.n. paracetamol. Anne was put on regular morphine with a small dose before dressing changes. Within a couple of days she was back to her old, interactive, happy self, and remained so until her death many weeks later.

2 Bennet D (2005) Consensus panel recommendations for the assessment and management of break-through pain. Part 1 assessment. *Pharmacy Therapeut* **30**, 296–301.

Dealing with persistent sedation from opioids

If sedation persists for more than a few days after starting opioids, or if severe:

- Does patient need so much analgesia? If they are in no pain you can reduce the dose.
- Is the pain likely to be opioid responsive? If not, change to the appropriate drug (📖 Chapter 8, Strong opioids, pp. 116–125).
- Can you use non-pharmacological techniques or adjuvant analgesics to reduce need for opioids? (📖 Chapter 8, Adjuvant analgesics, pp. 126–131.)
- Are there other reasons for drowsiness, e.g. UTI, low serum sodium?
- Occasionally, an opioid may need to be switched to another strong opioid to give a better adverse effect profile. This requires care and experience and is often best left to palliative care or pain specialists.
- Occasionally drugs may have to be used to reduce sedation. Drugs that have been used in this context include methylphenidate (an amphetamine), modafinil, and donepezil. RCT evidence is only available for the first, but the other two drugs may be safer to use in advanced dementia.

Further reading

Davis MP, Glare PA, Hardy J, Quigley C (2009) *Opioids in cancer pain*, 2nd edn. Oxford University Press, Oxford.

Flock P (2003) Pilot study to determine the effectiveness of diamorphine gel to control pressure ulcer pain. *J Pain Symptom Manage* **25**, 547–54.

Twycross R, Wilcock A, Charlesworth S, Dickman A (2009) *Palliative care formulary*, 3rd edn Radcliffe Publishing, Oxford.

Zeppetella G (2009) Impact and management of breakthrough pain in cancer. *Curr Opin Support Palliat Care* **3**, 1–6.

Adjuvant analgesics

Adjuvant analgesics are drugs whose primary indication is not pain, but which are useful for pain control in particular situations. Examples include antidepressants, anticonvulsants and benzodiazepines, which all have important roles in pain control in specific circumstances.

Number needed to treat and number needed to harm

In the following discussion, use will be made of number needed to treat for pain (NNT = number of patients needed to undergo treatment with a particular drug or other treatment modality, in order to achieve a 50% reduction in pain in one patient) and the number needed to harm for pain (NNH = number of patients treated with an analgesic for one patient to withdraw from taking the analgesic due to adverse effects). A good NNT is as close as possible to 1 (a NNT of 1 means the drug reduces pain by at least 50% in all patients, so NNTs cannot be lower than 1). On the other hand, the higher the NNH, the more acceptable a drug is. NNT and NNH are not of course the only measure of clinical utility. For example very severe but rare adverse effects can give a low NNH but still make one avoid using a particular drug.

Neuropathic pain

For a discussion of the mechanisms of neuropathic pain see 📖 Chapter 8, The biological wiring, pp. 98–103.

A number of drugs can be used to treat neuropathic pain. A recent consensus statement by most of the leading authorities in the field suggested that first-line treatment should consist of either a tricyclic antidepressant like nortriptyline, or a selective serotonin and norepinephrine reuptake inhibitor (SNRI) such as venlafaxine, or a calcium channel $\alpha 2$-δ ligand such as gabapentin.

Tricyclic antidepressants

These have the advantages of once daily administration, low cost, and concomitant effect on mood or sleep if desired.

- They have the best NNT of any drug class for this type of pain (depending on the type of neuropathic pain, generally 2–3, which is very good in this difficult pain area) but a fairly worrying NNH (14.7 in a recent large meta-analysis).
- The best evidence is for amitriptyline, but this has many hazards particularly in the elderly (Table 10.2 and 📖 Appendix 3). Nortriptyline and desipramine are safer as their anticholinergic profile is less pronounced.
- Start at 10mg at night if the patient is elderly, titrating up to the dose which controls pain (sometimes 75mg or more). Serum levels vary greatly between individuals, so titrate the dose to response.
- Response for pain is not due to an effect on mood. It is often seen within 4–7 days, well before any antidepressant effect, but may take many weeks.

SNRIs

An example is venlafaxine (NNT 5.1, NNH 16.0). Caution has to be used in the presence of cardiovascular disease.

SSRIs
An example is paroxetine. Current evidence suggests a low NNT of 7 for neuropathic pain.

Calcium channel α2-δ ligands
For example gabapentin and pregabalin:
- Gabapentin is sometimes used as an anticonvulsant or mood stabilizer in psychiatry, and should be considered particularly when this is needed as well as an agent for neuropathic pain.
- The main advantage of these drugs is their relative freedom from adverse effects. Drowsiness, dizziness, and peripheral oedema are common; of importance to palliative care patients, especially with dementia, myoclonus can be an adverse effect.
- The NNT for gabapentin averaged over the various types of neuropathic pain was 3.8 on 2400mg/day or more, but 5.1 if studies using lower doses were included. Gabapentin is significantly better tolerated than tricyclics (the combined NNH for all neuropathic pain conditions is 26.1). Questions have been raised over whether the drug company reported the evidence for gabapentin selectively to present it in a more favourable light.[2]
- Pregabalin had an NNT of 3.7 and an NNH of 7.4.

Opioids for neuropathic pain
Contrary to previous beliefs, neuropathic pain is opioid responsive, although opioids rarely give complete control of the pain.
- Opioid are second-line drugs in this situation. They are immediately effective, whereas other drugs will only work after an interval of days to weeks.
- Morphine and oxycodone have NNTs of around 2.5, with very low NNHs.
- There are theoretical reasons for believing that methadone (📖 Chapter 8, Strong opioids, pp. 116–125) is particularly useful in neuropathic pain, due to its NMDA antagonist properties (see below). However, no clinical trials have as yet substantiated this claim.

NMDA-receptor antagonists
NMDA and glutamate, the commonest excitatory neurotransmitter in the CNS, can both bind to NMDA receptors. NMDA receptors play an important role in central sensitization (📖 Chapter 8, The biological wiring, pp. 98–103.). Antagonists block elements of this central sensitization and can make some intractable pains much more responsive to treatment.
- Examples of NMDA antagonists include ketamine, dextromethorphan, memantine, methadone, phencyclidine, and pethidine.
- Low-dose (subanaesthetic) ketamine is sometimes used to treat intractable neuropathic and other pains. It can occasionally lessen the need for opioids so much that patients become opioid toxic unless the opioid dose is adjusted.

Other drugs for neuropathic pain
These include anticonvulsants such as valproate, carbamazepine (poorly tolerated by frail patients), phenytoin (rarely used due to the high

2 Landefeld CS, Steinman MA (2009) The neurontin legacy—marketing through misinformation and manipulation. *New Engl J Med* **360**, 103–6.

prevalence of drug interactions and narrow therapeutic index), and clonazepam (for which the evidence base is poor). Other potential drugs include sodium channel blockers such as mexiletine (rarely safe for frail patients often with a cardiac history; low NNT) and baclofen.

Muscle spasm pain

- Skeletal muscle spasm pain occurs, for example, in hemiparesis, where spastic muscles become very stiff and painful.
- It is an example of a poorly opioid-responsive pain.
- Drugs such as baclofen (5–30mg t.d.s.), diazepam in small doses, tizanadine, or dantrolene can be very effective.
- Botulinum toxin injection can be used in more intractable cases.
- Putting spastic muscles gently through a full range of movements on a daily basis may lessen discomfort. Good physiotherapy makes a major contribution to pain control.
- It is important not to overuse muscle relaxants, as converting a spastic leg to a floppy leg, for example, can convert someone who can stand and walk independently, albeit ungracefully, into someone who cannot stand or who runs a high risk of falls.

Colic (📖 Chapter 8, The biological wiring, pp. 98–103)

- Colic responds better to anticholinergic drugs such as hyoscine butylbromide than to opioids.
- Hyoscine butylbromide has poor oral bioavailability although it is very effective by injection.
- Hyoscine hydrobromide can also be used, but unlike the butylbromide, it crosses the BBB and can make people drowsy and more prone to seizures. It also has an anti-emetic effect, so may be considered if this is also needed. It can be administered as a skin patch.
- If a rapid response is wanted, s.l. hyoscine (Kwells® , used for travel sickness), can be very effective within minutes. As with all s.l. drugs, ensure the mouth is moist before administering (give a sip of water).
- Opioids can control pain due to constipation reasonably well, but at the cost of worsening the underlying problem, and should not be used for this purpose.

Pressure sore pain

- The pain of pressure sores can be very severe, often overshadowing pain from advanced cancer, for example.
- Superficial ulcers tend to be more painful, as in deep ulcers the nerve endings which transmit pain are often damaged.
- It is only partly responsive to systemic opioids.
- Non-drug measures used to prevent and relieve pressure sore pain must be used, alone or with medication.
- Topical morphine or diamorphine (applied in a vehicle such as Intrasite gel or the thermoreversible Lutrol gel) is useful in treating pressure sore ulcer pain. It is applied to the inflamed area at the edge of the ulcer particularly.

Routes of administration

The route of administration of drugs can have critical importance over their acceptability, practicality or usefulness.

Oral
- The preferred route as it is the easiest and the most convenient.
- Alternative routes may be needed if there are swallowing difficulties, vomiting, or impaired consciousness.
- First-pass metabolism may lessen the oral bioavailability of some drugs.

Rectal

Suppositories can be convenient ways of bypassing first-pass metabolism via a rapid transmucosal route.
- Insertion of the suppository reversed makes it more likely it will stay in place. It is important not to insert it into faeces with no mucosal contact.
- Some drugs, e.g. NSAIDs, can cause proctitis if given rectally.
- Some patients find suppositories unacceptable, especially if they are disorientated.

Subcutaneous
- Widely used in palliative care: convenient, easy to use, and reliable. Single s.c. injections are much less painful than i.m. injections.
- s.c. infusions via a syringe driver parallel serum levels of i.v. infusions with a time lag of a few hours. For this reason i.v. infusions, which are more difficult to maintain, are very rarely used in palliative care in the UK.

Transdermal
- TD patches are used for highly lipophilic analgesics such as fentanyl and buprenorphine, as well as other drugs such as hyoscine.
- Patches can be reservoir patches, where a membrane holds the drug in place, or matrix patches, where the drug is embedded in a reservoir which slowly releases it over time. The two types have different properties; patients must not be switched from one type to another without great care (📖 Chapter 8, Strong opioids, pp. 116–125).

Intramuscular
- The i.m. route is rarely used in palliative care because it is uncomfortable, especially for repeated injections, and rarely confers advantages over the much more acceptable, and less dangerous, s.c. route.
- A very few drugs can be given i.m. but not s.c.
- The other indication for the i.m. route is for patients in shock, where the peripheral circulation is shut down and absorption of s.c. injections becomes very erratic.

Intravenous
- This route is used only in exceptional circumstances in most palliative care practices. It is difficult to maintain, requires special training to use, depends on the availability of good venous access and may lead to life-threatening infections.
- In overwhelming pain, opioids can be titrated to pain i.v. until some control is again established; this carries a high risk of respiratory depression and should only be attempted by suitably qualified staff with facilities for drug reversal and resuscitation.

Non-pharmacological means of pain control

Non-drug means to prevent or manage pain at times have a greater effect on pain than drugs, and are often an important adjunct. However, in people with advanced dementia some treatment can be upsetting and distressing (one might not understand why one is being needled during a nerve block), patients may not cooperate with treatment which, for example, requires them to be still or is briefly painful, and treatment which requires ongoing education and skill development is not possible when memory is significantly impaired.

Physiotherapy

- Physiotherapy can contribute to pain control by improving mobility, reducing spasticity and stiffness, and reducing falls. Techniques such as splinting, provision of mobility aids, and ultrasound for joint disorders are also useful.
- However, people with advanced dementia will not be able to learn and practice exercises, nor will they be able to understand what the physiotherapist is doing and why (but see 📖 Chapter 11). Physiotherapy at this stage may become progressively more often done to the patient rather than with, and may become gradually more often passive than active for the patient.

Transcutaneous electrical nerve stimulation (TENS)

The pain gating theory of Wall and Melzack stated that traffic through touch pathways reaching the dorsal horn of the spinal cord would block traffic through pain pathways. TENS achieves this by producing slight skin tingling through electrical stimulation.

- There are various types of TENS—conventional, acupuncture-like, and pulsed—each with their own characteristics. Other related modalities such as percutaneous electrical nerve stimulation (PENS; where electrodes are embedded into the skin) also exist.
- TENS is useful in some neuropathic, musculoskeletal, and visceral pains.
- The effect of TENS often outlasts its application by several hours.
- TENS should not be used on patients with pacemakers, on areas of altered skin sensitivity, over tumours, over the neck, or where there is tissue bleeding.

Nerve blocks

- Nerve blocks are useful for localized pain.
- Many recipients of nerve blocks will still need to continue other analgesics, although the block may reduce the need to escalate analgesia and thus reduce adverse effects.
- Blocks can be axial (spinal or epidural injections—useful for pains with complex innervation below the level of injection, e.g. pain in both legs), peripheral (useful for pain originating from one or a small number of peripheral nerves, e.g. intercostal) or autonomic (for pain of autonomic origin for example visceral pain, e.g. superior hypogastric plexus blocks).
- Indwelling blocks, including implantable delivery systems, can sometimes be used when single injection blocks only provide brief respite from pain. However, the former are prone to displacement and the latter are expensive.
- Nerve blocks may have to be repeated every few weeks or months in some cases; in others the pain settles and there is no further indication for blocks.

Acupuncture
- Acupuncture may be useful in treating a number of conditions such as neck or back pain, nausea, and vomiting.
- However, recent reviews of the evidence suggest that analgesic effects are small, that it is currently impossible to separate out psychological from physical effects, and that effects tend to be short-lasting.

Kyphoplasty and vertebroplasty
These techniques involve the injection of bone cement into collapsed vertebrae, usually as a result of osteoporosis but also from malignancy or benign tumours, to reduce pain and regain height, which improves posture and may reduce risk of falling. They are useful in the acute phase of collapse but their applicability in later stages is unknown.

Radiotherapy and chemotherapy
- These are useful in cancer pain, e.g. metastatic bone pain.
- Palliative treatment will involve short courses and low doses with few adverse effects.

Further reading

Dworkin RH, O'Connor AB, Backonja M, Farrar JT, Finnerup NB, Jensen TS *et al.* (2007) Pharmacologic management of neuropathic pain: evidence-based recommendations. *Pain* **132**, 237–51.

Finnerup NB, Otto M, Jensen TS, Sindrup SH (2007) An evidence-based algorithm for the treatment of neuropathic pain. *Med Gen Med* **9**, 36.

Madsen MV, Gotzsche PC, Hrobjartsson A (2009) Acupuncture treatment for pain: systematic review of randomised clinical trials with acupuncture, placebo acupuncture, and no acupuncture groups. *Br Med J* **338**, a3115.

Chapter 9

Other physical symptoms

Introduction

A large number of physical symptoms other than pain can afflict people in the later stages of an illness. This chapter discusses a number of common symptoms, their origin, and their management, and frames these symptoms when possible in the context of advanced dementia.

There has been very little research into non-psychiatric symptoms in advanced dementia; there are no properly validated tools to measure symptom severity, nor is there much research-based knowledge on what symptoms are particularly prevalent. A recent survey of 130 people with advanced dementia followed up in Croydon in the UK showed that the common physical symptoms were weight loss, anorexia, fatigue, weakness, and drowsiness. However, other symptoms such as repeated seizures and myoclonus were also occasionally present.

Oral symptoms

Doctors, and to a lesser extent nurses, rarely look into patients' mouths, yet oral problems cause significant discomfort and contribute to other problems such as poor nutrition. The mouth is a mine of information about a person's day-to-day life. Regular dental checkups prevent many problems.

Routine inspection will take seconds (you need torch, gloves, and a tongue depressor). Look at:

- Lips, angles of mouth: lumps, redness, fissuring.
- Mucosa: moist or dry? Inflamed? Ulcers: appearance and distribution?
- Oral hygiene: thrush? Coating? Plaque? Pus? Blood? Often poor in debilitated or demented people who do not perform their own mouth care.
- Dentition: teeth missing or broken, loose, or tender? Is the person edentulous? Do dentures fit or do they come off during speech or eating?
- Gums: have they receded significantly? Is there a red line at the apex, indicating periodontal disease, which is associated with further tooth loss?
- Salivary gland orifices (parotid duct opposite the 2nd upper molar, submandibular and sublingual at midline under the tongue): pus?
- If abnormalities, check neck for lymph nodes.

Dry mouth

- Hyposalivation = underproduction of saliva.
- Xerostomia = sensation of dry mouth.

The two often go together, but may occur independently. The average person produces 0.5–1.5L of saliva a day. Saliva lubricates and cleans the mouth, dissolves food to permit taste, initiates digestion, facilitates mastication and bolus formation, washes away and dilutes bacterial matter, possesses antimicrobial activity, and cools down hot food. Its composition varies in response to need, from watery, large-volume, and electrolyte-rich to viscous, smaller-volume, and protein-rich. Salivary flow and composition is under autonomic control. Saliva can also cause discomfort through being too sticky and viscous.

Causes

- 30% of those aged >65 suffer from oral dryness.
- Dehydration, e.g. forgetting to drink, being unable to get a drink independently.
- Open-mouth breathing, especially during sleep, can rapidly dry the mouth.
- Anticholinergic drugs: tricyclic antidepressants, most traditional antipsychotics, drugs used for colic, some anti-emetics.
- Other drugs: clonidine, diuretics, octreotide.
- Past radiotherapy to head or neck.
- Oral sensory dysfunction: dry mouth sensation despite adequate saliva.
- Other illnesses, e.g. diabetes, late-stage renal failure.
- Replacement of salivary glandular acini with fibrous tissue in old age (probably an additional factor not a main cause).

Consequences
- Difficulty swallowing is probably the commonest effect.
- Loss of taste, reducing interest in food and contributing to malnutrition.
- Difficulty speaking clearly, making communication more difficult.
- Halitosis, often affecting social contact.
- Increased oral infections: poor oral hygiene and plaque accelerates tooth loss, making eating more difficult; it can cause oral pain; bacteria in plaque are a frequent cause of serious aspiration pneumonia.
- Higher risk of oral thrush.
- Dental caries.
- Poor adherence of dentures and dental prostheses, more pressure ulcers.

Management
- Ensure adequate hydration. Offer fluids regularly, in small repeated amounts if necessary.
- STOP or reduce the dose of offending drugs if possible: substitute another drug if practicable.
- Non-drug measures: cold drinks; sucking crushed ice; chewing pineapple chunks (fresh are best, but canned will do—they contain ananase, which cleanses mouth); sugar-free chewing gum. THIN coating of petroleum jelly to lips.
- Saliva substitutes, e.g. Saliva Orthana (contains pork-based mucin, unacceptable to some Muslims and Jews); Glandosane spray (contains methylcellulose); Biotene Oral Balance gel. NB: apply inside cheeks and *under* tongue, often many times a day to keep mouth moist.
- Pilocarpine, tablets 5mg t.d.s., or eye drops 4%, 2–3 drops t.d.s. given orally. May cause colic, diarrhoea, or sweating. May take days to weeks to work in resistant cases, e.g. after radiotherapy to the head.
- Bethanecol: 10mg t.d.s. with meals, titrate to response.
- For dealing with resistance to mouth care see 📖 Chapter 9, Oral symptoms, pp. 134–138.

Drooling
Drooling is often a sign of poor swallowing of saliva, poor head positioning (with the lips at the lowest point, e.g. flaccid neck), or a poor lip seal. It may indicate parkinsonism, sometimes induced by antipsychotics Occasionally overproduction of saliva (cholinesterase inhibitors, e.g. galantamine; lithium; cholinergic drugs, e.g. bethanecol, pilocarpine; intraoral mass, e.g. tongue tumour, ill-fitting dentures) or other fluids (pus) is responsible.

Management
- Positioning: often more upright is best, sometimes a lateral (recovery) position to aid drainage.
- Suction: rarely indicated unless obstructing breathing, as it might make salivation worse. Deep suctioning is ONLY indicated in total airways obstruction.
- Withdraw drugs with extrapyramidal adverse effects if causing parkinsonism.
- Anticholinergic drugs: usually drugs that do not cross the BBB are best, as they avoid central effects, e.g. glycopyrronium 0.2mg s.c. stat or 0.6–1.2mg/24 hours s.c. via syringe driver.

- Hyoscine transdermal patches (normally used for travel sickness) are also useful, and can be cut to reduce the dose, e.g. half a patch gives half the dose. However, they penetrate the BBB and may cause sedation, act as anti-emetics, and occasionally precipitate seizures.
- Antidepressants and other drugs with anticholinergic activity can also be used. Liquids allow the dose to be titrated more precisely than tablets.

Sore mouth

Causes

- Broken or damaged teeth: the commonest cause of an oral ulcer is a jagged tooth
- Hard food and poor dentition, e.g. crusty bread abrading oral mucosa
- Oral infections—herpetic ulcers are especially painful.
- Nutritional deficiencies: deficiencies of iron, riboflavin (vitamin B_2), or zinc can all present with red tongue or fissures at the lip angles (angular cheilitis).
- Foreign bodies in the mouth.

Consequences

- Food and drink avoidance, contributing to malnutrition.
- Agitation or withdrawal; disrupted mealtimes.

Findings

- A ragged ulcer next to a jagged tooth or under ill-fitting dentures suggests a traumatic origin.
- Small solitary shallow ulcers often in pairs or more, with a red rim, are aphthous ulcers. Usually heal spontaneously in a week.
- Herpetic ulcers are at first multiple small fluid-filled vesicles anywhere in the mouth, throat, or lips; these burst and ulcerate, then crust over.

Management

- Restore mouth moisture if impaired (see 📖 Chapter 9, Oral symptoms, pp. 134–138).
- Refer to dentist for jagged teeth (can be filed), tender or loose teeth, ill-fitting dentures (can be relined at the bedside or liners and adhesives can be used), or gum or tooth infections.
- Treat ulcers symptomatically. Warm saline mouthwashes are comforting. Local steroids, antihistamines, sucralfate, or other coating agents (carmellose paste—Orabase) may reduce pain. Benzydamine (Difflam) is a NSAID with local anaesthetic properties—give 15ml 3-hourly or as needed; dilute 1:1 if it stings (it contains alcohol).
- Specific ulcer treatments depend on the cause :
  - Hydrocortisone pellets to suck, or steroid plus Orabase ointment over aphthous ulcers.
  - Acyclovir 200mg 4-hourly for a week for herpetic ulcers if given within a day of onset.
- Assess and treat nutritional deficiencies: balanced diet, nutritional supplements.
- In people with no teeth, modify the diet accordingly.
- Once acute inflammation has subsided, institute gentle regular oral hygiene (see Box 'Mouth care for people with dementia').

Mouth care for people with dementia

Regular mouth care can prevent many problems. It needs to be done twice a day, in the bathroom, which carries visual cues to the procedure. Toothpaste should only be used in people with early dementia, still able to spit and swallow well; otherwise it can stimulate more saliva flow, may be inadvertently aspirated, and its taste may make some individuals more resistive to oral care. Sodium lauryl sulphate (the usual cleaning constituent of toothpaste) also tends to dry the mouth. Use a very soft toothbrush with a long handle, rubberized grip, and thin head, and water. Touching the face before you start can prepare them for what is to follow; as with all procedures, explain as you do things. To brush someone else's teeth, it may be easier to stand behind them, although standing in front of people on a chair or in bed can also work. Use a 'brush and mop' technique, cleaning up debris and saliva with a swab after every few brushes. In people with advanced dementia, a helper to gently immobilize their hands and to distract them can be helpful. Never use lemon glycerine swabs, as they can stimulate saliva flow and later dry the mouth. For people who can still operate a toothbrush, a hand-over hand technique, with you guiding them what to do, can be useful.

With resistive patients who refuse to open their mouth for care, you may want to try again later.[1] Consider also whether they have a painful mouth condition. Massaging the face and over the temporo-mandibular joints can lead to mouth opening. Using two toothbrushes, with them biting the rubberized handle of one as you clean the mouth with the other, is useful. Wear gloves, and never put your fingers between teeth, but only between teeth and cheek.

Oral and pharyngeal thrush (candidiasis)

This is a fungal infection caused by various species of *Candida*. It can take various forms:
- Pseudomembranous: dirty white film-like plaques.
  - Punctate: small deposits, with surrounding erythematous rim, easy to scrape off (unlike leukoplakia, a pre-cancerous condition).
  - Smooth red tongue and angular cheilitis (redness at angles of lips – can also be due to deficiency of iron, riboflavin (vitamin B_2), or zinc).
- Thrush makes the mouth uncomfortable, causes halitosis, dryness, and taste loss.
- Oesophageal thrush makes swallowing painful. It is suspected if there is oral thrush and painful swallowing. *Extremely* painful swallowing in a patient who is systemically unwell is often due to herpetic infections.

Predisposing conditions
- Dry mouth.
- Diabetes.
- Steroids.

---

1 van der Horst M-L, Scott D, McCoy B (2009) Oral health for frail older adults. Available at: http://www.rgpc.ca/best/BPC%20-%20Oral%20Care/Oral%20Health%20Webinar%20-%20 Feb.%202%2709/Oral%20Health%20and%20Dementia%20presentation%20Feb%202%202009.pdf

- Antibiotics.
- Poor nutrition.
- Dentures.
- Immunodeficiency, e.g. AIDS.

Management
- Treat predisposing conditions if possible.
- Nystatin 2–5mL (200,000 to 500,000U) q.d.s. or nystatin pastilles. The suspension has to be swished around the mouth for several minutes before swallowing, which makes it less practical for people with advanced dementia. The lozenges need to be left in the mouth to dissolve and not swallowed.
- Alternatively use miconazole gel or amphotericin lozenges (although these may occasionally cause oral inflammation).
- Systemic drugs: fluconazole 50–200mg daily or other imidazoles: useful for systemic infections or for oesophageal thrush. These are often easier to take than the above. However, there is resistance to any imidazole on the market, so send a swab for culture and sensitivity if response is poor. Remember that imidazoles are highly prone to significant drug interactions due to CYP450 (📖 Appendix 2).
- Continue antifungals until 2 days after the thrush disappears. If predisposing causes such as steroids or antibiotics operate, antifungals may need to be continued until these are stopped.

Further reading

Davies A, Finlay I (2005) *Oral care in advanced disease.* Oxford University Press, Oxford.
Napenas JJ, Brennan MT, Fox PC (2009) Diagnosis and treatment of xerostomia (dry mouth). *Odontology* **97**, 76–83.

GI symptoms

Weight loss, anorexia, cachexia

See also 📖 Chapter 13 for a discussion of the ethical issues of feeding and hydration.

- Weight loss and malnutrition are common in dementia.
- Women start to lose weight as much as 10 years before diagnosis, possibly a sign of early self-neglect. This suggests that the pathology starts much earlier than previously thought.
- In older people, weight loss of over 4% in a year is associated with increased morbidity and mortality.
- 30–40% of people with moderately severe to severe AD suffer clinically significant weight loss.
- One prospective population-based study found more weight loss than in patients with heart disease, congestive heart failure, or cancer, and that the dementia stage had no influence on the extent of weight loss. However, most studies show that weight loss accelerates in advanced dementia.
- Reduced food intake tends to be associated with behavioural disorders in early dementia (forgetting to shop for food). In the middle stages, apraxia (not being sure what to do with utensils), food hoarding in the mouth (forgetting to chew or swallow food), not finishing meals, and distractibility play a large part. In the late stages, problems with the oral stage of swallowing are more often the cause (📖 Chapter 9, GI problems, pp. 139–155).
- In AD, atrophy of the mesial temporal cortex, which is involved in both memory and feeding behaviour, correlates with loss of body mass index (BMI).
- A study of around 400 people, mostly with moderate or moderately severe AD, has described two patterns of weight loss. A third showed a gradual continuing weight loss of <4% of their body weight over a year. 10% had major weight loss (>5kg in 6 months), often associated with intercurrent medical or social upheaval. The authors hypothesized that when the stressful situation passed, the patients did not have a compensatory period of increased appetite to regain the weight they had lost, and that instituting extra feeding at these times will halt the accelerated weight loss.
- Some studies show that feeding in specialist units can stop weight loss, but other studies disagree.
- A number of studies show there is no increase in resting metabolic rate in AD, which would exclude a cachectic process.
- Malnourished patients deteriorate faster cognitively and functionally, and show more signs of BPSD. It is unclear whether this is a cause (poor nutrition worsens BPSD), effect (BPSD leads to poorer nutrition, e.g. lower food intake), or an epiphenomenon (one or more underlying mechanisms might be shared between both malnourishment and BPSD).
- However, in dementia, age and serum albumin levels are not predictive of survival, as they are in other nutritional problems in older people.

Dysphagia, swallowing problems, and aspiration

It is recommended that this section be read in conjunction with 📖 Chapter 13.

Difficulty swallowing affects many people with end-stage AD but is also present in other forms of dementia, sometimes much earlier. Aspiration of food contents into the lung setting up aspiration pneumonia is a common event in end-stage dementia, and gross aspiration is a sign that prognosis is probably measured in weeks, so the subject is addressed in detail.

Swallowing and its control

Swallowing has an oral and a pharyngeal phase.

In the oral phase:

- Food is chewed by the teeth.
- Pharynx opens voluntarily, the soft palate is elevated and the posterior tongue depressed.
- The tongue crushes food against the hard palate.
- The food bolus is pushed back into the pharynx.
- The soft palate closes off the nasopharynx, preventing nasal regurgitation.

The pharyngo-oesophageal phase follows the oral phase, transporting food from the pharynx into the stomach:

- The posterior tongue pushes the bolus into the pharynx.
- The larynx rises, and the pharyngeal muscles relax.
- The epiglottis closes off the larynx to prevent aspiration.
- The vocal folds (vocal cords) close to protect the trachea further.
- Peristalsis propels the bolus down to the stomach.
- The soft palate relaxes, and the larynx reopens.
- The gastro-oesophageal sphincter opens, allowing food to enter stomach.

The oral phase requires:

- A good lip seal to prevent liquids dribbling out.
- Adequate dentition for chewing.
- Adequate saliva to lubricate the mouth and prevent food sticking.
- A mobile tongue to produce and push back the food bolus.
- An intact palate.
- Functioning cheek musculature to prevent food collecting between cheek and gums.
- Intact innervation to oral structures. The lingual nerve (V), supplies sensation; the chorda tympani (VII) supplies taste to the anterior 2/3rds of the tongue; the glossopharyngeal (IX) supplies sensation and taste to the posterior 1/3rd of the tongue, and the hypoglossal (XII) supplies the tongue musculature. Loss of tongue sensation impairs swallowing more than an immobile tongue.

The pharyngeal phase requires

- A mobile posterior tongue.
- Intact innervation: neurological problems cause dysphagia to liquids first, then solids. Obstructive lesions cause dysphagia for solids before liquids.
- Intact innervation to epiglottis and vocal folds to prevent aspiration.
- Cranial nerves V, VII, IX–XII need to be intact for unhindered swallowing.

Central control of swallowing

This is only now being elucidated. Brainstem structures mostly control swallowing, but the cortex and other higher centres exert a strong modulatory influence.

- Before swallowing is initiated, the precuneus and cuneus in the parietal lobe are activated. They are important in memory for recognition, picking up cues for swallowing, e.g. sight of food.
- In reflex swallowing (e.g. of saliva) bilateral activation of primary somatosensory and motor cortices (particularly the areas representing face, tongue, and pharynx) and of the anterior cingulate cortex are prominent.
- In volitional swallowing, the cingulate cortex also appears to be involved in initiation and decision-making. Activation spreads into the insula and frontal gyri, which are concerned with motor control. Also involved are the frontal operculum, temporal cortex, and sometimes cerebellum, basal ganglia, and thalamus.
- In the brainstem, the nucleus of the tractus solitarius (taste and visceral sensation from cranial nerves VII, IX, X), the nucleus ambiguus (motor fibres of X to pharynx and larynx, motor IX to stylopharyngeus), and the reticular formation are interlinked with other cranial nerve nuclei which subserve muscles involved in the swallowing process. They are under descending cortical influences outlined above.
- Many of these structures are damaged in dementia, affecting swallowing.

Swallowing in the different dementias

- Recent fMRI studies suggest that subtle swallowing changes occur in early AD, rather than being a late feature as previously thought. In late AD, dysphagia is progressive. A recent endoscopic study found evidence of aspiration in 30% of people with moderate or advanced dementia. There was a trend for aspiration to penetrate below the vocal folds in advanced but not moderate dementia; although this did not reach statistical significance, this was probably due to the small numbers involved. Gradual, symmetrical, progressive damage to the temporal lobes in AD involving the insula (see above) and anterolateral and posterior parietal lobe, may well account for this.
- A recent publication has suggested that swallowing difficulties in AD arises predominantly from temporoparietal-dependent sensory dysfunctions while in VaD they are more often linked to motor corticobulbar tract disruptions. For example, while people with AD tend to have an oral transit delay for liquids, those affected by VaD will often have more problems with bolus formation.
- In DLB, dysphagia is associated with parkinsonism.
- In some people with frontotemporal dementia, excessive food leaks into the pharynx during rather than after mastication, suggesting a breakdown in control of swallowing. The compulsive eating behaviour sometimes seen may increase aspiration risk.
- Dysphagia is a common feature of other dementias, for example Huntington's disease and CJD.

Other contributory causes to dysphagia

- Feeding difficulties in advanced dementia can be due to a number of reasons (Table 9.1).

Table 9.1 Causes of feeding difficulties in advanced dementia

Apraxia: inability to recognize and use utensils	Food held in mouth
Insufficient time set aside for meals	Dentition problems: missing teeth, ill-fitting dentures
Interference by agitation or wandering	Dry mouth
Food refusal	Reduced oral sensitivity
Forgetting learned mealtime routine	Corticobulbar tract and cranial nerve nucleus damage in AD
Distractibility	
Agitated outbursts	Parkinsonism in DLB
Disrupted feeding ritual—patient or carer factors	Underlying disease, e.g. Huntington's, PSP

Natural history of swallowing problems

- Dysphagia supervenes in AD, usually as a result of damage to the corticobulbar tract and cranial nerve nuclei. Silent basal ganglia infarcts increase the risk, as does intake of neuroleptics, but not benzodiazepines.
- Dysphagia due to neurological damage from AD first affects liquids.
- At first, smaller volumes can be swallowed, using small sips and sometimes intricate manoeuvres to get them down.
- Drinking with a straw and later thickening liquids or using semi-liquids (e.g. ice cream) can preserve some swallowing function temporarily.
- Eventually dysphagia to solids becomes obvious. Changing over to soft solids, e.g. mashed or pureed food, helps. The former is said to be easier to swallow.
- Signs of aspiration supervene (Table 9.2).
- Increasing feeding difficulties correlate with increasing caregiver burden.
- Aspiration can be kept in check for a while by thickening fluids and using a number of techniques (Table 9.3), but eventually it becomes pronounced and repeated aspiration pneumonia becomes inevitable.
- Small amounts of oropharyngeal secretions are aspirated silently by about 50% of normal adults during sleep. The do not develop pneumonia due to a combination of lack of sufficiently pathogenic bacteria in the mouth, a good cellular and humoral immune response, and small volume of aspirate.

Table 9.2 Bedside signs suggestive of aspiration

Reduced alertness
Inattention
Drooling of secretions or food
Change in voice quality when eating
Cough or splutter during or after swallow
Wet or gurgly breathing
Pocketing of food in the oral cavity
Delay in triggering the swallow
Multiple swallows per mouthful
Avoidance of certain foods
Slow eating: how long does a meal take?

- In advanced dementia all of these elements can change. Poor oral hygiene increases the virulence of oral bacteria; frailty affects the immune response; and aspiration is more gross as the effects of neurological damage and frailty combine.
- Many episodes of aspiration pneumonia arise not from food that is aspirated but from aspiration of gastric contents (the acid in the stomach can set up a dangerous pneumonitis) or saliva, with its heavy bacterial load.
- Aspiration pneumonia tends to affect the (R) lower and middle lobes. If aspiration occurs while standing, it can affect both lower lobes. Those who aspirate while lying on their (L) side tend to have (L) lower lobe pneumonia. If aspiration occurs when lying flat on the back, it is most likely to affect the (R) upper lobe.
- Antibiotics should be directed at *Streptococcus pneumoniae*, *Haemophilus influenzae*, Gram-negative bacilli, and *Staphylococcus aureus*.

Table 9.3 Techniques to reduce risk of aspiration

Do not leave people who can still feed themselves alone when eating or drinking

Position upper body at 45° or more vertical

Tilt head forward during swallowing if possible

Minimize distractions: noise, moving objects

Use thickeners as needed

If there is unilateral pharyngeal paralysis, rotate the head towards the paralysed side to force the food to go down the normal side

Encourage the patient to cough after every swallow

Only put in the next bolus of food when the first one has been swallowed

Management options: hand-feeding (Table 9.4)

In people who can still feed themselves, several barriers still occur:

- The diurnal rhythm of people with AD changes, and they favour the main meal at breakfast, yet most institutions give the meals with fewest calories at breakfast, and heavier meals later when they are less likely to be eaten.
- Difficulties manipulating dishes, lids, and utensils may result in lower calorie intakes or missed meals. Attention to these details is essential.
- When a person is no longer able to manipulate feeding implements, substitution of finger foods will often allow them to continue eating independently for longer.
- There is a limit to the volumes consumed, but some evidence that more energy-rich foods allow people with dementia to have more calories in a volume they are happy to take.
- A large choice of foods at once may over-stimulate the individual and promote agitation, and less eating.
- An inability to bring food to the mouth or chew is strongly correlated to lower food intake. This needs to be identified and feeding by staff instituted.
- 'Healthy eating' options are rarely healthy in calorie-restricted states; high-fat, high-sugar foods are preferred (more calories per unit volume).

- In late-stage dementia, food may remain in the mouth as the patient forgets to chew and swallow, the patient may refuse to open their mouth at all, food may dribble out, swallowing may be delayed, or patients can lose their appetite and thirst sensation.
- Consider intercurrent conditions such as infection and depression.
- Feeding training for nurses and HCAs improves their attitudes but has no effect on the amount of food consumed.

Table 9.4 Simple tips for oral feeding

Sit at right angles to the person in an easily visible position (remember inattention or visual field defects)

Allow the person to see and smell the food before eating

Placing the person's hand on the spoon and moving their hand up to their mouth is useful

For those who refuse to open their mouth, try touching the lips with the spoon or placing some food on the lips—similarly when giving fluids

If food is held in the mouth, prompt the person to swallow

Remind the person to chew, as not chewing sufficiently is a common cause of choking

Stroking the throat can help induce swallowing

Watch the person's face for signs of distress

Take time: swallowing is delayed in late-stage AD

Keep the person upright for 20 minutes after meals.

Management options: enteral feeding

As oral feeding becomes unsafe, there has been a tendency to institute enteral feeding, either through a nasogastric tube (NGT) or through a gastrostomy. The easy availability of percutaneously or radiologically inserted gastrostomies (PEG or RIG, respectively) has made their use widespread.

- A number of questionnaires show that physicians believe that gastrostomies in dementia prolong life, improve quality of life, reduce aspiration pneumonia, reduce pressure sores, improve nutritional and functional status; and that they underestimate the short-term mortality of the procedure.
- A survey of speech and language therapists in the UK also suggested that many of them would recommend a PEG for advanced dementia, even though only a small minority would want one for themselves in such a situation.
- In the UK, the National Confidential Enquiry into Patient Deaths (NCEPOD) in 2004 reported on PEGs; they found that 12% of PEGs reported to them had been performed for dementia. In other countries such as the USA the use of enteral feeding in advanced dementia is even more common—over 50% of institutionalized people with dementia in some series. There is a wide variation in the use of enteral feeding between different countries.
- However, there has been a recent decline in use, for several reasons.

- There is no evidence that people with advanced dementia on enteral feeding survive longer than similar individuals who are not artificially fed—as recently confirmed by a Cochrane Review. Therefore in ethical terms, gastrostomy cannot be viewed as a life-prolonging treatment in this population.
- There is a high morbidity and mortality to gastrostomy insertion. A number of series show a 30–50% mortality within a month of the procedure—many may have died anyway, but almost no surgical procedure with such a high mortality would be considered acceptable in normal practice. Median survival of 60 days or less has often been reported. In contrast, a small number of series show longer survival with gastrostomies; but these are often inserted at an earlier stage of the illness.
- People who had concurrent infection and pressure sores when their PEG was inserted had a median prognosis of 32 days.
- An old series showed that general hospital patients aged over 75 with a UTI and a previous history of aspiration had a 67% mortality within a month of PEG insertion.
- Therefore if a PEG is to be inserted, concurrent conditions should be stabilized first.
- Proponents of gastrostomy are concerned that patients may feel hungry or thirsty without one, even if it does not prolong their life. A recent series of people in whom the decision to forgo enteral feeding had been taken showed few expressions of discomfort; these were mostly related to intercurrent symptoms such as breathlessness or myoclonus. The symptoms improved over the days after the decision to forgo artificial feeding had been taken
- Others find that gastrostomies and feeding tubes are well tolerated and cause minimal problems.
- There is no evidence that gastrostomies reduce the prevalence of aspiration pneumonias, that they reduce the prevalence of pressure sores, or improve functional and nutritional status in this patient group. Small series show no difference in these outcomes between gastrostomy patients and others.
- After insertion of gastrostomy, patients may sometimes suffer diarrhoea for a few days or bloating and vomiting if too much feed is infused or too rapidly.
- In one series, one in five nursing home residents with a PEG for dementia needed tube replacement or repositioning within a year; there was an average of one admission per patient lasting an average of 9 days; and one in three visited the emergency department without being admitted.
- A US study extrapolating a small sample calculated the costs of fixing dislodgment or malfunction of tubes through emergency at $11 million in 2003.
- NGTs carry a higher risk of aspiration and of dislodgement than gastrostomy tubes.
- To prevent the tubes being pulled out, restraint was used in 71% of patients in one study; NGT > PEG.

- Having said all this, it is important not to have a blanket policy which could leave some patients undertreated. Some people carry away the message that artificial feeding is bad in dementia, rather than that it is at best unhelpful in advanced dementia. The evidence for many of the above findings is not at a high level of certainty[1].
- People with dementia drink and eat less as illness progresses, and do not appear disturbed by this. Many think the sensations of thirst and hunger are blunted in late-stage disease, although there is no way of proving this.

Management of dysphagia

- Address common causes, e.g. dry mouth (☐ Chapter 9, Oral symptoms, pp. 134–138).
- A good assessment by a speech and language therapist is necessary if there is any evidence of aspiration, or if dysphagia is disabling or progressive.
- Dietary modification to suit the person's deficits will be needed.
- Drinks may need to be thickened. A number of safe swallowing techniques may be employed.
- Work in patients with stroke is showing that swallowing can be rehabilitated by utilizing the brain's capacity for plasticity. Using techniques like repetitive movements or actions, undamaged cortical areas can be recruited to take over the function of damaged areas. Whether such an approach has any place in a progressive, often symmetrical condition such as dementia is not yet clear.

Royal College of Physicians (London) recommendations

- Oral intake, modified as necessary, should be the main aim of treatment. Nutrient-dense foods or special provision of food (in hospital, the 'red tray' system) is helpful.
- Nil by mouth is a last resort.
- The evidence base for dementia is that tube feeding rarely prolongs life and may cause substantial morbidity.
- A multidisciplinary nutrition support team of health care professionals, ideally but not inevitably led by a doctor with special expertise in nutrition, should be available to work with patients and their families when oral feeding difficulties occur. A member of the team should be available on the telephone at weekends as well to provide advice.
- Such teams should be collaborative in nature and not be made up of independent professionals who are focused only on their area. The patient should be at the centre of their efforts.
- The first question should be 'what are we trying to achieve?'.
- Even when tube feeding is necessary, this should be additional whenever possible. At the end of life, even if deemed to have an 'unsafe swallow' a risk management approach may offer the patient the best quality of life.

Source: Royal College of Physicians (2010) *Oral feeding difficulties and dilemmas. A guide to practical care particularly towards the end of life.* Royal College of Physicians, London.

1 Regnard C, Leslie P *et al.* (2010) Gastrostomies in dementia: bad practice or bad evidence? *Age Ageing* **39**, 282–4.

Nausea and vomiting

Nausea is very distressing but difficult or impossible to diagnose in severe dementia. Proxy measures such as food refusal can make one suspect nausea, but one can never be sure of its presence without a clear statement from the person involved.

Physiologically, nausea and vomiting are distinct events. Nausea involves the hypothalamus and inferior frontal cortex and is accompanied by secretion of antidiuretic hormone (ADH) as well as changes in gastric electrical rhythms. Vomiting requires the coordination of a very complex chain of events, with changes in peristalsis, relaxation of some muscles and contraction of others, and protection of the airway from the vomitus. Failure to coordinate this sequence precisely may lead to aspiration, bleeding from gastric mucosal tears (Mallory–Weiss tears), or oesophageal perforation (Boerhaave's syndrome), all of which could be fatal. A vomiting pattern generator (VPG) therefore exists in the brainstem to coordinate this sequence. Various emetic sources stimulate the VPG to initiate the vomiting sequence. Blocking important neurotransmitters acting in an area will block vomiting originating from that area. Stimuli include:

- Chemical: sensed by the various chemoreceptor trigger zones (CTZs) in the body, the most important being the area postrema in the floor of the 4th ventricle in the midbrain. These sense chemical changes in the body and stimulate the VPG to produce vomiting. Chemical stimuli of nausea and vomiting include:
  - Biochemical changes: renal failure; hypercalcaemia; hyponatraemia.
  - Drugs: morphine and strong opioids; dopaminergic drugs, e.g. levodopa; chemotherapy agents, e.g. cisplatin; erythromycin; aminophylline; NSAIDs.
  - Radiotherapy especially to the L1 region, or large doses to the brain or to whole body.
- Nucleus of tractus solitarius: this conveys impulses from the GI tract or from structures embryologically derived from the GI tract. These include taste, secretions retained in the pharynx, the gut, e.g. gastritis, and the heart, e.g. myocardial infarction (i.e. cranial nerves VII—chorda tympani component, IX, X).
- Vestibular nuclei: nerve VIII. Often associated with autonomic symptoms (dizziness, nausea, palpitations) and cerebellar symptoms (nystagmus), e.g. motion sickness.
- Emotions and higher functions, e.g. fear, anxiety, severe pain, visual inputs, smells.

Diagnosis

A good history will often reveal the cause. Note medication and if necessary check blood levels (digoxin).

Distinguish *regurgitation* (food/fluid not actually swallowed—occurs within a short time of ingestion, no nausea, no bile, often little effort as vomitus is brought up) from vomiting. Regurgitation does not respond to anti-emetics, and there is a grave risk of major drug adverse effects as doses are increased repeatedly to overcome a perceived lack of response.

Delayed gastric emptying

Gastric emptying may be delayed by a tumour at the gastric outlet, scarring from ulceration, denervation, e.g. diabetic neuropathy, or a mass in the pancreatic head, e.g. tumour. Drugs such as anticholinergics and opioids can slow gastric emptying. The stomach is very distensible and secretes electrolyte-rich acidic fluid. Vomiting will therefore be of large volume, at least at first, often with little or no accompanying nausea; containing partly digested food eaten more than 4 hours previously; not containing bile if physical gastric outlet obstruction is complete (as the bile duct opens into the second part of duodenum); and leading to dehydration, hyponatraemia, and alkalosis which can all become so profound as to produce deep shock. NB: if the stomach is quite full, movement can set off vomiting; this is often erroneously interpreted as vestibular vomiting. Management involves rehydration with saline and potassium if needed, treating the offending cause if possible, and using a prokinetic drug: metoclopramide, domperidone or erythromycin (Table 9.5).

Squashed stomach syndrome

Pressure on the stomach, say from a large liver, produces a similar picture to delayed gastric emptying except that vomits are frequent and of small volume.

Raised intracranial pressure

This classically gives rise to early morning headaches, vomiting without nausea, and papilloedema.

Management

- Treat the underlying cause whenever possible.
- Avoid strong smells and tastes, which may precipitate vomiting.
- Rehydrate if necessary and appropriate: p.o., s.c., or if fluid loss is severe, i.v. There are various ways of assessing the degree of dehydration: by assessing fluid losses, e.g. volume of vomits; clinically (loss of tissue turgor, e.g. loss of elasticity of skin over the upper sternum; sunken eyes; dry mucosae; urine production; weight loss—1L = 1kg); and via blood tests especially full blood count (FBC), Na^+, urea, and protein levels.
- s.c. hydration can supply 2L of fluid a day (3L/day if two separate sites are used simultaneously). i.v. hydration should only be used if large volumes are required, if s.c. hydration encounters problems such as frequent tissuing, or if fluids unsafe to give s.c. are given, e.g. 40mmol/L of K^+. s.c. infusions are easier to insert and maintain, can be reinserted by nursing staff, carry less risk of fluid overload or septicaemia, and can be disconnected and reconnected for part of the day simply by capping the cannula. For a discussion of ethics of rehydration see 📖 Chapter 13.
- Anti-emetics: see Tables 9.5 and 9.6.

Hiccup

Hiccup is the involuntary sudden contraction of the diaphragm and other inspiratory muscles followed by closure of the glottis. It is a type of myoclonus (📖 Chapter 9, Neurological symptoms, pp. 163–166).

Causes

In general hiccup is caused by gastric or bowel distension or other subdiaphragmatic problem, or central causes. Drugs associated with hiccup include corticosteroids, benzodiazepines, megesterol, opioids, phenobarbitone, and co-trimoxazole. However, as cases of prolonged hiccupping are rare and sporadic, it is difficult to ascribe causation.

Management

The management of hiccup, like its causation, is hampered by the great difficulty in carrying out good controlled clinical trials. As always, try and reverse the underlying cause. Many non-pharmacological interventions have been suggested, including Valsalva manoeuvres, breath holding, swallowing granulated sugar, carotid sinus massage, and stimulating the pharynx with a catheter. The practicality of these in advanced dementia may be limited. Drugs which probably help control hiccups include:

- Baclofen.
- Metoclopramide.
- Chlorpromazine.
- Nifedipine.

Table 9.5 Choice of anti-emetic

Cause	Anti-emetic	Notes
Any cause: blocks neurotransmitters at VPG	Antihistamine, e.g. cyclizine 25–50mg t.d.s. p.o./s.c. Anticholinergic, e.g. hyoscine hydrobromide TD or 0.4mg s.c.	Useful general purpose anti-emetics or when choice unclear. NB: hyoscine butylbromide (Buscopan) does not cross the BBB and is hence not an anti-emetic
Chemical: block CTZ	Haloperidol 0.5–1.5mg daily or other phenothiazenes Levomepromazine 6–12.5mg p.o. or 3–6mg s.c. often used Ondansetron 4–8mg up to t.d.s. and other type 3 serotonin (5-HT3) inhibitors	Avoid haloperidol or levomepromazine in DLB or PD Large doses of levomepromazine cause b.p. drop—avoid, especially in old people with vascular disease
Nucleus tractus solitarius: taste, pharynx, heart	Hyoscine hydrobromide as above	Causes drowsiness, lowers seizure threshold
Delayed gastric emptying	Metoclopramide 10–30mg t.d.s. p.o./s.c. Domperidone 10mg 4-hourly p.o. Erythromycin 150mg t.d.s.	Watch for parkinsonism with metoclopramide, especially in conjunction with haloperidol Domperidone p.o. has poor bioavailability and is not a strong anti-emetic; p.r. it is much more effective Use erythromycin as anti-emetic very occasionally—valuable antibiotic
Vestibular	Cyclizine as above	
Emotional causes	Consider lorazepam 0.5–1mg s.l.	

Table 9.6 Anti-emetics: adverse effects

Anti-emetic	Main adverse effects
Hyoscine hydrobromide	Anticholinergic muscarinic: dry mouth, blurred vision, constipation, urinary retention, precipitation of acute closed-angle glaucoma. Sedation
Cyclizine	Drowsiness for first few days. Antimuscarinic, but less pronounced than hyoscine. Headache, psychomotor impairment, hypotension, arrhythmias are rare
Haloperidol	Sometimes lethal in DLB. Extrapyramidal symptoms, e.g. parkinsonism, dystonias (particularly common with haloperidol), akathisia, tardive dyskinesia. Less sedating than other antipsychotics. Few or no antimuscarinic effects. Prolonged QT interval may make interactions with other medication used in palliative care dangerous—risk of sudden death, e.g. methadone, erythromycin, tricyclic antidepressants. Neuroleptic malignant syndrome (NMS)
Levomepromazine	Significant postural hypotension, tachycardia, anti-muscarinic effects, drowsiness. NMS
Metoclopramide	Extrapyramidal effects (rarer in older adults), dystonias, akathisia, tardive dyskinesias. NMS
Domperidone	Cramps, colic, diarrhoea
Erythromycin	Nausea, vomiting, colic, antibiotic-associated colitis. Prolongs QT interval. Prone to drug interactions (📖 Appendix 2)
Ondansetron	Constipation, headaches, flushing, arrhythmias (rare)

Constipation

Constipation is difficult or painful defecation associated with passage of infrequent and hard, small faeces. However, patients or carers may also use to term to mean excessive straining at stool, a sense of incomplete evacuation, or spending too much time on the toilet. Constipation can lead to pain and discomfort, anal fissures, bowel obstruction, urinary retention, and restlessness in older people. Extreme constipation can even result in stercoral ulceration of the bowel or even perforation and peritonitis.

Causes

Constipation is explained by a combination of colonic dysmotility and pelvic floor dysfunction. Slow colonic transit means there is more time for fluid to be absorbed out of stool, yielding smaller, hard faeces. The causes of these changes are many.

- Aging: although some dispute that aging causes gut changes, others have found changes in the enteric nervous system associated with increasing age which contribute to faecal transit through the large bowel, with neuronal numbers decreasing by as much as a third and an increase in connective tissue. Rectal sensitivity, pelvic musculature, and anal function also change with age. The effect is more pronounced in women who have had vaginal deliveries.
- Low-residue diet.
- Immobility and inactivity.
- Low fluid intake/dehydration.
- Weakness and difficulty raising intra-abdominal pressure to defecate.
- Inability to get to the toilet on time.
- Lack of privacy leading to postponement of defecation.
- Painful defecation, e.g. anal fissure.
- Bowel obstruction.
- Drugs: diuretics, opioids, antimuscarinics, serotonin inhibitors.
- Biochemical: hypercalcaemia, hypokalaemia.

Management
- Keep a stool chart, otherwise you will not identify constipation until it becomes extreme.
- Treat the underlying condition if possible.
- Hydrate, mobilize, give a high-residue diet if possible.
- Make it easier to get to the toilet on time: raise the chair and toilet seat (easier to get off), assess and treat mobility problems (e.g. using a Zimmer frame), use commode rather than bedpan, assist getting to toilet, ensure privacy.
- Use laxatives (Table 9.7). Use these prophylactically if on opioids (90% of patients on opioids need laxatives); give them *regularly* not p.r.n. This avoids patients becoming constipated, then being given large doses of laxatives, subsequently developing diarrhoea, and stopping using laxatives until they become constipated again and the whole cycle restarts. Laxatives given p.o. are preferable to p.r. measures except when swallowing is not safe or in an effort to get some control over faecal incontinence by letting the patient become slightly constipated and using rectal measures every 3 days, e.g. in paraplegia.

Approach to the constipated patient
- Give laxatives regularly, titrate dose to effect.
- Macrogol is often a sensible choice, but requires a good fluid intake. A combination of a stimulant such as senna and an osmotic agent, e.g. magnesium salts with liquid paraffin (e.g. Milpar), can also be used. Lactulose is in general not popular because it causes flatulence and is very sweet.
- Do a rectal examination. If there is hard, impacted stool in the rectum, consider an arachis oil enema (the oil seeps into the stool, softening it). However, this needs to be retained overnight, which is unlikely to be practical in advanced dementia. A high-phosphate enema the next day clears the softened stool.
- If the rectum is full of soft stool, use rectal stimulant laxatives, e.g. glycerine or bisacodyl suppositories.

- If the rectum is empty, use osmotic laxatives or softeners with stimulants to encourage the gut to push the stool down.
- Occasionally, manual evacuation of very hard stool may need to be done. This should be done under sedation and analgesia as it is painful and very distressing. The distress can be much greater if one does not understand why it is happening.
- Suppositories must be placed in contact with the rectal mucosa. They are more likely to be retained if inserted the wrong way round, i.e. blunt end in.
- Occasionally, for intractable opioid-induced constipation, methylnaltrexone injections, which are specific to this condition, can be useful.
- Once impaction is resolved, institute regular oral laxatives to avoid a repeat.

Table 9.7 Common laxatives in palliative care

Laxative type	Notes
Bulk-formers, e.g. methylcellulose, ispaghula	Increase stool mass and stimulate peristalsis. Effect may take days to establish. However, with inadequate fluid intake may actually constipate, and are often unpalatable. Rarely used in palliative care
Stimulants, e.g. senna, bisacodyl, danthron, sodium picosulphate	Reduce stool transit time, ensuring less fluid reabsorption. Can cause colic in bowel obstruction or severe constipation. Danthron is licensed only for patients with terminal illness, as a component of codanthramer or codanthrusate. It can colour the urine orange or pink and cause excoriation perianally; it should be avoided in incontinence (faecal or urinary) to avoid skin damage
Osmotic agents, e.g. lactulose, macrogols, magnesium salts	Draw water into stool, making it easier to pass Lactulose is very sweet and can cause excessive flatulence, and is rarely used Macrogols (and all osmotic laxatives) require large volumes of fluid intake (2–3L/day) to be effective, which may be beyond most people under palliative care or with advanced dementia. Magnesium salts alone are useful on rare occasions in severely constipated patients to flush away the constipated stool. Useful In conjunction with liquid paraffin (e.g. Milpar), sometimes in conjunction with a stimulant
Faecal softeners, e.g. docusate	Used in combination with danthron (codanthrusate) or sometimes alone, e.g. in bowel obstruction. Probably also has some stimulant activity

Diarrhoea

Diarrhoea is defined as the passage of three or more unformed motions per day. Patients or carers may also define it as the passage of watery or soft stool, or frequent stool many times a day.

Water is reabsorbed from food and fluid through much of the course of the gut. Over 90% of the water is reabsorbed, mainly in the jejunum but also in the terminal ileum and colon. The latter has the capacity to more than double its water reabsorption capacity if necessary. Water and electrolytes are also secreted into the gut, so that the fluid content of the stool depends on the balance between secretion and reabsorption, which are separate processes.

Diarrhoea can be:

- Secretory: acute secretory diarrhoea occurs in many intestinal infections, due to viruses (e.g. rotavirus), bacteria (e.g. *Escherichia coli*) or parasites (e.g. *Giardia*). Chronic secretory diarrhoea occurs with inability to reabsorb bile salts due to terminal ileal resection; rare endocrine tumours (such as VIPomas); and rectal villous adenomas.
- Osmotic: due to the presence of osmotically active material in the gut lumen which prevents water reabsorption. This includes excessive osmotic laxative use; malabsorption due to intolerance of dietary sugars; vagotomy or gastrectomy; and the dumping syndrome.
- Rapid transit: rapid transit through the gut does not allow fluid reabsorption, causing diarrhoea. Causes include short bowel syndrome, fistulae, and thyrotoxicosis.
- Colonic diarrhoea: often profuse and watery; sometimes containing dark blood (e.g. dysentery).

Common causes of diarrhoea in people with dementia include:

- Drugs (laxatives, rivastigmine, donepezil, memantine, antibiotics, digoxin, B-blockers, NSAIDs, antimuscarinics).
- Faecal impaction: a period of constipation followed by sudden-onset diarrhoea. Diagnosis is by rectal examination; occasionally abdominal plain X-rays are needed to confirm high constipation. Treatment is by treating the constipation.
- Odd diets may be found in some people with dementia.

Management

- Treat the underlying cause.
- Rehydrate p.o., s.c., or i.v.
- If cause is unclear, send stool for microscopy, culture and sensitivity and *Clostridium difficile* toxin.
- Symptomatic treatment: loperamide 4mg p.r.n. p.o. up to 16mg/24 hours; weak (codeine) or strong (morphine) opioids.

Antibiotic-associated diarrhoea

Patients are often acutely unwell, with fever, abdominal cramps, pus and blood in the stool, which is very watery and may lead to severe dehydration. Due mostly to *C. difficile* superinfection. Spread is common on geriatric wards; handwashing with soap and water is better at getting rid of the spores than alcohol rubs. It can last for 2 weeks but recurs in up to a third of patients. Any current or recent antibiotic can cause this condition, but clindamycin, ampicillin, fluoroquinolones, e.g. ciprofloxacin, and cephalosporins are the most likely. Risk is higher in patients in institutions, older people on PPIs (e.g. omeprazole) or who have had GI surgery. PPIs also increase the risk of recurrence. Diagnosis is via detection of *C. difficile* toxin in the stool. Occasional false negatives occur. Treatment is with isolation, rehydration, stopping the offending antibiotic, and administering metronidazole or vancomycin. The most serious form, pseudomembranous colitis, is life threatening but rare. Seek microbiological advice.

Faecal incontinence

2–17% of community-dwelling older people suffer from faecal incontinence, and up to 65% of nursing home residents. In very advanced dementia, faecal incontinence is very common. Faecal incontinence increases the risk of UTI and decubitus ulcers and often leads to social isolation.

Faecal continence is maintained by the:

- Internal anal sphincter (IAS): a continuation of rectal circular smooth muscle (70–80% of anal resting tone—reduced by a third over age 70). Maintains continence at rest. Autonomic innervation.
- External anal sphincter (EAS): expansion of levator ani. Contributes 20–30% of resting tone. Pudendal nerve.
- EAS, puborectalis sling, and levator ani are recruited to further increase anal tone voluntarily when required.
- Nerve supply is via the pudendal nerve (S2–4), while puborectalis is supplied directly by S3/4.
- The pelvic floor and receptors in the anal transition zone detect distension.

Risk factors for faecal incontinence include:

- Dementia.
- Obstetric trauma, multiparity.
- Possibly female sex.
- Immobility.
- Diabetes.
- Anorectal surgery.
- Spinal cord lesions, e.g. cauda equina lesions.
- Stroke.
- Multiple sclerosis and other conditions causing neuropathic damage.
- Rectal/anal tumours.
- Rectal prolapse.
- Faecal impaction.

Diarrhoea and constipation both increase the likelihood of faecal incontinence. Faecal impaction is very frequently associated with loss of perianal sensation and often to an inability to distinguish faeces from liquid, with consequent unintentional leakage; it also often leads to reduced sphincter pressure. Anal hyper- or hyposensitivity may both lead to continence problems.

Dementia is a major factor in faecal incontinence, for reasons including:

- Neglect of the urge to open bowels (e.g. not associating a feeling of rectal distension with the need to open the bowel) leading to constipation and impaction.

- Poor fluid and food intake due to immobility, inability to obtain food and fluid for themselves, and food and fluid not being offered by others.
- Constipating or diarrhoea-inducing drugs. e.g. anticholinergics, cholinesterase inhibitors, amoxicillin.
- Loss of central inhibitory control.

Management
- Attention to diet, fibre, and fluid intake.
- Regular toileting; provision of commode or nursing close to toilet.
- Incontinence pads when appropriate.
- Physiotherapy may help mobility and enable faster transit to toilet.
- Treat diarrhoea or constipation.
- Bulking agents, e.g. ispaghula, may render it easier to distinguish solid from liquid (though evidence this is the case is poor).
- Loperamide can be useful but constipation is a risk.
- Skin barrier creams, e.g. zinc oxide, to reduce decubitus ulcer risk.

Further reading

The British Geriatric Society has a campaign called Dignity Behind Closed Doors, aimed at promoting provision of toilet facilities which provide privacy and maintain dignity: http://www.bgs.org.uk/campaigns/dignity.htm

Sampson EL, Candy B, Jones L (2009) Enteral tube feeding for older people with advanced dementia. *Cochrane Database Syst Rev* 2009(2):CD007209.

Whitehead WE, Borrud L, Goode PS, Meikle S, Mueller ER, Tuteja A et al. (2009) Fecal incontinence in US adults: epidemiology and risk factors. *Gastroenterology* **137**, 512–17, e1–2.

Respiratory symptoms

Breathlessness

Breathlessness can be extremely distressing for both patient and carer; at the extreme, it gives rise to severe panic and anxiety and a fear of not getting to the next breath. Severe breathlessness is always associated with major anxiety and psychological symptoms, which also need to be treated. Table 9.8 shows the common causes of breathlessness in older people.

Breathlessness is the *subjective* feeling of shortness of breath. Some people who look short of breath may not feel short of breath, e.g. many 'pink puffers' with chronic obstructive pulmonary disease (COPD) who maintain adequate oxygenation by breathing rapidly. Many will have adapted to this slowly developing state and not feel breathless; misguided attempts to control their breathing may push them into respiratory failure. The term for rapid breathing is *tachypnoea*. Not all tachypnoeic patients are breathless, and vice versa. This clearly poses a problem in severe dementia, where patients might not be able to say they feel breathless. One then has to rely on tachypnoea, laboured breathing, or other evidence for breathlessness, interpreted in the light of the causative condition coupled with signs of distress.

Assessment

From patient or, if impossible, from witnesses:

- Present at rest or on activity? What activity? How much activity, e.g. how far can one walk before having to stop due to breathlessness? How long does it take to recover?
- When did it start? How much change has there been recently?
- Is it constant or episodic? What precipitates episodes? What helps?
- Associated cough, wheeze, sputum, chest pain, or haemoptysis? How much sputum is produced? Has there been a change in the last few days? Is it easy to expectorate? What colour is the sputum?
- How distressed does patient become on average? At worst?
- History of smoking, childhood or adult pneumonia, bronchiectasis, allergies?
- Examination, occasionally chest X-ray may help elucidate cause.
- Pulse oximetry can be useful if hypoxia is suspected, e.g. to optimize oxygen or other therapies.
- Lung function tests are only possible in the early stages of dementia, but are rarely needed in people with advanced disease to guide treatment.

Assessing the extent of breathlessness is important in assessing the severity and in enabling later comparisons with the baseline to check for change. The MRC breathlessness scale is useful in quantification:

- Grade 1: Dyspnoea only with strenuous exercise.
- Grade 2: Dyspnoea walking up an incline or hurrying on the level.
- Grade 3: Walks slower than most on the level, or stops after 15 minutes of walking on the level.
- Grade 4: Stops after a few minutes of walking on the level.
- Grade 5: Dyspnoea on minimal activity or severe enough to stop one leaving one's house.

In palliative care many patients will have Grade 4 or 5 dyspnoea. Quantification of the number of steps a person can walk on the flat, or what activities make them breathless, and of the recovery time from the breathlessness, are particularly useful here. People with dementia, especially advanced dementia, may be able to give little or no detail about their dyspnoea.

Table 9.8 Common causes of breathlessness in older people

Cardiorespiratory	Asthma
	Bronchitis
	COPD
	Pneumonia
	Lung fibrosis or fibrosing alveolitis
	Lung volume changes: atelectasis, pleural effusion, pneumothorax
	Pulmonary oedema and cardiac failure
	Lung cancer
	Pulmonary embolism (PE)—acute or recurrent
Neuromuscular	Motor neuron disease
	Myasthenia gravis
Chest wall restriction	Kyphosis/scoliosis
	Obesity
Haematological	Anaemia
Metabolic	Metabolic acidosis
Emotional	Anxiety/panic attacks

Management
- Treat the underlying cause.
- Consider prevention, e.g. prophylactic heparin for those at high risk of PEs.
- Consider bronchodilators and anticholinergics if undiagnosed COPD is suspected, e.g. long-standing smokers.
- Often the cause is not amenable to treatment, and the symptoms of breathlessness itself have to be addressed.
- A fan in the room to make the air flow significantly reduces breathlessness.
- Physiotherapy to counter the deconditioning that results from disuse can improve exercise tolerance considerably. Teaching of exercises which are then self-initiated is only useful in early dementia, and supervision of exercises has to be ongoing in later illness. Encouraging

walking and exploration of the environment ('wandering') by making it interesting with lots of places to stop and things to look at can go some way to promote exercise.

- Relaxation techniques, including music, massage, and visualization, may be of use in this population.
- Explanation-based rehabilitation has a limited place in moderate to advanced dementia, as information is not retained and complex information may not be understood.
- Oxygen is useful in relieving the effects of hypoxia, particularly confusion, but its effect on the symptoms of breathlessness is much less predictable: some benefit significantly while the majority do no better than with a placebo. As British Thoracic Society guidelines on use of emergency oxygen put it: 'oxygen is a treatment for hypoxaemia, not breathlessness'. Its use is not risk-free: patients may become psychologically dependent on it even when it has little therapeutic effect; home supplies can run out, creating major anxieties; it dries mucous membranes in the mouth and nose if not humidified; face masks make communication difficult; and it carries a fire risk.
- Simple face masks give oxygen 40–60% at 5–10L/minute. Nasal cannulae can provide oxygen at rates of up to 5–6L/minute at concentrations of 24–40%. When there are worries about CO_2 retention, Venturi masks are employed to deliver particular oxygen concentrations (they are labelled and colour-coded) to keep oxygen and CO_2 levels within the target range. Other masks for specialized uses, e.g. rebreather reservoir masks for high oxygen concentrations, are available.
- People with COPD and chronic CO_2 retention can lose their sensitivity to CO_2 as the prime controller of respiration and become dependent on their hypoxic drive. In these patients a high oxygen flow which removes the hypoxia can precipitate respiratory failure and even arrest.
- In people with dementia, especially with moderate dementia, oxygen masks will often be removed. Nasal cannulae may be better tolerated but oxygen therapy may prove impossible without major restraint measures. These would rarely appear to be ethically justified, especially if the breathlessness is not due to a transient but dangerous condition from which recovery with treatment is expected.

Opioids

Opioids reduce the sense of breathlessness by reducing the ventilatory response to hypoxia and hypercapnia, but only very rarely lead to CO_2 retention. Morphine 2.5mg p.o. p.r.n. or 4-hourly (or equivalent s.c. doses if unable to swallow) is often a good starting dose, then titrated to response. A substantial minority of patients may not tolerate opioids if they have no pain.

Benzodiazepines

Diazepam 2–5mg nocte or b.d. may help patients who are chronically breathless, especially when there is associated severe anxiety. For emergency control of anxiety, lorazepam 0.5–1mg s.l. or midazolam 2.5–5mg s.c. can be very useful. When using s.l. drugs the mouth must be moist, and tachypnoea rapidly dries the mouth, so a sip of water first will help. However, benzodiazepines do induce drowsiness and a drop-off in performance, and may increase risk of falls and injury; short-acting benzodiazepines like lorazepam are quickly habit forming. Their use must be judged carefully. They are best reserved for patients who are non-ambulant, or in very severe distress and not responding to other measures.

Cough
The general principle in managing cough is that productive cough is trying to clear sputum that can block airways and cause lung collapse and should whenever possible be supported; whereas non-productive cough, with no sputum to bring up, serves no useful purpose and should be suppressed. As ever, the primary cause should be treated whenever possible and appropriate.

Productive cough
- Nebulized 0.9% saline can loosen thick sputum, as can steam inhalations (the latter may be risky in people whose comprehension is affected).
- Carbocisteine orally (500–750mg t.d.s.) may reduce sputum viscosity, but should be stopped if ineffective at 4 weeks. It can cause peptic ulceration.
- Physiotherapy (percussion, postural drainage) can dislodge sputum and open up atelectatic lung.
- If attempts at helping expectoration of very distressing cough fail, or if it is inappropriate to treat (e.g. patient too frail to cough up effectively), attempts at cough suppression should instead be made (Dry cough). At the same time, the secretions can be dried up with antimuscarinics, e.g. glycopyrronium s.c. or TD hyoscine.
- Corticosteroids can reduce bronchial inflammation and thus help cough.

Dry cough
- This can occasionally be due to mild asthma or left heart failure; appropriate treatment should be instituted.
- Cough suppressants include opioids (codeine 15mg, pholcodine 10mg, morphine 2.5mg) and non-opioids such as simple linctus. However, there is little evidence that non-opioids are effective.

Further reading
Abernethy AP, McDonald CF, Frith PA, Clark K, Herndon JE 2nd, Marcello J et al. (2010) Effect of palliative oxygen versus room air in relief of breathlessness in patients with refractory dyspnoea: a double-blind, randomised controlled trial. Lancet **376**, 784–93.

Urinary symptoms

Control of micturition

The detrusor is the smooth muscle layer in the bladder wall; its contraction expels urine. Continence is maintained by a combination of relaxed detrusor and closed urethral sphincters. The internal sphincter is a continuation of the bladder smooth muscle (and hence under autonomic control), and has the main role in maintaining continence in men but a less important role in females. The external sphincter is voluntary.

The *micturition centre in the frontal lobe* sends tonic inhibitory signals to the detrusor muscle in the bladder, inhibiting micturition until it becomes socially acceptable. The *pontine micturition centre* coordinates detrusor and sphincters so that they work in synergy: pontine centre activity makes the detrusor contract and the sphincter open. Bladder filling activates the pons, setting off the impulse to void, but the frontal cortex overrides this until it is socially acceptable, suppressing the urge until appropriate. The sacral spinal cord is the relay from brain to bladder, and in the absence of these modulating influences (infants, spinal cord damage), reflexly causes voiding as soon as the bladder starts to fill up. Under sympathetic control at rest, the detrusor is relaxed, so that as the bladder fills up, pressure does not rise and the urge to void is not initiated. Muscarinic cholinergic stimulation causes detrusor contraction and sphincter relaxation.

Incontinence and urge incontinence

Incontinence of urine occurs early in dementias affecting the frontal lobe, e.g. frontotemporal dementia. It also occurs earlier in DLB and VaD than in AD, where it tends to be a late feature. Prevalence figures for dementia vary from 11% in outpatient clinics to 90% for institutionalized patients. Risk factors for urinary incontinence in dementia include:

- Loss of social inhibition: voiding in inappropriate places (in frontal dementias).
- Inability to remember the way to the toilet and how to remove one's clothes.
- Physical inability to get to the toilet or a commode when the urge presents itself in patients with more advanced illness or gait abnormalities.
- Inability to express discomfort when passing urine so that urinary tract infections may pass unrecognized.
- Use of drugs which affect micturition: antimuscarinic effects, sedatives.
- Presence of relevant comorbidities, often multiple, especially among older people with dementia, e.g. prostate problems, congestive heart failure, diabetes. Treatment of some of these problems, e.g. surgery for prostate trouble, may be contraindicated because of the patient's physical condition.

Anteromedial frontal lobe damage, including damage to the nucleus of Meynert, a key area damaged in AD, leads to detrusor overactivity. If parkinsonian gait coexists with dementia, medial frontal lobe lesions often accompany the basal ganglia lesions; they overlap with the frontal micturition centre, contributing to incontinence. Loss of tonic frontal detrusor inhibition produces the detrusor syndrome (frequency, urgency, and incontinence).

Involuntary detrusor contractions may occur either because of local problems (e.g. in response to obstructive uropathy) or because of central influences. These may lead to incontinence or urgency and nocturnal frequency.

Management

- Reverse reversible causes, e.g. medication, infection, immobility.
- Mark the toilet clearly with a large picture on door, use wall rails and other walking aids, provide clear lighting, raise toilet seats, and dress in clothes that are easy to remove.
- Regular toileting (offered, e.g., every 2 hours, with the person only taken to the toilet if they agree), is useful particularly in people with lesser degrees of dementia.
- Anticholinergics will relax the detrusor and reduce urgency and incontinence, but may worsen cognition if they cross the BBB (e.g. oxybutinin). The more polar trospium is less prone to cause this problem.

Urinary retention

Urinary retention can present in various ways. Passing urine can be completely impossible (acute retention—can be extremely painful), a full bladder with overflow incontinence can be present (painless, but the smell and staining from urine is often detectable, and a full bladder can be found on examination), or voiding is possible but incomplete, leaving residual urine in the bladder. This may be asymptomatic but increase the risk of UTI or renal failure.

A good history and examination will often reveal the cause (Table 9.9). Ultrasound where appropriate can measure residual urine and exclude any hydronephrosis or kidney damage.

Management

Acute retention

Catheterization is required, usually a urethral catheter, although suprapubic catheters are better tolerated and have fewer complications.

- Starting an α-blocker, such as tamsulosin, at the same time, increases the chances of a successful trial without a catheter, which should be done 3 days later.
- If possible, avoid long-term indwelling catheters (UTI, septicaemia, prostatitis, urethral strictures, urethral trauma)—a long-term α-blocker will reduce the risk of repeated retention.
- Finasteride reduces prostate size, especially over the first 6 months of use, and improves flow rates and symptoms.
- For patients who again go into retention once the catheter is removed, referral to a urologist should be considered, as the alternative is permanent catheterization, with its risks.
- When catheterization proves impossible (stricture, large prostate, etc.), referral to a urology unit for the use of special catheters or suprapubic catheterization is indicated.
- Catheters may bypass or block. Bypassing is often due to bladder spasm caused by a large balloon or catheter, or by the underlying condition of the patient. Management includes treating the underlying condition if possible, replacing the catheter with a *smaller* catheter, and sometimes using antispasmodic drugs such as oxybutinin.

- Blockage is often due to infection by urease-splitting organisms such as *Proteus*, and sometimes *Pseudomonas*, *Klebsiella*, or *Staphylococcus*. The diagnosis is suspected by finding an alkaline pH (>7) on stix testing. Management is by adequate hydration, removal of the catheter if possible, and using acidic bladder washouts if not.

Table 9.9 Common causes of urinary retention in older people

Obstructive	Benign prostatic hypertrophy
	Bladder neck or urethral stricture
	Faecal impaction
	Pelvic mass, e.g. tumour
	Uterine prolapse
Drug induced	Antimuscarinics, e.g. tricyclic antidepressants, oxybutinin
	Carbamazepine
	NSAIDs
	Opioids
	Sympathomimetics, e.g. ephedrine
Neurological	Cauda equine lesions
	Diabetic neuropathy
	PD
	Prolapsed intervertebral disc
	Stroke
	Spinal stenosis
Infective	Acute prostatitis, urethritis, or vulvovaginitis

Overflow incontinence
This requires drug or surgical treatment if obstructive (prostate, cystocoele); if due to detrusor hypoactivity, the bladder regains its tone after temporary catheterization. Management is best conducted by a urologist, but in very frail patients, permanent catheterization is warranted.

Residual urine
This is treated by regular toileting and α-blockers. Ensuring privacy and lack of hurry is important. Sometimes, double toileting, with a return to the toilet very soon after the person has finished, is tried to reduce residual urine.

Further reading
Sakakibara R, Uchiyama T, Yamanishi T, Kishi M (2008) Dementia and lower urinary dysfunction: with a reference to anticholinergic use in elderly population. *Int J Urol* **15**, 778–88.

Neurological symptoms

Tremor

Tremor takes various forms, some associated with dementia.

- *Essential tremor* is the commonest tremor in the general population. It usually affects the upper limbs although it can also affect any other region of the body. It is symmetrical, regular, and stable over time. It is best brought out by asking the patient to hold a posture against gravity ('hold out your hands') or by activity. It may respond to β-blockers (especially propranolol, e.g. 40mg t.d.s.) or primidone. Gabapentin or alprazolam can also be tried.
- *Physiological tremor* is the normal tremor we all have, but can be increased in some conditions such as anxiety, tiredness, and difficult postures. Drugs commonly used in people with dementia that exaggerate physiological tremor include valproate, tricyclic antidepressants, SSRIs, lithium, and β-agonists.
- *Parkinsonian tremor* occurs at rest and improves on movement. It can also occur on walking, which is unusual for other tremors. Treatment of the PD particularly with levodopa may help. Antipsychotics may cause extrapyramidal effects; quetiapine is less likely to cause problems in this regard.
- *Cerebellar tremor* is an intention tremor, e.g. on trying to drink from a glass, or on the finger–nose test. It affects the upper half of the body predominantly and occurs at right angles to the direction of movement. Other cerebellar features (nystagmus, ataxia, dysdiadochokinesia, hypotonic reflexes) are present. Treatment is for the underlying lesion.
- *Dystonias* involve sustained spasmodic muscle movements, repetitive torsion, and abnormal posture involving head, neck, limbs, or trunk. Common causes in dementia include:
  - disease: PD, multisystem atrophy, CBD, progressive supranuclear palsy, Huntington's disease
  - drugs: neuroleptics, SSRIs, levodopa, metoclopramide, anticonvulsants.

Management

- Treat the cause.
- There is no specific treatment for dystonias. Some respond to levodopa or tetrabenazine.
- Botulinum toxin injected into the dystonic muscle.
- Physiotherapy to avoid contractures.

Choreas

Choreas are movement disorders where there is a continuous flow of sudden, random involuntary muscle movements. They are caused by dysfunction in the connection between the basal ganglia and motor cortex.

Causes in people with dementia

- Huntington's disease.
- Cerebrovascular disease.

- Drugs: phenothiazines and other antipsychotics, dopamine agonists, anticholinergics, phenytoin, carbamazepine, valproate, lithium, tricyclic antidepressants, baclofen, verapamil.
- Tumours around the basal ganglia or subthalamic nuclei—most commonly lymphoma.

Management
- Treat the cause when possible.
- Typical neuroleptics are much more effective than atypical at reducing choreiform movements, but run the risk of themselves inducing dystonias and extrapyramidal adverse effects.
- Risperidone and olanzapine have some activity.
- Tetrabenazine (pre-synaptic dopamine transporter inhibitor, i.e. depletes dopamine, and weakly blocks D2 receptors).

Myoclonus

Myoclonic jerks are quick involuntary movements due to sudden muscle contraction or inhibition. It may be localized or multifocal.

Common causes in people with dementia
- CJD (the commonest rapidly progressive dementia with myoclonus).
- Less often, AD or DLB.
- Some forms of PD.
- Progressive myoclonic epilepsy: rare, eventually produces dementia.
- Metabolic: renal failure, hepatic failure, electrolyte disturbances.
- Drugs: opioids, tramadol, gabapentin, carbamazepine, phenytoin, lamotrigine, tranexamic acid, dopamine agonists, dopamine antagonists.

Management
- Treat the underlying cause, e.g. by opioid substitution.
- Clonazepam—high doses may be required.
- Valproate—high doses may be required.
- Other drugs can be useful for specific causes, e.g. levetiracetam, primidone.

Seizures

Seizures in older people are most often symptomatic of cerebrovascular disease, toxic/metabolic causes, dementia, or brain tumours. Do not assume that seizures are related to the dementia, but consider investigation for other causes. In people with dementia seizures may occur in acute illness, or as a result of epilepsy. Seizures in the acutely ill elderly are particularly dangerous: a third present as status epilepticus, with a mortality of 40%. A recent prospective study suggested a seizure risk of 1% per year in people with AD, higher in younger people with AD, African Americans, in those with more severe illness, and those with focal EEG findings. Risk in many other types of dementia is also elevated. Subcortical dementias, such as Huntington's, are less likely to give rise to seizures.

Seizures can be partial (focal onset) or generalized. Partial seizures are simple if consciousness is preserved, and complex if the patient becomes unconscious. Diagnosis is initially made from history from patient and observers, but EEGs and brain scans may be needed.

Screen for hypo- or hyperglycaemia, hyponatraemia, renal failure, hypocalcaemia, hypothyroidism, pneumonia, UTI.

A number of conditions can mimic seizures, such as syncope (where myoclonus, tongue biting, and incontinence can all occur), transient ischaemic attacks, sleep disorders, and some cardiac conditions. Alcohol withdrawal can precipitate seizures.

Consequences of seizures in dementia
- Worsening of cognitive deficit.
- Reduced independence.
- Injury.
- More rapid loss of language skills.
- Adverse effects of anti-epileptics, risk of drug interactions.
- Earlier death than similar patients without seizures.

Management
- Treat the underlying cause.
- Seizures are very frightening to patients and carers—explain and reassure.
- Is the patient on drugs that lower the seizure threshold—neuroleptics, tricyclic antidepressants (rare), SSRIs (rare), penicillin or cephalosporins at high doses (risk higher in renal failure), drugs that lower serum sodium?
- Assess the balance of adverse effects from prophylactic anti-epileptic drugs (sedation, movement disorders, drug interactions) against the risk of not treating. In general, prophylaxis should be instituted if there are two or more seizures, though some recommend use even after a single seizure in high-risk scenarios.
- Assess risk to life or of injury from seizures, put in sensible preventive measures.
- Phenytoin, carbamazepine, phenobarbitone, primidone, and benzodiazepines are best avoided—sedative, movement disorder, and interaction risks.
- Valproate, gabapentin, oxcarbazepine, and lamotrigine are safest in older people.
- Maximize one drug before adding a second one—if this is needed, refer to an epilepsy specialist. Monotherapy makes adverse effects less likely.
- For focal seizures, consider gabapentin, lamotrigine, oxcarbazepine, valproate, or topiramate.
- For generalized seizures, consider valproate, lamotrigine, or topiramate.
- For indeterminate seizures, consider valproate, oxcarbazepine, lamotrigine, or topiramate.
- Some of these drugs, e.g. valproate, may also be useful mood stabilizers in people with dementia and agitation (📖 Chapter 10).

Management of status epilepticus
- Status epilepticus is defined as ongoing seizure activity lasting more than 30 minutes. Nowadays, many believe that seizures persisting for more than 5 minutes are unlikely to self-terminate and should also be classed as status epilepticus. Frequently recurring seizures without recovery are similarly termed.
- If status is prolonged it can cause irreversible brain damage.
- Protect the patient from injury, e.g. move away furniture they could hurt themselves against.
- Protect airway and breathing.

- Hospital admission may be very appropriate—weigh up risks and benefits.
- Give diazepam 10–20mg p.r., diazemuls i.v., or midazolam 10mg buccally. Repeat in 15 minutes if not settled.
- If not settling, give lorazepam 0.1mg/kg i.v., repeat after 20 minutes if necessary.
- If still uncontrolled, consider phenytoin 15–18mg/kg at 50mg/minute, under electrocardiogram (ECG) monitoring, phenobarbitone 10–15mg/kg at 100mg/minute, or general anaesthesia in ITU.

When unable to swallow

Very few anticonvulsants are available to maintain patients who become unable to swallow. In the UK the alternatives are carbamazepine p.r., s.c. midazolam or lorazepam, and s.c. phenobarbitone. Phenytoin can also be given by infusion but long-term use is not a realistic option in view of its narrow therapeutic index and serious toxicity risk, and the need for cardiac monitoring. Families, and when relevant patients, should be warned that the patient may become fairly heavily sedated, but that the alternative would be a serious risk of seizure.

Bruxism

Bruxism, or teeth clenching and grinding, is sometimes seen in people with dementia. It may occur both in wakefulness and in sleep. It can damage teeth, cause tooth sensitivity by wearing the enamel or fillings down, cause painful jaw spasm, facial pain, earache, and temporo-mandibular joint damage.

It is seen rarely in advanced AD, Huntington's diease, and PD. It has also been associated with SSRIs, antipsychotic drugs, amphetamines, and cocaine, as well as tardive dyskinesia and severe anxiety. It is thought to reflect abnormalities in dopaminergic systems, and in frontal lobe disease the striatopallidal tracts have been implicated.

Most cases do not need treatment. If the bruxism is causing pain a dental check-up is essential. Apart from dealing with damaged teeth, a dentist could also fashion acrylic mouth guards, which are highly effective, but the suitability and safety of these in someone with dementia need to be considered. Benzodiazepines, tricyclic antidepressants, and clonidine have been used in bruxism with moderate success. Botulinum toxin injection into the jaw muscles can give lasting relief—refer to a neurologist or rehabilitation specialist.

For further discussion of some neurological deficits resulting from dementia see 📖 Chapter 11.

Mental distress and psychobehavioural problems

Symptoms and signs of mental and psychological pain

We have already set out in Chapters 6–8 the signs of distress in advanced dementia. In those able to express themselves, it will be easier to identify whether or not the cause of distress is physical pain or mental. But as dementia progresses and the ability to speak is lost, this becomes difficult. A process of elimination of the various causes, starting with the more common, i.e. depression, pain, frustration, is required.

In non-verbal individuals, key signs of mental distress include:
- Anger/frustration.
- Aggression/agitation.
- Fear/anxiety.
- Tearfulness/misery.
- Restlessness.
- Insomnia.
- Calling out/vocalization.
- Wandering.
- Autonomic arousal, sweating, tachycardia, hypertension.

These are also symptoms that are often identified in pain rating scales.

Assessing the background
- Careful enquiry and observation may well help in beginning to identify the cause of distress.
- It is not possible to assess the significance of behavioural symptoms in someone with dementia without a good understanding of their background, the evolution and stage of the illness, how it has affected them, an appreciation of what is normal for them, and their social setup.
- Obtain as much detail as possible about the progression of the illness. How quickly have things changed? What disabilities are they showing? How well can they still carry out the ADLs and instrumental ADLs (IADLs) (Table 11.1)?
- Find out about recent changes in their behaviour.
- Build a picture of their personality, their normal behaviour patterns, and how they usually react to change or to difficulty.
- How long have they been in their current care setting? Have they recently arrived and are they still adapting to a new environment? Are they finding even the place they have lived in for much of their lives strange and difficult to find their way around?
- Elucidate their past medical history.

Understanding the causes of mental and psychological pain
- Information directly from the person with dementia is essential as they can often express their distress better than any observer.
- Gathering evidence from those closely involved in the care of the individual, observing and analysing behaviour, and integrating this with evidence from the patient's history and care setting, will enable at least a tentative diagnosis to be arrived at.

- Psychiatric unit staff may give a very different story from a carer with no psychiatric training or experience.
- Were any possible precipitating causes for the change noticed?
- Functional analysis of behaviour, looking at how a person with severe dementia responds to stimuli in their surroundings, can result in simple and effective interventions.
- A simple but very useful tool in functional analysis is the ABC chart (Antecedents, Behaviour, Consequences; Fig. 10.1). This lists what happened before the behaviour being studied (which may explain why it happened), describes the behaviour itself in detail, and what happened as a result of the behaviour.
- ABC charts can quickly clarify the origin of simple, repetitive patterns of behaviour. In such cases, the chart should only need to be filled in three to five times for the pattern to emerge. In more complex behaviours which vary considerably from one occasion to another, a longer period of observation may be needed.
- ABC charts should not be kept routinely, but only for specific behaviours which are proving difficult to understand; and their use should be brief and time-limited to maintain the effectiveness of the tool.

Patient's name: Date, time and location of reported behaviour:		
Antecedents	Behaviour	Consequences
Name and signature of person completing chart		

Fig. 10.1 An ABC chart

Assessing mental distress

When a patient shows evidence of distress a useful schedule of enquiry will include questions such as:
- Depressive symptoms:
  - Is the patient tearful or persistently miserable?
  - Does the patient have a poor appetite?
  - Is sleep poor?
  - Is the patient lethargic and withdrawn? Physical pain may masquerade as mental distress and is often missed.
- Psychotic symptoms:
  - Is the patient suspicious, fearful, or hallucinating?
- Symptoms of poor care or poor environments:
  - Is the patient fearful or do they appear afraid when approached?
  - Is the environment of sufficient quality and standard?
  - Are there signs of abuse or neglect ?
  - Are they hungry or malnourished?
- Symptoms of sleep–wake cycle disturbance:
  - Is the main difficulty sleep at night?
  - Is the patient worse in the evening (sundowning)?

- Is there an inverted sleep rhythm?
- Daytime occupation and spiritual issues:
  - Is there an adequate activity programme?
  - Are the patient's spiritual and social needs being met?

Having enquired of the broad range of symptoms and examined the patient, clinicians must conclude which they think is the most likely cause of distress and begin to deduce the best and most appropriate treatment.

BPSD

The concept of BPSD arose from the need to undertake better quality research into the treatment of dementia in the wake of the OBRA regulations in the USA.

Symptoms making up BPSD

- Agitation
- Elation
- Anxiety
- Irritability
- Depression
- Disinhibition
- Apathy
- Hallucinations
- Delusions
- Sleep and appetite disturbance

- BPSD are a collection of symptoms which arise from the many causes of mental distress and physical pain. It would therefore be surprising if one particular pattern emerged for all BPSD.
- Reports of the prevalence of BPSD vary from 20% in community dwellers to >80% in residential settings. Frequency increases with advancing dementia.
- Carer stress and burnout are closely related to BPSD, particularly aggression, paranoia, and sleep–wake disturbances.
- Undiagnosed dementia may present with BPSD.
- Care of people with BPSD is significantly more complex and costly. BPSD is a strong predictor of institutionalization.
- The presence of BPSD is a negative prognostic factor, correlated with faster disease progression and a shorter life span.

Principles of management of BPSD

- If you try to see things as the person with dementia sees them, the reasons for BPSD will often make sense; e.g. if one feels one is being given drugs by people one does not know for some reason one does not understand, agitation is a perfectly reasonable response.
- Look for patterns which often give clues to the origin: what precipitates the behaviour, what improves it?
- Current opinion suggests that identifying triggers and modifying behavioural response appropriately by non-pharmacological methods is the best first response (see Box 'Psychobehavioural approaches to BPSD').
- Drugs may have low effectiveness in this context and cause adverse effects. On the other hand, when used appropriately they can significantly improve quality of life. No one treatment is effective for all causes of BPSD.

Psychobehavioural approaches to BPSD

Correcting sensory impairment	Acceptance
Non-confrontation	Optimal autonomy
Simplification	Structuring
Multiple cueing	Repetition
Guiding and demonstration	Reinforcement
Reducing choices	Optimal stimulation
Avoiding new learning	Minimizing anxiety
Determining and using over-learned skills	Using redirection

Reprinted from: Zec RF, Burkett NR (2008) Non-pharmacological and pharmacological treatment of the cognitive and behavioral symptoms of Alzheimer disease. *NeuroRehabilitation* **23(5)**, 425–38, with permission from IOS Press.

BPSD and antipsychotics

There have been many attempts to curb the undoubted harms caused by antipsychotics.

- In 1987 the US OBRA regulations sought to limit antipsychotic use, prompting the study of BPSD as an entity.
- In March 2004, the Committee on Safety of Medicines in the UK advised that risperidone and olanzapine should not be used for BPSD.
- In 2007 NICE advised that antipsychotics should only be prescribed in people with significant distress, a view supported in the UK parliamentary report 'Always a last resort'. Recent Department of Health guidance reflects this intention.
- In a recent report by Professor Sube Banerjee for the Department of Health, it was estimated that 180,000 of the 700,000 people with dementia in the UK are on antipsychotics, and as many as 2/3 of these have them prescribed unnecessarily. The use of these drugs in this population is estimated to result in 1800 deaths and 1600 strokes a year.
- However, there continues to be little evidence as to whether or not these drugs effectively reduce distress.
- Antipsychotics should only be used after a careful analysis of the cause of BPSD, and consideration of pharmacological and non-pharmacological alternatives, with an assessment of the balance between side-effects and benefit. It is sensible to reach agreement with key relatives, carers, etc.
- Cholinesterase inhibitors may help BPSD in Parkinson's dementia. Rivastigmine can delay onset and decrease severity of neuropsychiatric symptoms and can therefore be used to treat mild or chronic BPSD, but the effect is small. Memantine may have a better effect size, but research is awaited on this. Memantine is, however, recommended by separate NICE guidance as first-line treatment for BPSD in DLB.
- The evidence base for the use of antidepressants in BPSD remains weak. Mirtazapine has been shown to be useful for both anxiety and

insomnia in dementia. Clinical experience suggests that antidepressant usage in dementia with agitation helps many patients and where anxiety or agitation is prominent a more sedative type of antidepressant appears sensible.

BPSD are symptoms of an underlying variety of causes. It is a serious error to consider only one treatment modality.

A bad case example

Horace has been wandering in the home and when approached by care staff tends to shout at them and can at times be aggressive. With some carers he reacts well but with others he is very cross. One morning he punches a carer whom he has not met before. Staff say they cannot accept what he did and he is prescribed haloperidol.

His family note that he has become flatter, unresponsive, and drowsy. He mobilizes less well and has a fall. Shortly after, he breaks his hip, goes to hospital, and dies soon after. His family are very upset and complain that he was sedated and died as a result of poor care.

A better case example

Rupert has dementia and is living in a care home. He is fearful and calls out. He also at times hits staff when they try to wash or dress him. He is not tearful, is eating well, and does not appear to be in pain. But staff note that he seems afraid and also seems to see people who are not there.

They discus with the GP and agree to try a small dose of antipsychotic. A discussion of risk and benefit is had with family and the family understand the risks but also that the purpose is to reduce Rupert's distress.

The dose is effective and reduces his distress. Several months later a trial reduction occurs, but again Rupert becomes distressed and agitated. It is decided to continue with the antipsychotic.

Further reading

Banerjee S (2009) *The use of antipsychotic medication for people with dementia: time for action*, p. 61. A report for the Minister of State for Care Services. Department of Health, London.

Ballard C, Day S, Sharp S, Wing G, Sorensen S (2008) Neuropsychiatric symptoms in dementia: importance and treatment considerations. *Int Rev Psychiat* **20**, 396–404.

Treloar A, Crugel M, Prasanna A, Solomons L, Fox C, Paton C, Katona C (2010) Ethical dilemmas: should antipsychotics ever be prescribed for people with dementia? *Br J Psychiat* **197**, 88–90.

Delirium

Definition and epidemiology
- Also known as acute confusional state, transient cognitive impairment.
- Occurs in 20–60% of all hospitalized elderly patients.
- Dementia is thought to double or treble the risk of delirium. A systematic review some years ago found prevalence rates of up to 89% in hospitalized dementia patients.
- In dementia patients in hospital, delirium affects the length of stay (doubling it in some series), increases cost of care, accelerates cognitive decline, has a higher morbidity (falls, pressure sores, serious infection) and mortality, and increases the likelihood of long-term institutional care.
- In people who are still at home, delirium doubles the risk of institutionalization within the next 2 years.
- Hospital admission with delirium carries a mortality rate of up to 25%. Development of delirium during hospitalization carries a much higher mortality rate, up to 75% in some series.

Pathophysiology
- A reversible change in cerebral oxidative metabolism is considered to be a common cause for delirium.
- Cholinergic neurotransmitter deficiency is also thought to play a key part in pathophysiology, brought about by changes in precursors, enzymes, or receptors. In AD this already exists, which might partly explain why such patients are more prone to develop delirium.
- Reciprocal excessive brain dopaminergic activity has been implicated. Anticholinergic drugs often precipitate delirium, and dopamine antagonists, such as haloperidol, control it.
- A role for serotonin, γ-amino butyric acid (GABA), endorphins, and cortisol has also been suggested.

Clinical picture
- Marked by rapid onset over hours to days of fluctuating global impairment in attention and cognition.
- Patients are very distractible and any change in their environment, e.g. someone entering the room or a loud noise, will break their concentration and make them focus on the immediate event. Conversely, attention can be difficult to shift, e.g. perseveration may occur with repetition of the same words over and over in response to a series of questions.
- Disorientation and disorders of perception (delusions, hallucinations) are common.
- Short-term memory is poor.
- Insight into the condition is often lacking.
- Patients can appear perplexed, suspicious, or irritable.
- Speech may be rambling and incoherent, and pressure of speech may occur.
- Some are agitated. Others may be withdrawn and their delirium is easily missed.

- The sleep–wake cycle may be disturbed, e.g. patients are up all night and asleep for much of the day.
- Autonomic features are common, e.g. tachycardia, sweating.
- Delirium and dementia can be mistaken for each other. DSM-IV does not allow dementia to be diagnosed while delirium is present, to prevent misattribution of the clinical picture.
- May be less reversible than previously thought; the prognosis of delirium is often that of institutionalization and worsened dementia.

Associated conditions

The degree of investigation for the underlying cause will depend on the degree of dementia, tolerance for intervention, and prognosis (Table 10.1).

Table 10.1 Some common conditions associated with delirium

Associated medical conditions	Dementia
	Infection: commonest are UTI, chest infection, septicaemia
	Intracranial causes: head injury, stroke, increased intracranial pressure, encephalitis or meningitis
	Associated with seizures, e.g. post-ictal
	Hypo- or hyperthyroidism
	Vitamin deficiencies, e.g. thiamine, B_{12}
	Anaemia
Metabolic abnormalities	Hypo- or hyperglycaemia, e.g. hyperosmolar non-ketotic coma (HONC)
	Hypercalcaemia
	Hyponatraemia
	Dehydration or starvation
Drugs	Anticholinergic drugs
	Opioids
	Antipsychotics
	Antidepressants
	Amphetamines
	Calcium-channel blockers
	Digoxin
	β-blockers
	H2 blockers (cimetidine)
	Corticosteroids
	Levodopa
Sensory impairment	Visual impairment
	Hearing impairment
Organ failures	Liver failure
	Renal failure
	Respiratory failure
	Congestive heart failure

(continued)

Table 10.1 Continued

Critical illness	Hypoxia
	Major trauma
	Post-operative
	Uncontrolled pain
	Heart block and other serious arrhythmias
Drug withdrawal	Alcohol
	Cigarettes: nicotine
	Sedatives, e.g. benzodiazepines
Other	Unfamiliar environment
	Use of restraints
	Sensory overload, e.g. very bright lights, loud environment
	Malnutrition
	Polypharmacy and drug interactions

Management

- Early diagnosis and management is associated with a more favourable outcome.
- In view of its significant mortality and morbidity, delirium should be treated as a medical emergency.
- Never leave delirious patients unattended.
- Moving to an unfamiliar environment, and being looked after by unfamiliar people, may worsen delirium. On the other hand, investigation and treatment may sometimes require hospitalization.
- In reaching a decision regarding transfer, weigh up the potential for treatability and long-term improvement of quality of life, burden of investigation and treatment, prognosis, patient's past wishes, the views of family and other carers, and the likelihood one can maintain comfort effectively in other ways. It is just as wrong to transfer someone with end-stage dementia who has developed a recurrent aspiration pneumonia as not to transfer someone with moderate dementia who is able to live with some degree of independence. See ▢ Chapter 13.
- Nurse in a single room. Avoid unnecessary room changes.
- Reduce risk of harm: for example, keep the patient in an environment where falls are less likely to be harmful (away from stairs); remove implements dangerous to self or others—replace glass by plastic glasses, remove sharp cutlery etc.
- Provide frequent, supportive contact with familiar people. Reduce new faces encountered to the barest minimum.
- Provide frequent reality orientation—explain gently where they are and what the time is, and what is happening. Have family photographs in the room where they can easily be seen.
- Enlist family, friends, and usual carers to assist in reality orientation and communication.
- Have a prominent large clock for ease of checking the time.

- Minimize distractions: do only one thing at a time, do not have staff members coming into and out of the room, or bleeps and mobile phones going off. Avoid loud noise.
- Avoid bright lights or subdued lighting—aim for even lighting without shadows so as to reduce misperceptions which may set off fears and feelings of paranoia.
- Give adequate food and fluid, by the least interventionist means possible.
- Encourage mobility within the limits of safety.
- Make sure glasses or hearing aids function properly and that they are used.
- Control pain with adequate, regular analgesia.
- Stop all medication that is not immediately vital. Review once the delirium has settled.
- Maintain bladder and bowel function (📖 Chapter 9).
- The draft NICE guidance on delirium recommends haloperidol (0.5–1mg p.o. up to t.d.s.) or olanzapine (2.5–5mg daily) to control acute symptoms. Risperidone is also frequently used (up to 1mg b.d.).
- Risks with antipsychotics include extrapyramidal symptoms, sedation, arrhythmias, and cerebrovascular events.
- Haloperidol can be lethal in DLB or Parkinson's associated conditions.
- A recent Cochrane review did not find good evidence for effectiveness of benzodiazepines outside the acute alcohol withdrawal situation. They may be used in withdrawal from other drugs of addiction.

Alcohol withdrawal

- This is a special situation, with a high risk of agitation, seizures, and delirium tremens (DT; severe limb tremors, misperceptions, visual hallucinations which are often frightening, and tactile hallucinations, e.g. formications—insects crawling up the body). DT has a mortality of 5% with treatment. Alcohol withdrawal may also lead to anxiety and panic attacks, alcoholic hallucinosis (more benign than DT), and autonomic symptoms, e.g. tremors, sweating, fever, nausea, and vomiting.
- Chronic alcohol intake produces GABA receptor downregulation.
- Treatment is with high doses of benzodiazepines, ideally titrated to response. Common regimes include chlordiazepoxide 10–30mg q.d.s., gradually reducing over 7–14 days, and diazepam 5–15mg q.d.s. p.o. reducing over a similar time scale.
- Treat vitamin deficiencies, especially thiamine (common).

Specialist advice should be sought regarding patients already on benzo-diazepines or those who continue to drink, where benzodiazepines are not safe.

Further reading

Lonergan E, Luxenberg J, Areosa Sastre A, Wyller TB (2009) Benzodiazepines for delirium. *Cochrane Database Syst Rev* (Online) 2009(1):CD006379.
Taylor D, Paton C, Kapur S (2009) Delirium. In: *The Maudsley prescribing guidelines*, 10th edn, pp. 445–50. Informa Healthcare, London.

Depression

- Depression affects up to 40% of dementia sufferers.
- Some have suggested that depression can increase the risk of developing AD, but this is not proven.
- Depression is a key differential diagnosis for dementia as it is easy for the elderly depressed patient to be misdiagnosed as having cognitive difficulties (Table 2.2). Cognitive impairment due to depression may be reversible with treatment.
- The commonly accepted criteria for diagnosing depression are the DSM-IV criteria (see Box)
- Diagnosis of depression in people with dementia is often not easy. Many features of depression mimic dementia: poor concentration may make intake of information patchy, giving rise to a suspicion of cognitive loss; responses may be delayed and stereotyped ('I don't know'); abstract thought and executive function may be impaired; the patient may be very distractible and sometimes disorientated. Sadness and feelings of hopelessness and guilt may help differentiate depression from the apathy common in dementia, though this is more difficult in advanced dementia. Fatigue is common in advanced dementia and the value of this and other somatic symptoms (poor appetite, sleep disruption) in diagnosis is confined to providing additional supporting evidence for other criteria already met.
- In order to aid diagnosis, a number of scales have been proposed. Perhaps the most widely used is the Cornell Scale for Depression in Dementia (see Box). Another scale that is often used is the Neuropsychiatric Inventory (NPI).
- Depression in dementia is commoner soon after diagnosis, and immediately after admission to a care facility, such as nursing home.
- Depression in AD may fluctuate but recur frequently.
- A recent review showed that in AD depression is associated with poorer quality of life, greater disability in ADLs, faster cognitive decline, a high rate of nursing home placement, relatively higher mortality, and a higher frequency of depression and burden in caregivers.
- Management of depression in dementia can be non-pharmacological or pharmacological.
- There are various forms of non-pharmacological management, though the evidence for their usefulness in this situation is very limited. They include:
  - Maintaining a stable, caring environment with clear routines.
  - Sensory input: there is evidence that Snoezelen therapy, using multisensory rooms, has some impact on mood.
  - Bright light therapy has been suggested, but ambient bright light has not been shown to impact on dementia, although individual bright light therapy might be more efficacious.
- The evidence for the effectiveness of pharmacological treatment is limited but there is widespread agreement among clinicians that it is very important to ensure that those who appear to be depressed get treatment.
- SSRI antidepressants such as fluoxetine have a favourable side-effect profile and do not appear to be associated with increased mortality. While a Cochrane Review demonstrated only weak evidence for the practice of prescribing antidepressants in depression and dementia,[1] there is good quality evidence that citalopram is an effective, non-sedating

SSRI in depression in mild to moderate dementia. Such drugs are safer than antipsychotics and are a far more rational treatment if the underlying causes include depression. Research studies to clarify the benefit of such treatment have yet to be concluded.

- If agitation is a prominent feature, mirtazapine or other more relaxing antidepressants may be best.

Why is diagnosing depression in dementia difficult?

To diagnose a major depressive episode, DSM-IV criteria require:	In dementia:
A depressed mood lasting most of the day	May be difficult to gauge especially in non-verbal patients
and/or anhedonia (loss of pleasure) in most activities	Passivity may be misread as anhedonia
Plus some of the following:	
Weight loss or gain > 5% of body weight in a month	Weight loss is common, usually from poor feeding (📖 Chapters 9, 13)
Change in appetite	May be affected in dementia
Sleep disturbance	Changes in sleep patterns are frequent (📖 Chapter 10, Sleep disturbance, pp. 196–199)
Feelings of worthlessness or guilt	May be precipitated by feeling out of one's depth or by the way one is treated by others. May be delusional
Psychomotor agitation or retardation	Common BPSD; may be signs of delirium
Fatigue	May result from poor nutrition, loss of muscle mass
Poor thinking and concentration and inability to decide	Deterioration of thinking and executive function are common features of many dementias, e.g. damage to brain association areas
Morbid thoughts or suicidal ideation	

For more details see American Psychiatric Association (2000) *Diagnostic and statistical manual of mental disorders*, 4th edn, text revision. American Psychiatric Publishing Inc., Arlington, VA.

- Older (tricyclic) antidepressants, e.g. amitriptyline, have serious side-effects such as increased confusion, increased risk of falls, and constipation, and are therefore less desirable. In bedbound patients, some of the adverse effects, e.g. postural hypotension, may be less relevant. However, effects such as confusion and arrhythmias could still be an issue.

1 Bains J, Birks JS, Dening TD (2002) Antidepressant for treating depression in dementia. *Cochrane Database Syst Rev*, Issue 4, CD003944.

Cornell Scale for Depression in Dementia

Administered through semi-structured interviews with the patient and an informant. Many items can be completed by observation of the patient. Scoring reflects the rater's clinical impression based on the interviews and observation rather than the views of the patient or informant.

Score ≥12 suggests depression requiring treatment.

Score 8–11 suggests depression which requires monitoring.

Scoring: a 7 unable to evaluate; 0 = absent; 1 = mild to intermittent; 2 = severe.

A: Mood-related signs
  1. Anxiety; anxious expression, rumination, worrying.
  2. Sadness; sad expression, sad voice, tearfulness.
  3. Lack of reaction to pleasant events.
  4. Irritability; annoyed, short tempered.

B. Behavioural disturbance
  5. Agitation; restlessness, hand wringing, hair pulling.
  6. Retardation; slow movements, slow speech, slow reactions.
  7. Multiple physical complaints (score 0 if GI symptoms only).
  8. Loss of interest; less involved in usual activities (score 0 only if change occurred acutely, i.e., in less than 1 month).

C. Physical signs
  9. Appetite loss; eating less than usual.
  10. Weight loss (score 2 if greater than 5lb/2.3kg in 1 month).
  11. Lack of energy; fatigues easily, unable to sustain activities.

D. Cyclic functions
  12. Diurnal variation of mood; symptoms worse in the morning.
  13. Difficulty falling asleep; later than usual for this individual.
  14. Multiple awakenings during sleep.
  15. Early morning awakening; earlier than usual for this individual.

E. Ideational disturbance
  16. Suicidal; feels life is not worth living.
  17. Poor self-esteem; self-blame, self-depreciation, feelings of failure.
  18. Pessimism; anticipation of the worst.
  19. Mood-congruent delusions; delusions of poverty, illness or loss.

Reproduced from Alexopoulos GS, Abrams RC et al. (1988). Cornell Scale for Depression in Dementia. *Biol Psychiat* **23(3)**, 271–84. with permission from Elsevier.

Case example

Gladys has severe dementia and lives in a nursing home. Care staff have noted that she is somewhat withdrawn, agitated, and restless. The GP reviews her and it turns out that she has poor sleep, is distressed during the night, and tearful during the day. She does not appear to enjoy seeing her family very much. Although she is agitated it is considered best to try an antidepressant. Through the proper discussion with care staff about identifying the possibility of depression, care staff became better at recognizing the possible causes of distress in dementia.

Antidepressant treatment options (Tables 10.2 and 10.3)

A SSRI is probably the best first choice (favourable side-effect profile). If agitation is prominent a more sedating antidepressant such as mirtazapine might be chosen. If the patient is bedbound and falls are not likely to be a risk and the first two options do not work, a tricyclic antidepressant might be a possibility.

- A response to an antidepressant takes 2–6 weeks at therapeutic dose level, although a recent meta-analysis in the non-dementia population has shown that response can occur after a week. Perhaps the commonest reason for failure to respond is taking the drugs inconsistently, common in dementia, and even more so in dementia with depression. Another frequent reason for non-response is that too low a dose of antidepressant is used. For example, with amitriptyline or nortriptyline, doses below 75mg daily are unlikely to improve depression.

- In general, in a depressive episode, continue antidepressants for 6 months and then review. If the depression is a recurrence, continue treatment for 2 years and then review. If the patient's general condition changes, the risk/benefit of antidepressants may alter, and their use would have to be re-evaluated.

- Antidepressants must be withdrawn gradually or a discontinuation syndrome may result. This takes the form of a flu-like illness with chills, muscle pains, headaches, and nausea, with dizziness, anxiety, irritability, insomnia, and vivid dreams. Cognitive function may be temporarily worsened.

- If there is no response to a SSRI, strategies include increasing the dose, changing to another SSRI, or switching to a non-SSRI antidepressant. A recent meta-analysis in a non-dementia population found a clinically small but statistically significant advantage to the latter course of action. However, resistant cases should be reviewed by a psychiatrist.

Table 10.2 Antidepressant drugs

Group	Examples and doses	Adverse effects	Notes
SSRIs. First-line treatment	Fluoxetine 20–40mg daily Paroxetine 20–40mg daily Sertraline 50–200mg daily Citalopram 20–40mg daily Escitalopram 5–20mg daily	Nausea, vomiting, dyspepsia, abdominal pain, diarrhoea, constipation, headache, sexual dysfunction, fatigue, restlessness. SSRIs carry a significant risk of gastric bleeding and hyponatraemia	Dosage is simple. Less toxic in overdose than tricyclic antidepressants (TCAs)
Selective serotonin/nor-epinephrine reuptake inhibitors (SNRIs)	Venlafaxine 75–150mg in 2 divided doses Duloxetine 30–60mg daily	Similar to SSRIs. Can occasionally produce sustained hypertension but occasionally hypotension; can cause insomnia or somnolence	May be useful first line in patients with significant fatigue or pain Introduction of venlafaxine requires a baseline ECG and blood pressure measurement

(continued)

Table 10.2 Continued

Group	Examples and doses	Adverse effects	Notes
TCAs	Amitriptyline 75–150mg (build up from 10–25mg) Imipramine 50–75mg (start at 10mg) Dosulepin 75–150mg (build up from 25mg) Nortriptyline 75–100mg	Toxic drugs with many side-effects. Postural hypotension (can cause strokes, falls, fractures!). Confusion, sedation Antimuscarinic: dry mouth, constipation, blurred vision, tachycardia/arrhythmias, urinary retention, precipitation of acute closed-angle glaucoma Use with caution in the elderly Avoid in bipolar disorder (can precipitate mania)	Start at low dose, e.g. nortriptyline 10–25mg, build up to therapeutic dose, e.g. 75mg Nortriptyline, desipramine have fewer antimuscarinic effects and are generally safer TCAs may give highly variable serum levels for the same dose, and measuring serum levels may at times be necessary. Dry mouth is said to be a good surrogate marker of an effective dose
Serotonin antagonist/ reuptake inhibitors (SARI)	Trazodone 300mg	Sedation, dizziness, headache	Start at 100mg nocte
Noradrenergic and specific serotonergic antidepressant (NaSSA)	Mirtazapine 15–30mg daily	Increased appetite, weight gain, postural hypotension, sedation with initial use, oedema, fatigue	Useful especially with agitation, when some sedation is required
MAOIs	Phenelzine Tranylcypromine	Hypertensive crises with tyramine-containing foods	Almost never used nowadays due to risks including many dangerous drug interactions

Table 10.3 Which antidepressant?

Sedation required, e.g. sleep disturbance	SARI, e.g. trazodone NaSSA, e.g. mirtazapine
Sedation not wanted	Some SSRIs, e.g. fluoxetine SNRI, e.g. venlafaxine

Table 10.3 Continued

High anxiety component	SSRI, e.g. citalopram
	SNRI, e.g. venlafaxine
Concomitant pain	TCA, e.g. nortriptyline
	SNRI, e.g. duloxetine

Suicide risk in dementia

- A recent systematic review found that the risk of suicide in dementia is similar to or smaller than that of the general population.
- However, it is higher soon after diagnosis, in patients diagnosed with dementia during hospitalization, and in Huntington's disease.
- Factors that increase risk include depression, hopelessness, mild cognitive impairment, preserved insight, younger age, and failure to respond to antidementia drugs.

Further reading

Haw C, Harwood D, Hawton K (2009) Dementia and suicidal behavior: a review of the literature. *Int Psychogeriatr* **21**, 440–53.

Korczyn AD, Halperin I (2009) Depression and dementia. *J Neurol Sci* **283**, 139–42.

Tagariello P, Girardi P, Amore M (2009) Depression and apathy in dementia: same syndrome or different constructs? A critical review. *Arch Gerontol Geriatr* **49**, 246–9.

Switching antidepressants if patient has been on antidepressant for 6 weeks or longer

Cross-tapering means the cautious withdrawal of one antidepressant, usually over 4 weeks or longer depending on tolerance of the process, while gradually building up the new antidepressant over the same time period.

NB: Fluoxetine has a very long half-life and (up to 16 days in some individuals), and slow withdrawal over 1–3 months may be needed. Fluoxetine is also particularly prone to drug interactions (CYP450, see 📖 Appendix 2).

SSRI to TCA

STOP the SSRI, build up the TCA dose cautiously from a low dose. With fluoxetine, wait for 4–7 days before starting the TCA.

SSRI to trazodone

Withdraw the SSRI, then start trazodone. If fluoxetine, wait 4–7 days before starting trazodone.

SSRI to mirtazapine

Cross-taper cautiously.

SSRI to venlafaxine

Cross-taper cautiously over many weeks, starting venlafaxine at 37.5mg daily, increasing dose very slowly over weeks. Withdraw fluoxetine before starting venlafaxine.

(continued)

TCA to SSRI

Halve the dose of TCA, introduce SSRI while tapering down the TCA.

TCA to mirtazapine

Cautious cross-tapering.

TCA to venlafaxine

Cross-taper cautiously, starting with 37.5mg venlafaxine.

Mirtazapine to SSRI

Withdraw mirtazapine over 4 weeks, then start SSRI.

Mirtazapine to venlafaxine

Cross-taper cautiously.

Based on Taylor D, Paton C, Kapur S (2009) *The Maudsley prescribing guidelines*, 10th edn, pp. 216–19. Informa Healthcare, London.

Psychosis

- Psychosis affects up to 70% of dementia sufferers during the course of their illness.
- Psychotic features take many forms: delusions (often paranoid and short-lived); misidentification (e.g. being convinced that a relative is somebody else, or that people on television are actually present), and hallucinations (most commonly visual; 📖 Chapter 2, Symptoms of dementia, pp. 15–19). Most patients with hallucinations also have delusions.
- Psychosis may be associated with a more rapid course, worse general health, and more cognitive impairment even at the stage of mild cognitive impairment.
- Psychotic features are also associated with greater carer stress.
- There is genetic, neurochemical, and histopathological evidence of a subtype or subtypes of AD more commonly associated with psychotic features.
- People with AD are at higher risk of delusions if their insight into their deficit is limited, if they are depressed, if their cognitive deficits are global, and if their mood is elevated.
- Psychotic features are commoner in some forms of dementia.
- In DLB, visual hallucinations and delusions occur early and are prominent. Patients sometimes gesture at and conduct an argument with someone who is not present. The presence of visual hallucinations may be associated with a greater likelihood of response to cholinesterase inhibitors.
- In AD and VaD, hallucinations and delusions also occur. A review of 10 studies looking at the psychotic features in AD found no association with disease severity in any of them.
- In people with very advanced AD, delusions and hallucinations have to be inferred from behaviour, and may go unrecognized.
- Figures regarding the persistence of psychotic features in AD vary from very low (5% or less) to very high (>85%). The persistence of these symptoms has implications for drug use; drugs may be deemed effective if psychotic symptoms are short-lived and do not persist after initiation of medication.

Management of psychotic features in dementia

- The effective treatment for psychosis is antipsychotic medication (Tables 10.4 and 10.5).
- Antipsychotic drugs are broadly classified into two groups: the typical antipsychotics (e.g. chlorpromazine, haloperidol, trifluoperazine) and the newer atypical antipsychotics (e.g. risperidone, olanzapine, quetiapine). The term 'atypical' denotes the relative lack of extrapyramidal adverse effects (dystonias, parkinsonian features, akathisia, tardive dyskinesia) from the newer drugs.
- While high doses are required to treat acute schizophrenic episodes, the doses required to treat psychotic symptoms in dementia and delirium are generally much smaller.

- The effectiveness of typical antipsychotics for a particular patient is similar, but is much more variable between atypicals.
- Both typical and atypical antipsychotics carry significant risks.
- Extrapyramidal effects and sedation are common with the former. Antipsychotic use is known to be associated with more chest infections, accelerated cognitive decline, an increased risk of strokes (odds ratio 2.5–3.0 for atypical antipsychotics), and a higher mortality (1.5–1.7 times increased all-cause mortality with atypical antipsychotics during the 6–12 week period of treatment in drug trials). This has led the FDA in the USA and European Medicines Agency (EMEA) in Europe to advise against using atypical antipsychotics for the treatment of BPSD in people with dementia.
- The recent DART-AD trial demonstrated that the excess mortality does not fall with longer-term use (⊞ Chapter 10, Agitation and aggression, pp. 193–195).
- Evidence for mortality from typical antipsychotic use is less well established and comes mainly from observational studies of people with delirium. Such studies suggest an equal or even higher mortality than with atypical antipsychotics.
- Over the years, antipsychotic drugs have been increasingly used to treat not just psychotic symptoms but also BPSD. This has led to significant overuse of these drugs and an emerging backlash against their liberal use for behaviour control.
- The evidence of effectiveness of both typical and atypical antipsychotics in the treatment of psychosis in dementia is limited. There is only evidence for aripiprazole, an atypical antipsychotic, which carries a very low NNT of 13.8.
- Extrapyramidal effects can cause death (particularly in DLB). As a result clinicians frequently prefer to use atypical drugs in low dose.
- The recommendation not to use atypical antipsychotics in dementia in BPSD and an appreciation of their risks and evidence for effectiveness should cause one to approach their use for psychotic symptoms in this condition with caution. However, a small number of patients who have been psychotic will deteriorate when the antipsychotic is stopped, although there is good evidence that stopping antipsychotics is often not associated with deterioration. A sensible guide is to use antipsychotics at low dose, to review that dose, and make attempts to reduce or discontinue treatment when possible.
- Perhaps the key ethical reason for continuation of treatment is when discontinuation causes a return of distress.

Some serious adverse effects of antipsychotic drugs

A number of serious adverse effects may result from the use of antipsychotic drugs. The drug data sheet will give a complete list, but the adverse effects listed here are particularly linked to typical antipsychotics (see also Table 10.6).

Table 10.4 Some commonly used antipsychotic drugs

Drug	Normal dosage in dementia	Adverse effects	Notes
(1) Typical antipsychotics			
Haloperidol	Start at 0.5mg daily. Final dose in elderly usually 1–3mg daily in 1 or 2 doses	Extrapyramidal symptoms, particularly dystonic reactions and akathisia. QT interval prolongation	AVOID in DLB, other extrapyramidal disorders
(2) Atypical antipsychotics			
Olanzapine	Start at 5mg daily, increase up to 10mg daily	Hyperglycaemia. Weight gain. Nausea and vomiting. Anticholinergic effects. Sedation. Postural hypotension and extrapyramidal effects less common. Peripheral oedema	Women may need slightly lower doses as they clear olanzapine more slowly
Quetiapine	25–100mg b.d. Start low, titrate up over a few days	Sedation common. Anticholinergic effects. Postural hypotension less common. Extrapyramidal effects rare. Hyperglycaemia. Weight gain	May be drug of choice in Parkinson's and DLB. More sedating than many other antipsychotics, but is a very weak antipsychotic
Risperidone	0.5mg nocte to b.d. for 1 week, then double if necessary	Insomnia, postural hypotension, less commonly, extrapyramidal side-effects, sedation, nausea and vomiting	The only antipsychotic licensed in the UK for short-term treatment of agitation in dementia. Greater extrapyramidal risk than quetiapine

Table 10.5 Comparison of typical and atypical antipsychotics

Drug	Extra-pyramidal	Anti-cholinergic	Postural hypotension	Sedation
(1) Typical antipsychotics				
Chlorpromazine	++	++	+++(i.m. > p.o.)	+++
Trifluoperazine	+++	+	+	+
Haloperidol	+++. (i.v. < i.m./p.o.)	+/–	+	+
Levomepromazine	++	++	+++	+++

(continued)

Table 10.5 Continued

Drug	Extra-pyramidal	Anti-cholinergic	Postural hypotension	Sedation
2) Atypical antipsychotics				
Olanzapine	+/–	+	+	++
Risperidone	+	+	++	+/– (often insomnia)
Quetiapine	+/–	+	++	++

Postural hypotension
- Defined as fall in systolic b.p. >20mmHg on standing, a decrease in diastolic b.p. >10 mm Hg, or an increase in heart rate of 20 beats per minute (b.p.m.) on standing, or a systolic b.p.< 90mmHg with symptoms indicative of postural hypotension.
- Probably due to α-blockade, inhibiting reflex vasoconstriction on standing.
- Aliphatic phenothiazines (chlorpromazine, levomepromazine) are most prone to cause this.
- The elderly are both more susceptible to postural hypotension and more likely to develop serious complications, e.g. falls leading to injury (fractures, subdural, or intracranial bleeds), strokes.
- Management: check for other drugs affecting b.p., e.g. diuretics, β-blockers, TCAs.
- Substitute a less hypotensive antipsychotic.

NB: Postural hypotension is dangerous in the elderly and must be treated decisively!

NMS
- Syndrome consists of generalized muscle rigidity (lead pipe), pyrexia usually >38°C, altered consciousness and autonomic dysfunction (e.g. b.p. changes, tachycardia, arrhythmias, sweating, tremor). The picture develops over 1–3 days.
- Apart from antipsychotics, can also be caused by metoclopramide, amphetamines, lithium.
- Common lab findings are high CK, myoglobinuria, leukocytosis, metabolic acidosis.
- NMS can continue for days or weeks after discontinuation of the offending drug.
- May be fatal especially if significance of symptoms is not appreciated.
- Management: discontinue causative drug; treat hyperthermia (paracetamol); parenteral hydration. Get advice from a neurologist or intensive care specialist, consider transfer. Consider ventilation in ITU if seriously hypoxic. A variety of drugs have been used, the evidence for which is patchy. These include bromocriptine, levodopa, dantrolene, and benzodiazepines.

NB: Restarting the offending drug may re-precipitate NMS.

Extrapyramidal side-effects

Movement disorders in this category can occur acutely (usually within the first 5 days of treatment, mostly within the first 4 weeks) or delayed (tardive), after 6 months of treatment or more. They include:

- Parkinsonian symptoms: tremor, rigidity, bradykinesia. A pill-rolling tremor at rest, also seen with outstretched arms, is often accompanied by a more subtle, fine, high-frequency tremor. Rigidity can be lead pipe (similar throughout the range of motion) or cogwheel (on/off/ on throughout the range of movement, due to tremor superimposed on rigidity), and is best seen by flexing and extending the wrist. Bradykinesia means slowness of movement. Loss of facial expression, small handwriting, and slow, quiet speech are other aspects of bradykinesia. Rigidity can be made more obvious by getting the patient to move the contralateral limb. Late in the disease, postural instability occurs, with falls being common. This is most obvious when turning in a tight circle.
- Akathisia literally means an inability to sit. It is defined as a subjective feeling of motor restlessness. Patients complain of an inability to sit or stand still and feel compelled to pace around. It is more likely if a patient is also on morphine or valproate.
- Dystonias present as twisting movements or abnormal posture, or both, of any voluntary muscle group in the body. Common dystonias include involuntary movements of the limbs, facial grimacing, tics, trismus (inability to open the mouth wide due to muscle spasm), cervical dystonia (torticollis—spasmodic positioning of the head sideways—or retrocollis—backward spasmodic positioning of the head), oculogyric crisis (spasmodic upward rolling of the eyes), rhythmic tongue protrusion, jaw opening or closing, and occasionally spasmodic dysphonia, or stridor and dyspnoea.

Management

Parkinsonian symptoms

Stop or substitute the offending drug, e.g. switch from a typical to an atypical antipsychotic. Ideally one would give an anticholinergic drug—see dystonias below but also the warning.

Akathisia

Stop or substitute the causative drugs. Antimuscarinic drugs (see dystonias below) may help, but response is often delayed by 3–7 days; the same strictures apply as for dystonias. Propranolol 20–80mg daily and benzodiazepines (diazepam 5–10mg/day, clonazepam 0.5–1mg/day, lorazepam 1–3mg/day) are also sometimes used, although both are probably less effective than antimuscarinics; akathisia can recur when the benzodiazepine is stopped. However, propranolol can be continued for 6 months without tolerance developing. Selective β_1-adrenergic blockers, e.g. atenolol, are less effective and should not be used.

Dystonias

Treat acute-onset dystonias as soon as possible, as persisting with the offending drug occasionally causes life-threatening laryngeal spasm and is intensely uncomfortable. Stop the offending drug, substituting an alternative if necessary. If antipsychotics are impossible to stop or substitute without precipitating psychotic symptoms again, reduce the dose as much as possible. However, most acute dystonias settle anyway within a week or two, and occasionally it may be possible to continue the drug if absolutely necessary unless it precipitates recurrent episodes.

Consider an antimuscarinic antiparkinsonian drug (but see NB; avoid or use very sparingly), e.g.

- Benztropine 1–2mg i.v./i.m., then continue with 2mg p.o. daily–b.d. for 1 week OR
- Procyclidine 5–10mg i.v./i.m, then continue with 2.5–5mg p.o. t.d.s. for 1 week OR
- Orphenadrine 50mg p.o. b.d.–t.d.s.
- Benefit is seen within 10-20 minutes; the parenteral drug may be repeated after 30 minutes if necessary.
- Diazepam 5mg i.v. has also been used.
- Tardive dyskinesias may be made worse by withdrawing the causative drug.

NB: Antimuscarinic drugs can worsen confusion in people with dementia; their use should be carefully weighed up, and, if used, they should be discontinued as soon as possible.

Table 10.6 Time of greatest risk for appearance of major adverse effects of antipsychotic drugs—however, symptoms can appear outside these times

Adverse effect	Timing
Postural hypotension	Hours to days
Acute dystonia	1–5 days
Akathisia	5 days–2 months
Parkinsonism	3 days–1 month
NMS	1 day–several weeks
Tardive dyskinesia	Years of treatment

Further reading

Ropacki SA, Jeste DV (2005) Epidemiology of and risk factors for psychosis of Alzheimer's disease: a review of 55 studies published from 1990 to 2003. *Am J Psychiat* **162**, 2022–30.

Anxiety and poor understanding

- Dementia is an illness in which understanding is lost. There are important ways of improving understanding and engaging those with severe cognitive difficulties so that they collaborate with treatment and care more easily with reduced distress (Chapter 11). Good care, with an engaging, non-confrontational approach, with the specific aim of minimizing the challenges caused by poor understanding, is essential to reduce fear and anxiety.

- It is not difficult to imagine how hard it must be for some patients with dementia when they find complete strangers coming up to them and washing and dressing them. Perhaps the greatest surprise of all of this is that, most commonly, patients with dementia are remarkably tolerant with such personal care and accept it with very little resistance. It is in fact only the minority who appear to resist and be severely distressed by such care.

- Explanation of any procedure in simple terms should always be used, even in patients whose ability to comprehend is very limited. Poor understanding compounded by the inability to communicate needs leads to frustration and behaviour that is often perceived as challenging. The real challenge is identifying the person's needs such that their distress is relieved.

Anxiety as a specific condition

Not all fear and anxiety is caused by poor understanding. Some will be caused by depression, some by psychosis and some by the knowledge that (for example) pain will be caused by the process of addressing washing and personal care.

- Anxiety disorder can take several forms: *generalized anxiety disorder* (GAD) is long-standing anxiety not focused on a particular object or event; in *panic disorder*, sudden attacks of severe anxiety occur, sometimes but not always triggered by a known cause or stress, with shaking, weakness, tremor, sweating, palpitations, dizziness, nausea, and hyperventilation; in *phobias*, fear and anxiety are triggered by a specific object or situation. Anxiety symptoms are much less long-lasting and haphazard.

- Anxiety symptoms have been found in 8–71% of patients with dementia, more than in the general population. Prevalence is linked to diagnosis (higher for VaD and frontotemporal dementia) and method of screening (lower if structured clinical interviews are used). Anxiety disorder has been found in 1 in 20 to 1 in 5 people with dementia.

- No correlation with sex, age, or educational attainment has been demonstrated.

- Anxiety in people with dementia is associated with poorer quality of life, more problem behaviour, poorer performance on ADLs, more awakenings at night, and more care home placement.

- Anxiety is not always easy to diagnose in dementia. Elderly patients tend to somatize their psychiatric symptoms, reporting more physical symptoms instead. People with dementia verbalize less with disease progression. Many symptoms of anxiety overlap with symptoms of dementia itself (e.g. poor concentration) or BPSD (e.g. agitation).

- Anxiety and depression often co-exist (up to 75% of anxious patients have been found to be depressed in studies involving AD). However, a recent study showed that in many of the current assessment scales, there is overlap between anxiety and depression indicators, so that a spurious correlation might account for some of this.
- Anxiety levels remain the same at all stages of dementia, but fall off in advanced dementia.
- There are some suggestions that environmental variables, e.g. lack of daytime activities, are correlated with levels of anxiety in dementia; however, this has not yet been adequately demonstrated.
- In assessing for anxiety, take the views of as many informants as possible, including the patient whenever they are able to express themselves, carers, and professionals involved in care.
- One study found a correlation between anxiety and restlessness, irritability, muscle tension, fear, and respiratory symptoms of anxiety e.g. hyperventilation. Difficulty in concentrating, fatigue, and sleep disturbance, all common in dementia, were not found to be correlated.
- A number of assessment scales can be used to detect the presence of anxiety in people with dementia, e.g. general psychiatric assessment scales for people with dementia such as the NPI and the Behavioral Pathology in Alzheimer's Disease (BEHAVE-AD) scale; and anxiety-specific scales: the Rating Anxiety in Dementia (RAID) scale and the Worry Scale. The latter is only suitable for use in mild dementia.

Management

Non-pharmacological treatments are first line and include approach, staff skills, activities, spiritual care, etc. Where anxiety is very prominent it has been successfully treated with atypical antipsychotics, SSRIs, and cholinesterase inhibitors.

- Olanzapine in low doses (2.5–5mg daily) has been found to be useful, but will be no less harmful than when it is when used for psychosis.
- Mirtazapine is useful for both anxiety and insomnia in dementia.
- Benzodiazepines can further depress cognition and increase risk of falls, and should rarely be used those with dementia who are still mobile.
- Non-pharmacological interventions include anxiety management techniques, modified and simplified for their use with dementia patients, as well as 'touch with verbalization', which continues having a soothing effect for several days after the intervention is stopped.
- Benzodiazepines may disinhibit patients at night, with the result that they become more agitated, disinhibited, wander, and may injure themselves seriously.
- There are times when dealing with the sleep disturbance may be particularly important, perhaps when the patient is living at home with family and the carer will not cope without some good sleep.

Further reading

Seignourel PJ, Kunik ME, Snow L, Wilson N, Stanley M (2008) Anxiety in dementia: a critical review. *Clin Psychol Rev* **28**, 1071–82.

Agitation and aggression

- Agitation is a frequent and very important form of BPSD, being responsible for great carer stress, more institutionalization, increased staff burden, and potentially resulting in increased isolation for the patient.
- Cohen-Mansfield recognized four types of agitated behaviour in dementia:
  - Physically non-aggressive: restlessness, pacing, hiding or hoarding things, dressing or undressing inappropriately, repetitive mannerisms, handling things, inappropriate eating or drinking, seeking to exit.
  - Physically aggressive, e.g. hitting, hurting oneself or others, biting, scratching, spitting, pushing, grabbing, falling intentionally, kicking, physical sexual advances, tearing or throwing things.
  - Verbally non-aggressive: negativism, attention-seeking behaviour, complaining, interruptions, repetitive sentences or questions.
  - Verbally aggressive: screaming, angry outbursts, cursing, making strange noises, verbal sexual advances.
- Women show more verbal agitation. Physical agitation is commoner as dementia advances and verbal ability is lost.
- Agitation is more frequent in the presence of depression, psychosis, more advanced illness, and sleep disturbances.
- The frequency of agitation depends on how one defines it. One survey found aggression to be present in 20% of their sample of AD patients despite defining it narrowly as behaviour that could cause physical injury to others.
- The Cohen-Mansfield Agitation Inventory (CMAI) is the most widely used clinical measure of agitation in dementia, and is extensively used in studies of the condition. It is a 29-item checklist, each rated 1–7 according to frequency (1 = never, 7 = several times an hour). Other measures which include agitation, such as the NPI, are sometimes used, but the results may be contaminated by the other variables. For example it has been claimed that some of the improvements in trials for cholinesterase inhibitors for aggression in dementia are due to improvements in other elements of the NPI, not aggression.

Aetiology

- Agitation can result from any cause of distress.
- *People become agitated when they feel under threat.* Understanding the perceived threat can often lead to non-drug means of reducing the agitation. Such means should always be used in preference to drugs if there is a reasonable chance that they will be effective.
- People with dementia are often very stressed. They may feel lost, unable to understand what is going on around them, unable to predict what will happen next, and feel they are surrounded by strangers.
- In assessing agitation look at various factors, e.g.
  - Physical factors: infection, hunger, pain, drugs, poor eyesight.
  - Mental state: depression, anxiety, psychosis, paranoid ideation.
  - Relationships: with family, with staff, with other residents.

- Environment: lack of privacy, too much or too little light, too much or too little noise, boredom.
- Psychological makeup: personality, past history and coping strategies, culture, habits.

Management

- Assess the immediate risk to the patient and to others, and if the risk is high, take steps to reduce this risk before proceeding further, e.g. move potential means for self-harm out of the patient's surroundings.
- When practicable, work out the origins of the agitation, talking to family and staff, and if necessary using an ABC chart.
- As far as possible, treat non-pharmacologically, as the effectiveness of drugs in this context is often limited and the short- and long-term effects may be quite negative.
- Assess the appropriateness of the environment for care and modify accordingly. In extreme cases, rehousing may be needed if a highly unsuitable environment cannot be improved.
- Refer to an old-age psychiatry team if there are complex problems or dangerous behaviour, but in the meantime take steps to understand and manage the cause of distress.
- Correct causative factors, e.g. make snacks available if agitation is precipitated by hunger; provide a calm environment without confusing visual or auditory stimulation (📖 Chapter 11).
- Considering the situation jointly with other team members may suggest useful avenues of intervention.
- Enlist family members in planning and implementing non-pharmacological responses, and sharing the rationale. Behavioural management techniques have been shown to be as effective as haloperidol or trazodone for agitation. In each case the effect was modest but statistically significant.
- There is weak randomized controlled trial (RCT) evidence that aromatherapy, music therapy, physical exercise, sensory stimulation, and bright light therapy (see 📖 Chapter 10, Sleep disturbance, pp. 196–199) can all reduce agitation in people with severe dementia. However, with some of these, e.g. music therapy, the effect does not outlast the intervention.

Jean's son, when washing and dressing his mum at home, used to play her favourite songs. This would distract her and she was less resistive to care. He conveyed this to the carers looking after her when they said they would need to give her a sedative. Once they tried this, she was much more relaxed.

- A multicentre randomized trial of training and supportive intervention with nursing home staff in the UK showed a reduction in neuroleptic use of 19.1%. There was no worsening of agitation and disruptive behaviour in the homes using fewer neuroleptics, and the results were still in evidence after 10 months. However, this study did have methodological weaknesses. The randomization was at the level of homes not individuals, and 95% confidence intervals (0.5% to 37.7%) were broad and straddled 1.0, suggesting weakness of the evidence.

- Pharmacological management of agitation in dementia is often fraught with problems. It is important to differentiate the response of agitation from the response of psychotic symptoms to these drugs.
- Trials of both typical (e.g. haloperidol) and atypical (e.g. risperidone) antipsychotics have shown a significant but small effect on aggression in dementia over 6–12 weeks of treatment. Typical antipsychotics have more frequent, and more severe, adverse effects (Table 10.5).
- Risperidone is the only drug licensed in the UK for short-term (up to 6 weeks) management of continued aggression in moderate to severe AD which carries a risk to self or others, and which has not responded to non-drug measures. Other drugs can of course be used, but outside the terms of their licence.
- Both groups of drugs cause serious problems in this population, varying from the adverse effects listed in Table 10.4, to an increase in morbidity and mortality. For example, there is good evidence that sedation and chest infections are commoner, cognitive decline is more rapid, and strokes occur up to 3 times as frequently in people with dementia on atypical antipsychotics. The evidence is less established for typical antipsychotics, but the problem may be even more serious.
- A meta-analysis shows a 1.5–1.7-fold increased mortality in people with dementia taking atypical antipsychotics for 6–12 weeks. This increased mortality does not settle with continued use; the DART-AD trial recently demonstrated that at 24 months of antipsychotic drug use, survival in the atypical antipsychotic group was 46% vs 71% in the placebo group, and at 36 months, 30% vs 59%.
- Cholinesterase inhibitors (donepezil, rivastigmine, galantamine) slightly reduce behavioural disturbance in dementia but only after weeks of use. Trial data also suggested that such behaviours were less likely to emerge on cholinesterase inhibitors. However, in those with severe disturbance who had not responded to 4 weeks of psychosocial treatment, the CALM-AD multicentre trial of donepezil showed no advantage of the drug against placebo after 12 weeks of use.
- Mood stabilizers used in bipolar disorder (carbamazepine, valproate, gabapentin, lamotrigine, oxcarbazepine, topiramate) have been used to reduce agitation and aggression in people with dementia. Carbamazepine has been shown to be effective but poorly tolerated in three controlled studies in BPSD. Valproate showed promise in open studies but none of the five controlled studies carried out confirmed its effectiveness. No controlled studies have been published to date with any of the other drugs. Although many psychiatrists use these drugs, until further evidence of their effectiveness emerges one cannot recommend their routine use.

Further reading

Ballard C, Hanney ML, Theodoulou M, Douglas S, McShane R, Kossakowski K et al. (2009) The dementia antipsychotic withdrawal trial (DART-AD): long-term follow-up of a randomised placebo-controlled trial. *Lancet Neurol* **8**, 151–7.

Cohen-Mansfield J (2008) Agitated behavior in persons with dementia: the relationship between type of behavior, its frequency, and its disruptiveness. *J Psychiatr Res* **43**, 64–9.

Sleep disturbance

Sleeping disorders are common in dementias. This can arise from the dementia itself (Table 10.7), including problems such as sundowning, from obstructive sleep apnoea (OSA), which is commoner in AD, from associated conditions, e.g. depression, anxiety, or from other medical conditions such as heart failure, COPD, or prostate problems causing nocturia.

Table 10.7 Dementias associated with sleep disorders

AD
DLB
VaD
Frontotemporal dementia
PD dementia
PSP
Huntington's disease
CJD

- Normal sleep has four non-rapid eye movement (NREM) stages, with increasing depth of sleep, followed by rapid eye movement (REM) sleep. Most sleep is spent in Stage 2, where the individual is rousable, though with some difficulty. Stages 3 and 4 of NREM are known as slow wave sleep (SWS; from the EEG) and are phases of deep sleep. In REM sleep, the brain is highly active, muscles are atonic, and observers can notice rapid movements of the eyes.
- In young adults, there are 4–6 cycles through the various sleep phases each night. SWS dominates the first half of the night, while REM sleep dominates the last half.
- As one ages, one tends to experience less total sleep time and reduced sleep efficiency (time asleep as a percentage of time in bed).
- SWS decreases significantly with age, especially in men, where by age 60 it may no longer be present. REM sleep is also decreased, and more of the night is spent in Stage 1 and 2 sleep. Predictably, the number of arousals from sleep each night increases with age. Napping in the daytime increases. There is great individual variability in sleep patterns in the elderly.
- SSRI and SNRI antidepressants reduce SWS sleep.
- People with AD show less SWS sleep and more Stage 1 NREM sleep. REM sleep is also reduced.
- Thus AD patients will rouse more easily.
- Circadian rhythm disorders are common, especially as more disorientation to time occurs. The clue lies in unusual sleep times—excessive daytime sleep, odd times to go to sleep at night. Damage to the suprachiasmatic nucleus of the hypothalamus and the pineal gland may account for these changes.

- REM-sleep behaviour disorder (RBD) is characterized by violent movements and unpleasant dreams during REM sleep. It can occur in PD and the Parkinson-plus syndromes, DLB, and cerebellar degenerations.
- Restless legs syndrome is an almost irresistible urge to move the legs, sometimes accompanied by paraesthesiae or dysaesthesiae, occurring mostly in quiet periods and therefore especially sleep. It can lead to broken sleep and increased stress, as well as problems sleeping for a sleeping partner. It is common in AD, PD, DLB, VaD, and frontotemporal dementia. It can produce interference with sleep. It is commonly due to low dopamine states.

Assessment

- Enquire regularly about sleep from patients or witnesses.
- Exclude pain and other medical disorders as factors contributing to poor sleep.
- Look for drugs which may worsen insomnia (Table 10.8)
- Check about excessive daytime sleepiness. This can be part of AD, PD, DLB, and frontotemporal dementia. Always exclude other causes.

Table 10.8 Some drugs which can contribute to insomnia

Alcohol
SSRIs
SNRIs
Cholinesterase inhibitors, e.g. donepezil
Bronchodilators
Sympathomimetic drugs, e.g. cold remedies: pseudoephedrine
Steroids
Levodopa and dopaminergic drugs
Medications containing caffeine e.g. some antimigraine drugs; coffee or tea
Smoking, drugs containing nicotine, e.g. TD patches

Management

Non-pharmacological measures are safe and easy ways of helping with sleep disturbance and disruption of the sleep–wake cycle. A sleep hygiene programme should be instituted (Table 10.9).

- Circadian rhythm problems are worse if one is not exposed to daylight regularly. Bright light therapy in the evenings, using special lamps, can reverse these. Melatonin, produced by the pineal gland, acts on the suprachiasmatic nucleus of the hypothalamus and plays an important role in establishing circadian rhythms. It is a useful drug in circadian rhythm problems—start 3mg nocte, increase gradually up to 12mg nocte if needed. (Note: in the UK only 2mg tablets are currently

available on general prescription, and use as outlined above has to be on an off-licence basis).
- Re-evaluate the need for any medication which can cause insomnia (see Table 10.8). Giving some of these medications earlier, e.g. early in the day for steroids, cholinesterase inhibitors by early evening, may help.

Table 10.9 Sleep hygiene measures

Avoid spending too much time in bed during the day
Exercise during the day.
Avoid caffeine, alcohol, smoking, and heavy meals before bedtime. A light snack may be useful
Avoid daytime sleeping
Develop a regular time for going to bed
Develop a regular routine for going to bed, e.g. a cup of Horlicks or a malt drink, a quiet comfortable room without intrusive interruptions at an appropriate temperature and with gentle lighting
Avoid watching television in bed or before going to sleep
White noise can help people who still have difficulty sleeping

- Mirtazapine and quetiapine may improve sleep, probably through their histaminergic activity, and could be good choices when combined antidepressant and hypnotic activity, or antipsychotic and hypnotic activity, is required.
- Gabapentin, pregabalin, and trazodone improve SWS.
- In excessive daytime sleepiness, modafinil or small doses of methylphenidate, both psychostimulants, can be useful. Cholinesterase inhibitors drugs can have similar effects.
- OSA if suspected (witnessed by spouse, excessive daytime tiredness, excessive snoring, obesity) may need to be confirmed by sleep studies, which can to some extent be done in a person's own environment. There is some evidence of improvement of OSA with donepezil in AD. It is unclear whether continuous positive airways pressure (CPAP) ventilation, normally used in OSA, has any impact on cognition in AD.
- RBD often responds to nocturnal clonazepam 0.25–1.5mg nocte.
- Restless legs syndrome can respond to dopaminergic drugs, e.g. co-carbidopa, ropinirole, pramipexole—but in some patients these increase psychosis or insomnia. Anticonvulsants and benzodiazepines are also sometimes of use.
- Hypnotics such as zopiclone or zolpidem or short-acting benzodiazepines can be tried if no cause for the insomnia can be found. If short-acting drugs do not work then a slightly longer-acting benzodiazepine may help. However, benzodiazepines carry some risk of hangover into the daytime, resulting in an increase in falls, and this is especially the case with longer-acting benzodiazepines. On the other hand, short-acting benzodiazepines are more often associated with rebound insomnia

when stopped, which may make them harder to stop. Zopiclone is metabolized by phase I oxidative pathways in the liver, and metabolism may be affected by age. Hypnotics metabolized by phase II conjugation pathways, e.g. lorazepam, temazepam, are not handled markedly differently in old age and are therefore preferred. It is preferable for hypnotics to be used on a p.r.n. basis, and for them to be used for up to a few weeks at a time if possible. It is far too easy to prescribe a benzodiazepine instead of working through what underlies the poor sleep.

Case example

Ernest is living at home with his wife and has severe dementia. During the day he potters around and goes out with his wife, being somewhat resistive to care at times but manageable with difficulty. He may well have a nap during the afternoon and then goes to bed at about 9 pm. But at night he is restless, wakes up, and is really quite disturbed. His wife becomes exhausted as a result, and without a good night's sleep will no longer be able to care for him at home.

There are several options:
- Exercise during the day may help.
- Avoid caffeine in the evening.
- Allow him to sleep in a separate room for at least some of the night so that his wife is not woken up by his moving.
- Consider one or two nights a week in a residential home so that his wife gets a really good night's sleep.
- Try short-acting hypnotics.

Further reading

Bloom HG, Ahmed I, Alessi CA, Ancoli-Israel S, Buysse DJ, Kryger MH et al. (2009) Evidence-based recommendations for the assessment and management of sleep disorders in older persons. J Am Geriatr Soc 57, 761–89.

Petit D, Montplaisir J, Boeve BF (2005) Alzheimer's disease and other dementias In: Kryger M, Roth T, Dement WC (eds) Principles and practice of sleep medicine, pp. 853–62. Saunders, Philadelphia.

Specific symptoms

Wandering

• People with dementia often wander. This used to be viewed with suspicion, and in the past medication was often used to suppress it. Now the view is that wandering is natural, a perfectly common thing for people to want to do when they are distressed, and healthy as long as it is safe.

• However, wandering can cause difficulty for a number of reasons. Wanderers can get lost, go out poorly dressed, or fall. It is often more of a challenge when people are living at home.

• Wandering can also become problematic when the need to stop makes the person angry or distressed. Feeling confined by others at home or in a ward environment can lead to great frustration.

• Care may be much easier to provide in a setting other than an acute ward. The lack of places to wander in acute hospital settings may lead the patient to interfere with another patient's bed or care. In psychiatric or residential settings, where the corridors are longer and the exits secure, wandering can be allowed in greater safety, thus reducing distress.

• It is important to try and understand why someone wanders. This could be due to a feeling of being lost and looking for something or someone familiar, the perceived need to get to work, looking vainly for a toilet, hunger and searching for food, as well as physical pain, psychosis, depression, akathisia, or other causes of distress.

Management

• Look for, and treat, an underlying cause.

• Assess mobility (preferably through a physiotherapist): is it safe, and can it be made safer?

• Provide a safe environment (handrails, plenty of places to sit on the way, good, even lighting), and make it engaging and interesting with things to stop to look at, touch, and handle.

• Antipsychotics and sedatives increase the risk of falling without suppressing wandering and are best avoided.

Calling out

• Calling out most often indicates distress and requires an analysis of the cause.

• The greatest therapeutic effect will come from good quality care and human interaction with sympathetic, communicative care staff who will support and tend the person in their distress.

Resistiveness to care

• Patients who lack understanding and feel rushed, threatened, or put upon are likely to react in ways similar to any other normal person. It is perfectly normal to become aggressive or to resist the demands of others when you cannot see why they are making demands, or understand why it is necessary for you to do something you do not wish to do.

- Patients may resist taking tasteless medication, having a bath, or getting dressed.
- There are many techniques to allow this to be resolved.
- Perhaps the first response to resistance is to have a short break and then to try again. If somebody refuses a bath at 9 o'clock they may well accept one if they are offered in the right way at 10 or 11 o'clock. Patients may refuse to eat at lunchtime but if offered food a little while later may well eat quite well. Patients may decline the set meal, but may then eat cake or biscuits.
- An informal approach with ongoing chatter may allay anxieties and make people feel better about undergoing personal care. One carer reported that singing to a patient while offering medication and food was effective.
- Resistiveness during dressing changes or movement is often caused by pain. A prophylactic painkiller 20 minutes before the procedure will often settle this quickly (📖 Chapter 8, Strong opioids, pp. 116–125)
- Resistance to care may also be triggered by paranoia. At such times antipsychotic medication may be the treatment of choice, using the lowest dose for the shortest time.

Neglect
- It is quite unacceptable to leave someone sitting in urine and faeces, or to leave them hungry when in fact they are not choosing to be so, lacking the capacity to understand the consequences and sometimes basing their choices on delusional beliefs. If patients are soiled and uncomfortable, appropriate care should be imposed upon them in their best interests (📖 Chapter 18). Restraint may occasionally be required, and clinicians have a duty to use this proportionately if necessary to avoid harm.
- Gentle persuasion is often successful and far preferable.

Sundowning
- Sundowning is a description given to patients who become agitated usually in the late afternoon. It has very little to do with oncoming darkness; increasing agitation and distress appears to be associated with fatigue, and comes on and has an impact earlier in people with dementia than those without it.
- At times it may be better to allow distress for a period each day rather than use other treatments, so as to ensure that the patient has a better experience for the other parts of the day.
- A variety of treatments have been suggested and include:
  - Restriction of daytime sleep.
  - Walking for 2 hours in the early morning and an hour in the afternoon (gave a 30% reduction in aggressive events).
  - Controlling light exposure.
  - The use of memory notebooks.
  - Adding visual, auditory, or olfactory stimuli to the nursing home.
  - Touch, massage, etc.
- Neuroleptics are frequently prescribed, but the evidence base is weak.

- Benzodiazepines are the second most frequently used group of drugs, and although they can show significant sleep improvement they are probably not very useful for sundowning behaviour.
- Propranolol may have some benefit and melatonin has been tried but again with little clear evidence of benefit.

Case example

Alice, 90, was referred because she was agitated and calling out at night. She had been treated with haloperidol but upon questioning it turned out that she had become very frail, forgetful, and very depressed. She was fearful and called out at night for comfort as she felt alone and frightened. Appropriate antidepressant treatment was given along with advice to staff to provide better support and greater understanding. Staff sat with her in the early night and held her hand until she fell asleep. She died peacefully 3 weeks later.

Pain and the differential diagnosis of BPSD

We have pointed out elsewhere (📖 Chapter 8) that physical pain is common in dementia and must be considered. It may easily present as BPSD.

'Wild card' diagnoses and thinking 'outside the box'

The differential diagnosis of distress and BPSD must be wide and detailed. Psychiatrists, for example, may see several patients present with BPSD due to scabies. This is only one example that reminds us of the need for a detailed and careful analysis of the cause of all BPSD and distress in dementia—always think 'outside the box'.

Case example: scabies

Alan had been admitted 18 months ago for a medical condition and also had dementia. Since discharge he has been sleeping poorly, is restless, and keeps itching. Haloperidol had been tried and failed. Examination led to a diagnosis of scabies and appropriate treatment saw a substantial reduction in his distress and improved sleep pattern.

Chapter 11

Managing disability in dementia

Basic concepts

Dementia produces a multiplicity of functional deficits and disabilities which are important to understand in order to manage people affected properly.

Impairment and disability

The WHO looks at disability not as an intrinsic feature of an individual but as a result of interaction between an individual and the environment. It points out that every human being will at some point suffer a reduction in health and thus experience disability. We are all disabled at some time in our lives. It considers disability to be the effect of the interaction between

- Impairment in bodily function: a problem in body function or structure.
- Limitations in activity: a difficulty encountered by an individual in executing a task or action.
- Restriction in participation: a problem experienced by an individual in involvement in life situations.

Thus disability is a complex phenomenon, reflecting an interaction between features of a person's body and features of the society in which he or she lives.

It is clear from these definitions that disability is a social construct, and that the environment can be disabling or facilitative. Disability is not the product of the impairment, but of an environment that does not allow someone with that impairment to function. There is no denying that people with dementia suffer from a wide array of impairments and disabilities, caused by the profound effects of the pathology on the brain, which deeply affect their interaction with other people, objects, and their perceptions of the outside world. Equally, a difficult physical or social environment can deeply impair function and undermine self-confidence, greatly magnifying disability.

ADLs

One way of defining the degree and type of disability, at least in mild to moderate disease, is to examine how a person copes with the ADLs and IADLs. From the above definitions, it will be clear that improvement in functioning in ADLs and IADLs can be brought about by improvement in one's physical impairment, a reduction in one's restriction in activity, and an enhancement in the possibility of participation in activity. Thus, physical, environmental, and social factors all need to be brought into play. Few things are more disabling than an introjection of the idea that one is not good enough to participate in normal society. And yet this is what many people with dementia experience on a daily basis. Attitudes, and a restitution of a sense of belonging and self-worth, are key.

- ADLs represent a minimal level of independence and require a basic level of functioning; IADLs are more complex and allow for more independent living (Table 11.1). They require a correspondingly more sophisticated level of health.
- In AD there may be some loss of ability to perform IADLs at an early stage, related partly to memory problems, to impairment in executive function (mainly due to frontal lobe dysfunction), and to depression.

- There is then a sharp fall-off in ability to perform IADLs in moderate dementia (MMSE ≤ 16), particularly pronounced if behavioural disturbance is marked. ADLs then start to decline, and most are lost in the following year or two.
- In VaD impairment may for a long time affect some skills more than others, and some ADLs may be relatively preserved while others are severely affected.
- IADL and ADL performance declines more slowly in VaD than in AD. However, in a cohort of over 250 people with dementia, those with VaD were impaired in more ADLs which than those with AD. In general, VaD affects predominantly executive psychomotor speed while AD has a greater impact on memory and verbal ability.
- Apathy correlates particularly strongly with performance. It is linked to damage to connections between the frontal lobes and subcortical circuits.

Table 11.1 ADLs and IADLs

ADLs	Feeding
	Continence
	Transferring and mobility
	Toileting
	Dressing and undressing
	Bathing
IADLs	Preparing food and cleaning up after meals
	Doing light housework and housekeeping, e.g. laundry
	Using the telephone
	Handling medications and maintaining health
	Using public transport, e.g. a bus or train
	Shopping
	Managing money and finances
	Care of others (including selecting and supervising caregivers)
	Care of pets
	Safety procedures and emergency responses

Preserving ability

It is widely believed that the exclusion of people with dementia from much day-to-day interaction and activity increases the impairment due to the illness itself. By keeping people with dementia actively involved, cognitive and physical deterioration may be slowed down and skills better preserved. On top of this, specialized techniques and adaptations can help to preserve ability and function.

Cognitive rehabilitation

- There is a lively interest in cognitive rehabilitation for early dementia, using techniques aimed at specific modalities which are impaired, e.g. particular aspects of memory or problem solving. Clients set their own goals, and the approach is holistic, aiming to encompass cognitive, emotional, and social aspects of the person. Rehabilitation is personalized, working on those areas most meaningful for the person concerned.
- Cognitive rehabilitation is also possible in the later stages of the illness, although using modalities and techniques applicable to the stage.
- The underlying principle is that while there is inevitable loss from the illness itself, the disability is greatly increased by the depersonalization, social attitudes, and lack of self-worth resulting from the way our society views dementia (📖 Chapter 17). This is akin to the idea that in wasting diseases, the inevitable muscle loss is compounded by loss from deconditioning due to disuse, stemming from fatigue or anxiety, which then become self-perpetuating. The individual programme is based on a neuropsychological profile and a study of functional ability.
- Cognitive rehabilitation has been employed with AD as well as with other dementias such as frontotemporal dementia. Results are encouraging, but it is a novel concept that is still developing and remains unproven.

Physical preservation of function

- Increasing physical dependence in AD is associated with a higher risk of accidents, increased burden on carers as well as increased cost of direct medical care and informal care.
- The level of daily activity is correlated with the degree of cognitive impairment.
- Dementia is associated with physical deterioration and loss of muscle and bone mass. Changes in muscle and bone mass start very early in dementia. Functional loss occurs in parallel with the progression of dementia.
- A number of clinical tests of function have been validated in people with various dementias. These include the up and go test, the 6-minute walk test and gait speed in AD, and similar tests in other dementias such as Huntington's.
- There is evidence that exercise reduces the risk of dementia in individuals, and that a programme of exercise treatment in early dementia helps improve physical condition and slow cognitive decline.
- A Cochrane Review in 2008 found insufficient evidence that physical activity programmes stabilize or improve cognition, function, behaviour,

depression, and mortality in people with dementia. The need for well-designed studies that examine these questions is obvious.

- A nihilistic attitude to physical rehabilitation in dementia is not justified by the evidence.
- It has been shown that after femoral fracture, a rehabilitation programme allows people with dementia to make the same progress as people with normal cognitive function.
- A 6-month trial of a physiotherapy-led or multidisciplinary balance training programme produced improvements of balance in people with mixed dementia compared with controls.
- A recent meta-analysis showed that people with mild or moderate dementia obtain similar outcomes from strength and endurance training as age- and gender-matched cognitively intact older participants.
- Balance and eye movement training is of benefit in people with moderate PSP.
- The best programmes and methods for use are still being worked out in this very young field.

Further reading

Clare L (2008) *Neuropsychological rehabilitation and people with dementia*. Psychology Press, Hove.
Marshall M (2005) *Perspectives on rehabilitation and dementia*. Jessica Kingsley, London.

Cognitive disabilities

Memory and cognitive changes in dementia

📖 Chapter 4 charts the progression of these changes over time.

Implications for practice

Memory loss and orientation can be helped in a number of ways:
- Do not do things for people but with them. Gently guide the person without imposing or giving them too many bewildering choices.
- Establish (or better, maintain pre-existing) daily routines.
- Keep things in set places to facilitate finding them.
- Important objects need to be easily visible: what cannot be seen will be considered lost and cause much stress. Glass-fronted cupboards which show their contents, prominent places to hang keys and clothes, good lighting and contrasting colours facilitate easy location.
- Try particularly to maintain routines and keep objects that matter to the person involved.
- Encourage independence within safe boundaries and encourage people with dementia to make everyday choices, as long as this does not paralyse them.
- Early on, written reminders can help, but they become meaningless later.
- Have a large easily read clock with an analogue clockface in a clearly visible position.
- Windows looking to the outside also help with time orientation.
- Simplify and adapt activities as memory loss advances so as to work within the person's capacities, avoiding frustration from failure to do simple tasks.
- Do not test people ('What is this?') but gently explain.
- Guide people into doing things they are good at—success makes one feel good.
- Photographs of a person's past can be a good anchor for discussion and reminiscence.

Visuospatial and constructional problems

- Visual problems are common in dementia. They can be divided into:
  - *Visuoperceptual problems:* impaired discrimination of form and pattern.
  - *Visual agnosia:* the inability to recognize familiar objects despite adequate perception, i.e. there are no problems with the eyes etc. Affected persons will still be able to name an object by its feel in *apperceptive visual agnosia*. In *associative visual agnosia*, however, there is a disorder of internal language, causing naming to be lost in all modalities.
- Usually due to bilateral occipitotemporal lesions; aetiologies other than dementia are rare.
- Disturbances of form and pattern recognition are common. They lead to problems such as being unable to make out a form that is partly in shadow, being unable to recognize shapes which overlap or are partly obscured, and being unable to construct a visual whole from complex parts.

- *Prosopagnosia* is the inability to recognize familiar faces, even though the person may still be recognized by their voice or other qualities.
- Colour vision changes include lower contrast sensitivity in AD, often with a reduced ability to see colour.

Visuospatial disorders (visual orientation or location in space)
- Unilateral visual neglect, more commonly left-sided, is common in AD. This can result in a person only combing half of his hair, applying makeup to only half her face, dressing one half of his body, or leaving one side of her plate of food untouched. Individuals with visual neglect will turn only in one direction, which contributes to their disorientation.
- Neglect may affect half the field of vision or half of each object. It may also affect modalities other than vision, e.g. touch.
- Judging distances, e.g. extending a hand to touch something, may be affected.
- Unilateral neglect, failure of object recognition and memory disorders all contribute to individuals often getting lost in familiar surroundings.
- Visuospatial ability is often preserved in frontotemporal dementia.
- In Huntington's disease, it is often severely affected.

Constructional ability
- In AD, drawing a clockface is progressively impaired as disease progresses. Copying from another drawing improves accuracy.
- In DLB, constructional ability suffers significantly early on.

Implications for practice
- Allowing the person to handle and touch as well as look at objects may aid recognition. Recruit as many senses as possible.
- Talking to individuals who suffer from prosopagnosia, and giving them other non-visual cues, helps them identify individual carers. Do not assume that because someone can see you, they know who you are, or that if they stare at you blankly, they will have no other way of recognizing you. Do not just rely on their sight; introduce yourself and engage them in other ways. Explain to families about prosopagnosia, as it can be very distressing for them.
- Avoid your face being partly shadowed when talking to people with dementia.
- Place objects you want people to see well into the non-neglected side of their field of vision, and sit on their non-neglected side to talk to them. However, this effect can be limited as the person can turn their head to the object in question.
- In stroke, it is possible to gradually re-educate people into perceiving objects just inside the ignored area of their visual field by, for example, making them follow trajectories of objects moving into these areas. It is not known whether the same can happen with dementia.
- In stroke, the use of prism glasses to shift the field of vision has been shown to extend rehabilitation of neglect when used with tracking techniques. It is unclear whether this has a role in dementia.
- Designing buildings appropriate to the needs of residents with dementia can compensate to some extent for perceptual deficits. Particularly useful in this regard has been the work of the Dementia

Services Development Centre at the University of Stirling, Scotland (http://www.dementia.stir.ac.uk/).

- Even lighting with little shadow improves recognition. High contrast in flooring between rooms can give a sense of a visual barrier and increase anxiety and a sense of entrapment, whereas continuity of flooring promotes free movement.
- Dark corridors and reflective flooring are very disorientating for people with dementia.
- Toilet seats of the same colour as the toilet hinder recognition; high contrast helps orientation and reduces voiding in inappropriate places. High contrast between walls and floors may help reduce falls.
- Intelligent assistive technology being trialled will allow, for example, GPS-linked mobile phones that learn to track somebody's usual route outside the home and warn them when they deviate from this before they get lost, and technology which helps people stick to a particular route inside the house when they are at risk of being lost. GPS shoes have also been developed.

Further reading

Bharucha AJ, Anand V, Forlizzi J, Dew MA, Reynolds CF, 3rd, Stevens S *et al.* (2009) Intelligent assistive technology applications to dementia care: current capabilities, limitations, and future challenges. *Am J Geriatr Psychiat* **17**, 88–104.

Dementia Services Development Centre (2007). *Best practice in design for people with dementia.* Dementia Services Development Centre, Stirling. Available at: http://www.dementia.stir.ac.uk/

Physical disabilities

A good assessment by an occupational therapist or other suitably trained professional is essential to maximize independence and safety with physical disability. These notes aim to provide some understanding of the important factors when choosing equipment and techniques.

Dysphasia and dysarthria

- Dysphasia is a partial or total loss of the ability to use or understand language as a result of brain damage. A total loss of speech or language is called aphasia. The loss can involve verbal or written language.
- Dysphasias are widely referred to as aphasias to distinguish them in conversation from the dysphagias.
- Speech is lost early in many cases of frontotemporal dementia, either with a non-fluent difficulty in naming objects or with a fluent aphasia where the meaning of words is lost.
- In AD, word-finding difficulties are first covered up by circumlocutions ('Where is that thing I drink?' meaning, 'Where is my glass?'). Difficulty naming objects (nominal aphasia), at first unusual ones and later everyday ones, appears, and eventually is joined by receptive aphasia, where comprehension of speech becomes impaired. Perseveration, echolalia, palilalia, reduced fluency, and non-speech verbalizations follow. Finally, very few words are used and the patient with far advanced dementia may descend into a mute state.
- Reading ability declines progressively, but people with dementia may continue to read fluently although they can no longer understand the meaning.
- See also 📖 Chapter 2, Symptoms of dementia, pp. 15–19, 📖 Chapter 4, Cognitive changes in advanced dementia, pp. 52–55, and 📖 Chapter 9, GI problems, pp. 139–155.

Implications for practice

- Remember that while aphasias arise from difficulties with language, in dementias some speech problems are the consequence of difficulties in concept formation. Aphasics with speech-finding difficulties will try different words and cues around the subject of conversation, and one can feel them working their way until they cue themselves into the correct word. In language difficulties due to conceptual problems, there is no central theme for words to coalesce around, and it may be very difficult for a listener to follow a thread of conversation. In trying to improve communication, concentration on language rather than concept formation can miss the point.
- When talking to a person with dementia, find a quiet place. It has been said that a noisy environment for someone with dementia is the equivalent of stairs for someone with a wheelchair.
- Aim for clear, even lighting.
- Attention wanders easily: remove distractions (television!) to concentrate on talking. Be attentive to the person yourself—distractedness breeds distraction.
- Make and keep eye contact. This helps reduce diversion by other events, and gives the person other cues apart from words to

understand your meaning. Remember that emotional responsiveness is
retained until late.
- Do not cover your face with your hands or mumble.
- Use a person's name often in conversation, and touch them.
- Take time. Allow long silences if the person with dementia is not
  clearly getting your meaning quickly—it may just take longer. This has
  been called the 15-second rule—wait for 15 seconds before going on.
- When getting to know a person with dementia, pay attention to
  the fluency of their speech, the breadth and expressiveness of the
  vocabulary they use, the degree of preservation of grammar, the
  precision of their words, and the presence of circumlocutions, non-
  fluent speech, or abnormal speech patterns. Modify your own speech
  patterns accordingly, e.g. simplify your vocabulary bearing in mind the
  level they express.
- Keep concepts simple. Speak in short, clear sentences with one
  concrete theme. Give information in bite-sized pieces, with enough
  time to process and absorb it.
- Sentences with two or more parts will confuse people with dementia.
  Give one instruction per sentence.
- Speak slowly and clearly but naturally and without affectation or over-
  emphasis.
- Use words they would use.
- Involve people with dementia in frequent therapies and exchanges
  which involve language use, e.g. listening to speakers, art therapy. This
  stimulates involvement with speech without concentrating directly on it.
- Be aware that speech-finding difficulties reduce one's ability to get
  involved in group conversation, as by the time the words are found
  the conversation will have moved on. Keep groups small, conversation
  slow with many silences, and keep one single thread of conversation.
- With dementia, understanding becomes very literal. Do not use
  euphemisms or metaphors, but say what you mean simply and clearly.
  Avoid jokes—they will be hard to get.
- Do not ask open-ended questions, but go for yes/no questions or at
  most two choices.
- In responding, do not say just 'yes' or 'no', but repeat the idea: 'Yes, it
  is time for lunch'. This helps those with memory problems retain the
  train of thought.
- Do not interrupt the person—they may lose their thread.
- If they are not understanding, do not repeat—rephrase in different
  words.
- Focus on abilities, and don't use negatives—don't say 'Don't do that!'
  but 'Why don't we do this?'. Arguing or contradicting may precipitate
  anger, frustration, or withdrawal.
- Listen for and respond to the underlying emotion. Someone asking for
  their mother may well miss her comfort and reassurance—provide
  these yourself.
- Keep conversations short.

Mobility problems
- Falls, unsteadiness, and difficulty with mobility are features of most
  advanced dementias. Most people with dementia are older and

movement may be slow and painful. In dementias with prominent extrapyramidal symptoms problems may occur much earlier. Visuospatial problems accentuate poor balance. The poor judgment of distance may lead to a nervousness about mobility, which is further intensified by deconditioning from apathy and pain.

- Communication about these problems needs to be adapted as described above, using many sensory modalities, e.g. touch as well as speech. Physiotherapists are used to employing touch to help them direct movement and posture—watch them and learn.
- When moving, allay fears by walking with or behind the person with dementia, on occasion with a chair for them to sit on should they tire. Rhythmic sounds, e.g. a song to sing, can assist regular pacing.
- Demonstrate exercises rather than just describing them.
- For people who can still read, memory sheets detailing the right procedure are useful. Involve carers, even more so at later stages.
- Tailor any interventions to the abilities and personality of the person.
- A recent systematic review found some evidence that people with cognitive impairment who fracture their hip can be rehabilitated as inpatients as effectively as others who are cognitively intact, although it did not find sufficient evidence to make specific recommendations regarding the type of rehabilitation to be employed.
- Moderate-intensity exercise in moderate to severe AD can reduce depression and anxiety after the session over a 12-week period.
- Studies also suggest that cognitively impaired individuals benefit from endurance and strength training as much as cognitively intact ones, and that upper body strength, balance, gait flexibility, and agility are increased by a short exercise programme.
- A simple twice-weekly exercise programme slows down deterioration of ADLs in AD over a 1-year period.
- Group exercise sessions for rehabilitation of people with AD are feasible.

Aids and adaptations for mobility

Footwear

- Safe footwear is well-fitting and comfortable, slip-resistant, and with a wide-based heel. Slippers and open-heeled sandals, as well as painful or worn footwear, increase the risk of falls.
- Slippers must be properly put on. Walking on the heel turns the slipper into an open heel shoe, increases the risk of pressure sores and makes twists and sprains more likely.
- Velcro straps and soft slip-ons are easy to put on and take off, reducing the risk of falls.
- Thick but flexible heels and insoles keep the feet warm and cushion painful feet when walking.
- For insensitive feet (e.g. diabetic neuropathy) sturdy, well-fitting shoes are necessary. The recommended daily inspection of the feet with prompt treatment of any cuts and bruises, as well as putting one's hand into the shoe before putting it on to check for foreign bodies, is particularly important for people with dementia, to prevent neuropathic ulcers.
- Toenails need to be cut regularly and with skill, by a chiropodist if necessary. Long nails interfere with walking. Attention to foot hygiene is vital.

Furniture and flooring

- Getting out of or sitting down on low chairs or beds is difficult— getting up from a chair is one of the most dangerous mobility manoeuvres. A high enough chair is infinitely safer, but chairs which are so high that the feet do not touch the ground comfortably are tiring to sit in. A properly fitted chair will have hips and knees at right angles and feet square on the ground. Chair cushions need to be firm enough to push against to stand up.
- Riser chairs assist the person to stand if they find standing from sitting difficult. However, in dementia they may have to be used with close supervision in order not to increase falls risk, and can be very frightening when the person can no longer understand why they are being tipped forward. Riser chairs are dangerous in people unable to reposition themselves and their feet as the chair rises. In choosing a riser chair, ensure it cannot entrap parts of the person's body or clothes. Riser chairs should be reserved for those with enough leg power and truncal balance to stand.
- Arm rests and high backs allow for whole body support. Arm rests for prolonged sitting should be padded, as ulnar nerve palsies (numbness in ulnar 1½ fingers, claw-hand, weakness of the small muscles, i.e. fine movements of the hand) are not uncommon from resting the elbows on a hard surface.
- Carers should be taught techniques that enable the person to stand up and sit, transfer, and dress and undress safely.
- Floors and stairs should be free of clutter, wires, and slippery materials.
- Carpets and rugs must be secured with non-skid tape.
- Low-pile carpets or smooth flooring reduce the risk of falls and enable wheeled walking aids to be pushed easily around—but some surfaces, such as vinyl, become slippery when wet and should be avoided.
- Thresholds between rooms should not be raised, again to reduce falls risk.
- Hand rails fitted to walls in bathrooms and showers help the person safely get up from sitting, and can be held on to when tired or unsteady on their feet.
- If the person holds on to furniture to walk, ensure the furniture is sturdy and of the right height, and that there are firm, fixed places to hold—not potentially mobile ones such as drawer handles.
- Good lighting and use of colour and contrast helps prevent falls and makes walking safer (📖 Chapter 11, Cognitive disabilities, pp. 209–211).

Walking sticks and walking frames

- Walking sticks increase stability by changing a biped into a triped. They also drastically reduce the weight transmitted to painful or diseased joints.
- If there is one-sided leg pain or weakness, the stick needs to be held in the contralateral arm.
- A walking stick should be of the right height (generally, this equals the distance from the proximal wrist crease to the ground, but should be slightly longer if a lot of weight is put through the stick).
- The rubber tip at the bottom of the stick is essential to its stability on dry ground, and needs to be changed as it gets worn down. The

rubber tip, becomes dangerous in slippery conditions. Use of walking sticks should be avoided on wet ground or ice.
- Tripods, and frames with four legs, or two legs and two wheels or four wheels (trolleys) can be used. Tripods are quicker and more manoeuvrable through narrow spaces, but less stable.
- Four-legged frames need to be lifted, wheeled frames can be pushed along. Having to lift a frame may be unsafe in many people with dementia who lack the coordination to do this properly. Larger wheels enable walking with less effort over flooring such as carpeting. Trolleys can be particularly useful as the person can carry a tray or shopping basket to transport things, or a seat to sit on when tired.

Wheelchairs
- Wheelchairs greatly increase the mobility of those who are too weak to walk or those who tire easily.
- With many people with dementia, muscle weakness and perceptual difficulties mean that attendant-propelled wheelchairs (with small hind wheels) are needed. However, each assessment has to be individualized.
- A wheelchair base needs to be long enough to support the thighs, to prevent buttock pressure sores developing from poor weight distribution. Too long a wheelchair base will abut into the back of the knees, again causing discomfort and risking pressure ulcers.
- The base of the wheelchair must be horizontal, as a sagging wheelchair will throw the thighs together and create bad posture and pressure areas. A pressure-relieving cushion, regularly changed, is important in people who sit in their wheelchair for long stretches of time.
- Footrests, if slightly angled, reduce the tendency to fall.
- When standing from a wheelchair remember to swivel the footrests out and put on the brakes.
- Tyre pressures on wheelchairs need to be checked weekly.
- Ramps assist wheelchair users to get out of or into buildings. Ramps need to have a gentle enough gradient to be safe. The recommended gradient for self-propelled wheelchairs is 1:12, meaning that climbing a single 15cm stair will require a 1.8m ramp.

Managing incontinence
- Many people with dementia are doubly incontinent. Some simple changes may make their management easier.
- Seats should have surfaces that are easily washable while not slippery or shiny. Similarly, floors need to be easy to clean but not slippery. A number of materials achieve this (see Further reading).
- Clothing needs to be kept simple and minimal, loose so it can be taken on and off easily, with few and easy to operate fasteners, e.g. by using zips with tags.
- Access is easier in emergency is easier if nightdresses are kept short (knee length).
- Women who need transferring to the toilet or commode frequently can find open crotch or drop-front knickers handy.
- Long vests can take time to put on and off, and get soaked during incontinent episodes, so should be avoided.

- Elasticated trousers and skirts are faster to put on or off; braces are faster to take off than belts.
- However, people with dementia who can still choose their own clothes should be encouraged to do so.
- Local continence advisors can advise on pads and other continence aids.

Bathing equipment

- Bathing may require a walk-in shower or a bath.
- A bath board or bath chair is useful for bathing people with mobility problems. Slip-resistant mats also reduce accidents.
- Bath lifts and bath hoists can be used to transfer people with mobility difficulties into and out of baths. They require a lot of space in the bathroom and will often require the operator to be fit enough themselves to lift the person's legs safely over the sides of the bath. They are more likely to be found in care homes than at home.
- Specially fitted showers require enough space to put in a mobile chair; even if the person is still currently mobile, it is very likely that future deterioration may require this.

Hoists

- Hoists are needed to move individuals who cannot safely bear weight.
- Lifting and handling regulations in the European Union make the use of hoists mandatory in many nursing situations.
- Using hoists at home can present problems with space, especially in bathrooms or toilets, movement if the flooring is unsuitable, and storage. In assessing space requirements remember where the hoist operators need to stand and what manoeuvres they have to perform. The working height for the tasks required and the size of the person being transferred must also be borne in mind.
- Most hoists require two carers to use, and thought needs to be given to who will perform the tasks and when.
- There are various types of slings available and the right sling should be selected for the job in hand.
- Care homes may have overhead hoists, which free up floor space and are stronger and more flexible. However, standing hoists usually allow more dignity and are preferred.

Beds

- Beds must fulfil different requirements at different times in an illness. When someone is still mobile, a bed is a place to sleep at night and rest in the daytime when desired. When one is bedbound, or nearly so, the bed is occupied most or all of the time, except for short periods when transferred to a toilet or commode, or perhaps to an armchair. It also becomes the place where most care is given.
- The height of the bed should make it easy to get out of and into safely. Low beds make rising difficult, beds that are too high risk falls when a person attempts to stand.
- When one spends much time in bed, the ability to change the position of the head can enable different tasks to be carried out, e.g. feeding or watching television. They may also enable the occupant to watch what goes on outside through a window, breaking the monotony of facing a

wall all day. A rising section under the knees stops the occupant from sliding down if the head is raised. Beds with adjustable heights allow both the occupier to get on and off easily and carers to provide care without risking back injury.

- Adjustable hospital beds are therefore often insisted on by nursing staff when a person has to be looked after in bed. At earlier stages, however, especially while some memory is preserved, sleeping in one's own bed is much more personal and links in with one's past. This is especially important for couples who share a bed, and affection.

Alarms

- Telephones with pre-programmed fast-dial numbers (e.g. to family, carer, doctor) can be helpful in early dementia. Telephones which emit a flashing light as well as a sound when a phone call comes in can help some people with dementia locate the call more easily.
- Pendant autodialler alarms allow the person with dementia to summon help should they for example fall and become unable to get up. The alarm will phone a pre-selected telephone number, e.g. a relative who lives close by, to request assistance. Some systems can work their way through a list of phone numbers, and then call a care centre if no one is available on these lines.
- One-way intercom systems (e.g. baby alarms) enable a carer to monitor what is happening with the person with dementia from other parts of the house, leaving them free to do essential housework, have a rest etc.
- Two-way alarms are also available which allow interaction between person and carer. Their use is of course limited in people with communication problems as well as in people who may be delusional or unable to connect a disembodied voice with a real person.

Food and drink (see Chapters 9 and 13)

- Feeding for people with dementia should not be in large, noisy dining rooms. Noise is very disorientating for them and activity is very distracting, increasing the risk of interrupted feeds leading to poor nutrition, and aspiration.
- Feeding must not be rushed—it takes a long time.
- Assistance must be provided when needed, but independence, even if limited, should be promoted. For example, when someone is unable to feed themselves with a spoon, holding their hand and helping them use the spoon is preferable to feeding them passively.
- Food needs to be eaten in the same place every day, with good even lighting. Plates, utensils, cups, and salt and pepper should always be placed in the same place and in the same order.
- Poor colour and contrast perception and visuospatial problems can lead to food not being seen on a plate. Aim for plates with one colour, which contrast with the food on top, e.g. dark coloured not white plates with chicken. Glasses and cups should similarly be easily visible, contrasting with the table or tablecloth. Coloured drinks also aid perception, and hence hydration.
- Remember visual inattention when placing food or utensils on a table.
- Placing plates on non-slip mats aids those who have little dexterity.

- Knives, forks, and spoons with an expanded handle may allow self-feeding when manual dexterity deteriorates. When even that becomes impossible, use of finger foods allows independent eating to continue for longer.
- Food that is already in bite size pieces, e.g. casseroles, is much more likely to be eaten than food that needs to be cut up.
- Suitably designed bibs allow feeding to take place without massively increasing laundry load, especially important for older lone carers.
- Cups with one or two handles are easier if muscle weakness is present or manual dexterity is impaired. Plastic cups are lighter than glass and will not cause cuts if they fall and break. Half-full glasses are lighter and reduce spillage risk compared with full ones.
- On the other hand, weighted cups may reduce the risk of spillage due to tremor. Weighted cutlery can also be useful in tremor.
- Cups with lids also reduce spillage.
- Thick liquids are easier to swallow and reduce spillage. They also keep hotter for longer, which can lead to scalding if too hot.
- Larger spouts permit drinking even with a poor lip seal.
- Straws are useful in people who are unable to bring a cup to their lips. Non-return valves can help those who do not produce enough suction to pull fluid up through a straw.
- Gas cookers may be accidentally left on, or the gas turned on without a flame. This can be prevented by changing to electric cookers; using gas alarms; or installing a device that will turn off the gas if levels are high.

Assistive technology

- Body alarms can detect a wandering person getting into a dangerous location, e.g. emitters on the body set off alarms located at the front door to alert the carer when the person wanders out.
- An intercom can be used to control door entry.
- Alarms for smoke, carbon monoxide, gas, and hypothermia can be set up, and can be connected to telecare systems which alert the individual about the action he or she needs to take.
- Smart technology can now monitor the environment in a home and allow it to be controlled remotely from a distant site.
- Alarms can be set to warn if someone falls or if activity is reduced.
- GPS tracking devices are in development which may make the care of people who get lost or wander safer.
- It is important to use such technology to maximize opportunity for safe independence, not to restrict the choices of what a person can do.

Funding issues

- Adaptations costing under £1000 are provided free of charge in England from the discretionary social fund, aimed at keeping people at home and avoiding admission (http://www.disabilityalliance.org/f41. htm). Details of grants in Wales, Northern Ireland, and Scotland can be found at the same website on http://www.disabilityalliance.org/f49.htm. Grants may be available for other adaptations, but are often means tested.
- Carers are also entitled to an assessment of their own needs (📖 Chapter 22, Support for carers, pp. 381–382).

- Disabled Facilities Grants (DFGs; http://www.disabilityalliance.org/
f51.htm) are available from local authorities to improve access of a
disabled person to and from or within their home, facilitate bathroom
use, improve heating or lighting, and for mobility within the house.
Local authorities are obliged to give a DFG if one fulfils the conditions.
- Under the Regulatory Reform (Housing Assistance) (England and
Wales) Order 2002, local authority assistance can also take the shape
of loans, labour, materials, or advice.
- Up to date advice on eligibility to grants can be obtained from the
Alzheimer's Society (http://www.alzheimers.org.uk/), the Citizens
Advice Bureau (http://www.citizensadvice.org.uk/), or the Disability
Alliance (http://www.disabilityalliance.org), all of whom publish
useful fact sheets.

Further reading

Heyn PC, Johnson KE, Kramer AF (2008) Endurance and strength training outcomes on cognitively
impaired and cognitively intact older adults: a meta-analysis. *J Nutr Health Aging* **12**, 401–9.

Disabled Living Foundation fact sheets are a very valuable source of up-to-date information on
equipment and adaptations, and were used as one of the sources for this chapter. See http://
www.dlf.org.uk/content/full-list-factsheets .

A number of groups working with the elderly have mounted a joint campaign called Dignity 2010,
to increase the dignity with which people receiving care are treated, e.g. by appropriate choices
in technology and technique. See http://www.bgs.org.uk/index.php?option=com_content&view=
article&id=307&Itemid=179

Intercurrent illness in advanced dementia

Introduction

It is important in advanced dementia to use a high index of suspicion but also common sense when managing a physical illness. Chronic pre-morbid conditions which often sit alongside the dementia still need to be managed to maintain control, though rationalization of medication with regular review is important. Acute problems can benefit from prompt intervention, but in every case the human cost of the intervention in relation to the benefit for the individual should be carefully considered from all perspectives (Chapter 13). Carers and family may have more insight into the impact of treatments on a person who is unable to decide for themselves than health care professionals, and so their views are at the core of informing the decision-making process.

- There comes a time when symptom relief and comfort are the priorities of treatment when caring for individuals with an advanced incurable disease of whatever nature.
- This philosophy does not, however, equate to no treatment. Active management in a patient with advanced dementia can have a significant positive impact on both the patient and their carers.
- This group of patients often carry with them a multitude of other diagnoses along with their dementia which need managing and controlling.

Optimizing physical abilities every day

Most people with advanced dementia are unable to let others know that their physical abilities have deteriorated, and so carers and health care professionals have to be alert to possible changes and have a system that involves a schedule of review. Optimizing the following physical dimensions is crucial to reduce the likelihood of an intercurrent illness developing. Key things that must be dealt with include:

- Vision (📖 Chapter 16).
- Hearing (📖 Chapter 16).
- Urinary function (📖 Chapter 9).
- Bowel care (📖 Chapter 9).
- Mouth care (📖 Chapter 9).
- Nutrition and weight (📖 Chapter 9).
- Preventing and managing contractures (📖 Chapter 9).

Skin care

- Up to 95% of people with advanced dementia in nursing homes have skin problems.
- Common challenges are dry skin, itch, skin trauma, venous skin disease, oedema, skin infections, and pressure damage.
- Many problems can be prevented by maintaining hydration of the skin (using bath emollients, soap substitutes, and moisturizers), attending to hygiene, and taking measures to avoid damage.
- If a skin injury takes place it is important not only to manage the wound, but also to consider how it came about and whether preventative measures such as equipment padding would be helpful.
- Attention to foot hygiene is particularly important, including watching for and treating fungal skin infections and nail problems that can easily lead to skin infections such as cellulitis.

Contractures

- Fixed contractures of the limbs are common in end-stage dementia and most of these are so-called static contractures. These occur due to immobility and the increasing development of paratonia ('gegenhalten'). Paratonia is an involuntary resistance to passive movement which appears to be a direct consequence of brain changes and worsens with the severity of the dementia.
- Immobility leads to changes in the connective tissues, including cross-linkages and fibrous adhesions which lead to reduced joint flexibility.
- Immobility may be both a cause and consequence of muscle weakness, leading to a vicious cycle.
- Once developed, contractures can cause significant problems in providing personal care and positioning, and can lead to pain and skin problems such as infection and pressure sores.
- Considering that over 80% of people with end-stage dementia have this problem, it is surprising that little research has been done to identify causes or prevention strategies.
- A recent Cochrane Review showed that stretch does not lead to lessened contractures if maintained for less than 7 months.

- If there is any dynamic element to the contractures (spasticity), other treatments, such as serial casting, muscle relaxants or botulinum toxin injections could be considered, but this would normally be appropriate when there is a co-morbidity (such as stroke or multiple sclerosis) contributing to the contracture.
- Despite the lack of research in this area, the principle of promoting and encouraging maximal mobility and normal posture remains unchallenged.
- When giving personal care to persons with paratonia and contractures, the less force applied and the slower the movements made, the less resistance there is.
- Warming the tissues also increases the amount of passive stretching possible.
- Both fear and pain probably have a role in the development of contractures in dementia, leading to a protective huddled posture.

Pressure sores

- Pressure sores are a complication of immobility and are exacerbated by nutritional problems, skin problems, and continence issues.
- Persons with AD have more than double the risk of the general population of developing a pressure ulcer.
- Probably the most effective prevention strategy is awareness and constant vigilance for pressure ulcers amongst carers and health professionals.
- Clinical experience shows that attention to pressure surfaces, using pressure-relieving devices, repositioning (either self or assisted), and maximizing nutrition are effective in reducing the rates of pressure sores, although the evidence base in terms of randomized, controlled trials is surprisingly thin. This is probably because in a trial situation vigilance levels in both the intervention and the control group are likely to be high. Guidance for the prevention and treatment of pressure ulcers has been given by NICE and are due for review in 2011.

Acute presentations of physical illness

- The later stages of dementia can be accompanied by episodes of intercurrent illness. The physical challenges of dementia make certain illnesses much more common, especially infection and electrolyte imbalance.
- Communication difficulties mean that people with dementia often present much later in the course of the illness, and that diagnosis can be more difficult.
- Advanced dementia is associated with increased 'frailty', which means that relatively small physical insults can lead to dramatic deterioration. Such older adults have little physiological reserve, and so are living day to day near the threshold for decompensation. But while this means deteriorations are likely to happen, it also means that relatively small, simple interventions could lead to improvement again, if instituted in a timely manner.
- Dealing with acute illness in advanced dementia does not usually require complex invasive management—every intervention should be assessed in terms of whether it will improve symptoms and quality of life and what burdens it poses (📖 Chapter 13).

Some common presenting complaints

Sometimes people with advanced dementia present in a typical way, e.g. cough and shortness of breath with a pneumonia, or chest pain in the case of an acute coronary syndrome. In these cases, getting to the root of the problem and deciding on treatment are relatively simple. However, more often people with advanced dementia become unwell in a non-specific way which can be a challenge to carers and health professionals. One problem can soon snow-ball into others, which all have to be unravelled and treated before the patient's optimal health is restored. What follows is a series of vignettes which illustrate common presentations of intercurrent illness in advanced dementia.

Pain (📖 Chapter 8)

Mr Jones has PD with dementia and osteoarthritis. He still lives in his flat and is cared for by carers who visit four times a day to help him get in and out of bed, and manage all his ADLs. One morning his carer had difficulty getting him out of bed and he seemed very unwilling to be moved but wouldn't say what was wrong and didn't want any breakfast. He was examined by his GP who found that he had a hot and tender knee with an effusion. The GP learned from the carer that there was no history of trauma, and looking in his case notes saw that he had previously been treated for pseudogout in his knee. The GP gave Mr Jones some analgesia, and, with his carer present, explained to him that he would feel better if the fluid was removed from his knee. She aspirated 30ml of fluid; after this he was able to bend his knee without much pain. She sent the fluid urgently to the hospital for microscopy which confirmed pseudogout. With analgesia, Mr Jones was able to get up, have breakfast, and take his normal medications.

Learning points

It is easy to see how Mr Jones could have deteriorated further. Without timely treatment, he might have missed his Parkinson's medications. This could lead to further stiffness and immobility which could have worsened the gout and put him at risk of constipation and chest infection. His unwillingness to eat and drink could have led to dehydration.

Increased confusion

Mr Patel lives at home with his wife. He has cerebrovascular disease, atrial fibrillation, and heart failure. The chronic cerebrovascular disease has left him with a significant VaD. Mrs Patel notices that her husband has become more confused over a period of 5 days. He has gone off his food and she is having difficulty getting him to take his usual medication. Due to increasing confusion Mr Patel wanders outside and falls over the back step. The emergency services attend and take him to the Emergency Department to rule out a fracture. He has not broken any bones but blood tests reveal him to be dehydrated with a high digoxin level of 2.4ng/mL. Following review of his medication his digoxin is discontinued and a couple of days of rehydration soon restore Mr Patel back to his previous level of functioning.

Learning points

- Worsening confusion may represent a deterioration in the underlying dementia, but can also be an indication of underlying pathology.
- Underlying pathologies include infection, drug toxicity, and dehydration.
- There may be more than one cause for increased confusion.

Incontinence

Peggy lives in a care home and has severe AD; she needs the help of two carers and a standing hoist to get out of bed. She has a history of constipation and is given regular lactulose. Over the last few days she has developed faecal incontinence with diarrhoea. She has also had reduced appetite and started calling out more and hitting out. She was seen by an older person's specialist nurse who examined her. p.r. examination revealed stool impaction with overflow diarrhoea. He prescribed an enema followed by a regime of regular, timed, prompted voiding, after suppositories in the beginning. After a few days Peggy stopped having faecal incontinence and her behaviour calmed. The specialist nurse was able to run through the management of constipation in dementia with the care home's staff.

Learning points

- Sometimes constipation does not respond to normal laxatives, which only lead to faecal incontinence.
- Constipation is particularly common in DLB and dementia in PD and may well pre-date the dementia.
- Constipation is linked with physical and verbal aggression, and antipsychotic medication can worsen constipation.

See 📖 Chapter 9 for details of management

Acute abdomen

Mr Wallis has severe AD and has been cared for by his wife for the last 10 years. One day he develops repeated vomiting and his belly becomes distended. He becomes agitated and distressed. Mrs Wallis calls an ambulance. The accident and emergency doctor examines Mr Wallis and finds that he has a tender irreducible left inguinal hernia and signs of abdominal obstruction. He is continuing to vomit and is not responding to anti-emetics. He is becoming dehydrated despite i.v. fluids and there is a risk of aspiration. The surgical doctors assess him and find that he is unable to take on any information to decide what to do next. They discuss the pros and cons of surgery with his wife, and together opt for surgery as the best chance of improving his symptoms. The surgery is successful and the day after the operation he is much more comfortable and responds to his wife.

Learning points
- Even in advanced dementia, invasive treatment including surgery is sometimes the only way to ensure good palliative care.
- Often this will necessitate a best interest decision under the Mental Capacity Act (MCA) (📖 Chapter 18).
- Delirium is common after surgery. It is important that nursing staff on the surgical wards are briefed as to the management of delirium.

Agitation/distress (📖 Chapters 6 and 10)

Miss Smith is a resident of a nursing home for people with dementia. She has been there for 5 years and the staff know her well. She is doubly incontinent and usually managed with pads. The staff have noticed that Miss Smith has become more agitated and seems in pain. It is difficult to localize the pain as she is unable to communicate. An ambulance is called and Miss Smith is transferred to the local Emergency Department; fortunately one of the carers accompanies her. The doctor identifies localized pain in her lower abdomen and asked whether she has been passing urine or opening her bowels lately. It strikes the carer that although she has had wet pads they have not been as wet as usual and her bowels have not been open for a couple of days. The doctor suspects urinary retention and a catheter is passed. 1L of cloudy concentrated urine drains and a specimen is sent to the laboratory for analysis. Miss Smith appears relieved. Rectal examination reveals a rectum loaded with soft stool. A suppository is given which produces a good result. 1L of fluid is given overnight and in the morning Miss Smith has the catheter removed as is able to return to the nursing home.

Learning points
- Constipation and UTI are common causes of urinary retention, so look for both.
- If continence expertise is available to care homes, this sort of presentation could be entirely managed in the care home, avoiding

the need for transfer to a new place of care. This is only possible if care home staff are alert to the possibility and have access to specialist advice.
• In this situation getting information from the carer was vital, so remember the collateral history! A home can always be telephoned if the patient arrives unaccompanied.

Off food and drink

Mary Robinson has severe dementia and is cared for at home by her husband Harry. She remains mobile around the house and usually keeps a good diet with a bit of encouragement. Two weeks previously she had required a course of antibiotics from the GP for a chest infection. Mary has started to refuse to take her biscuits and cake at tea time, which she usually loves, and also her dinner. Harry has managed to encourage her to take some soup and a little porridge at breakfast time. He remains worried about this development and calls the GP in again. On examination the GP finds that Mary has extensive oral candidiasis. He prescribes some oral medication which rapidly resolves the problem and Mary returns to her previous eating habits

Learning points
• Sudden unexpected reluctance to take food and drink may have an acute cause. A local problem such as candida, mouth ulcers, or ill-fitting dentures may be enough to put a person off their food (📖 Chapter 9).
• Soft foods or nutrient drinks/soups may be useful in maintaining nutrition while the underlying cause is treated as they will be better tolerated.
• Local preparations for candida may not be so well tolerated in patients with dementia as they may not grasp the logistics of using a mouth wash, so a systemic preparation may be more effective.

Drowsiness

Mrs Black is in hospital following a fall and fractured neck of femur. This has been repaired surgically and she is making progress with mobility. Due to her underlying dementia she gets a little restless particularly at night; she is disorientated, tries to get out of bed, and calls for her husband. One night the nurses find her on the floor. The doctor is called; he cannot identify any new problems but the hip is X-rayed again to check for further damage. In the morning Mrs Black is reviewed by the day staff; they are concerned that she seems more drowsy and difficult to rouse and will not eat her breakfast. Medical review reveals no focal neurological signs but drowsiness. Blood is taken to look for infection and dehydration and fluids are started as Mrs Black looks dehydrated. A CT brain scan is arranged which confirms the presence of an acute subdural haematoma. Discussions follow as to whether intervention is indicated or appropriate.

Learning points
- If there has been an unwitnessed fall a person with dementia may have struck their head, and relying on that person's own memory will be inaccurate.
- Following a fall, regular neurological observations should be considered so that any change in neurological status can be identified quickly.
- Increased drowsiness can also be caused by other things such as intercurrent infection, the overuse of analgesics (especially opiates and their derivatives), and dehydration/electrolyte imbalance, all of which can occur on a post-operative surgical or a medical, ward.
- If considering neurosurgical intervention in a patient with advanced dementia, careful discussion needs to occur with the family and neurosurgeons. Active intervention may not be beneficial or appropriate (📖 Chapter 13).

Falls

- Falls are extremely common in patients with dementia, particularly those who are still independently mobile as often they get up and mobilize with no thought to safety, i.e. they lose their ability to anticipate falls risk.
- These falls are difficult to prevent as it is difficult to supervise someone for 24 hours a day. Furthermore, advice given to patients in an attempt to prevent falls is not retained for any length of time.
- In a residential setting it is important that the carers are appraised of individual clients' falls risks and have a strategy to try to avoid them.
- There are numerous falls risks assessments available to identify fallers.
- If a usually stable patient becomes suddenly less stable and has increasing falls there may be a new underlying cause rather than the dementia alone.

Fred White lives at home with his wife Winnie. She cares for Fred but recently Fred has been having problems with his urine. He is calling several times at night for Winnie to take him to the toilet and is getting occasional incontinence. He also makes increasing visits to the bathroom during the day. Winnie is finding this difficult to manage as she is not getting any sleep. Having ruled out an infection, the GP thinks this may be prostatism so he starts indoramin to see whether this improves the symptoms. After a few days Winnie finds that Fred is beginning to stumble when he stands up and has a fall when going to the bathroom during the day. The GP realizes that this may be postural hypotension induced by the indoramin and stops it. He refers Mr White to a urologist for advice on his urinary problems.

Learning points
- Many drugs can induce falls, either by causing unsteadiness (e.g. tranquillizers, pain killers, anti-emetics) or postural hypotension (e.g. antihypertensives and Parkinson's medication).
- Falls in patients with dementia may prove impossible to completely eliminate, so environmental factors (such as flooring and bed heights), extra vigilance, hip protectors, and bone protection may be the only options.
- Seeking a second opinion regarding the management of Fred's urinary symptom may not only help this but also reduce his falls risk.

Weakness/fatigue

Mrs Cotton lives in a residential home. She is usually mobile around the home and often likes to help with the dusting. The carers in the home notice that she has stopped doing this and is now found sitting in the conservatory or in her room. She also seems a bit more breathless when mobilizing. She continues to eat and drink as normal. Due to this change in behaviour the GP is called, and on examining Mrs Cotton can find no obvious abnormalities. He arranges a blood test which confirms her haemoglobin to be only 6g/dL (normal >11.6g/dL for a woman). He arranges for her to attend the local day unit for a transfusion and after this Mrs Cotton returns to her usual level of function.

Learning points
- It is important to check haematinics in these patients as iron and folate deficiency is common. Thyroid problems are also common causes, and often not clinically obvious.
- If the anaemia is due to iron deficiency it may be due to occult GI blood loss. It is then time to take a very individual approach to whether further investigation into this would be helpful or appropriate. Symptomatic treatment with transfusion and iron supplements may be the best way forward. If upper GI pathology is suspected then a pre-emptive PPI may be justified. If further investigation is considered then CT enema may be better tolerated than colonoscopy or barium enema
- When a person with end-stage dementia develops cancer, symptom control remains the priority, and careful decisions will need to be made regarding intensity of intervention. A painful bony metastasis may respond well to a single fraction of radiotherapy, but the potential risks of intensive radiotherapy or chemotherapy may outweigh the benefits. Intensive investigations may also be too onerous. Sensitive discussions with carers and the patient (if possible) should be had before embarking on such a path because if no further intervention is planned then undergoing sometimes frightening procedures for the patient may not be necessary or contributory.

Injury

Minnie Brown lives at home with her husband Wilf. She has advanced dementia and Wilf is her main carer. Minnie likes to go out to the bird table, which is on the balcony of their flat, to feed the birds. One day, Wilf hears a crash and finds Minnie on the floor on the balcony. She has no recollection of the fall and appears to be in pain. He tries to help her to her feet but is unable to do so. He calls their life line and an ambulance comes. Minnie is taken to the local A&E. She is distressed and agitated in the unfamiliar environment with bright lights and noise. The doctor has difficulty examining her as she appears to be in pain and is uncooperative. He feels that she might be better managed in the local intermediate care centre but when the physiotherapist assesses her she finds her unable to stand due to pain. She suggests X-ray of the pelvis. This confirms a fractured hip. Minnie is then referred to the orthopaedic surgeons for repair.

Learning points
- Localizing pain in this scenario may prove difficult, but it is important to consider significant injury in such a patient.
- The fact that a patient is uncooperative is not an excuse for an incomplete assessment.
- It is always important to consider non-accidental injury, particularly if there is evidence of bruises of various ages and if the patient appears fearful of their carer.

Things to consider in the management of chronic illness

- Patients with advanced dementia often carry with them a range of other comorbidities such as diabetes, heart failure, arthritis, COPD, and epilepsy which may have preceded their dementia diagnosis. Many of these may exist simultaneously in one individual.
- These conditions often require the patient to take an assortment of medication, some of which can be vital in keeping their symptoms under control. This can sometimes lead to confusion with medication (too often or forgotten) and thought needs to be applied to help compliance, e.g. prompting, 'dosette' boxes and modes of delivery.
- It is important to keep medication to a minimum to keep the patient well. Regular review of the necessity and importance of medication is crucial.

COPD

Mrs S lives in a care home. She has mixed dementia and has had three hospital admissions in the last year for exacerbations of COPD. She also has long-standing back pain secondary to osteoporosis. She has always had a strident personality and now that her dementia has got worse she has had more difficult behaviour. Last week she was refusing her tablets by spitting them out. The doctor therefore prescribed an equivalent dose buprenophine patch instead of oral pain killers. Today her daughter has come to visit and has alerted the care staff because she is not herself. She does not recognise her, and normally she perks up at the sight of her granddaughter but today she has not. She is assessed by the duty doctor who hears crackles in her left base and arranges for her to be admitted to A&E. In A&E she is found to be drowsy with significant respiratory acidosis which requires non-invasive ventilation. There does not seem to be any sign of infection. Her daughter knows when she is getting better as she pulls the mask off.

Learning points
- Delirium doesn't only mean difficult behaviour (📖 Chapter 10, Delirium, pp. 174–177). Over half of delirium cases are hypoactive delirium. In this case Mrs B's behaviour became easier for her carers as she became delirious. Her daughter, however, noted the change.
- Opiate pain relief can cause type II respiratory failure in patients with COPD—use with care.
- Take care when changing routes of medications, as compliance with the oral medication may have been much less than realized.
- Nebulized B-agonists and anticholinergic bronchodilator medication give symptomatic improvement in COPD but may have variable tolerance in patients with dementia.
- Non-invasive ventilation (NIV) can be tried if tolerated, but usually in this situation admission for full ventilation to an ICU would not prolong life and is rarely appropriate in a patient with end-stage dementia.

Careful discussion would need to be had with any family members/carers in order for them to understand the reasons for this.

- It would be appropriate to have discussions with carers about ceilings of treatment for such patients prior to any deterioration in the chest in order to prepare for how best to manage such a situation.

Diabetes

- Diabetes may be dependent on insulin injections, treated by diet alone, or oral hypogylcaemic drugs.
- As dementia progresses robust control of blood sugar becomes less of a priority.
- It is important to avoid hypoglycaemia as the patient may be unable to identify the symptoms and slip rapidly into a coma.
- As appetite and oral intake and weight reduce with the progression of dementia it is important to review patients' requirements for hypoglycaemics as this may change.
- Occasionally oral medications can be discontinued completely.
- It is thought that a normal diabetic may experience symptoms of hyperglycaemia with a blood glucose >15mmol/L, but it is difficult to ascertain whether this is the case in any dying person.
- Diabetes management is a good example of how the priorities of treatment change when face with a person at the end of life. Much of the treatment in diabetes in the general population is about preventing long-term complications. So where the life expectancy is shortened from the dementia, the benefits of rigorous control of blood sugars will never come to fruition, but the risks will still be faced.

Heart failure

- Patients who have heart failure often need medication to stop them becoming breathless. However, this must be kept under review, as when the activity of the patient declines, such regular or high doses of medication may be no longer required. When oral fluid intake declines the patient can become dehydrated if still taking regular diuretics.
- Assessment of any valve lesions and the degree of ventricular dysfunction may be useful as it gives information on the severity of the underlying problem and hence prognosis.
- Atrial fibrillation can be associated with heart failure or exist independently. It is associated with an increased incidence of stroke. The use of warfarin can reduce this risk. The risk of bleeding on warfarin in patients with dementia may be increased by confusion around dosages, missed appointments at the anticoagulation clinic, and increased risk of trauma due to falls.
- Hence processes must be in place to mitigate these risks if warfarin is used. Regular review of the use of warfarin in such patients is important to monitor the risk versus benefit, the balance of which may change over time as the dementia progresses.

Further reading

Allen SC (1997) Competence thresholds for the use of inhalers in people with dementia. *Age Ageing* **26**, 83–6.

Close JC (2005) Prevention of falls – a time to translate evidence into practice. *Age Ageing* **34**, 98–100.

Katalinic OM, Harvey LA, Herbert RD, Moseley AM, Lannin NA, Schurr K (2010) Stretch for the treatment and prevention of contractures. *Cochrane Database Syst Rev* 9:CD007455.

Kim EA et al. (2007) Evaluation of three fall-risk assessment tools in an acute care setting. *J Adv Nurs* **60**, 427–35.

National Institute for Clinical Excellence and Royal College of Nursing (2003) *The use of pressure-relieving devices (beds, mattresses and overlays)for the prevention of pressure ulcers in primary and secondary care*. NICE, London.

National Institute for Clinical Excellence and Royal College of Nursing (2005) *The management of pressure ulcers in primary and secondary care: a clinical practice guideline*. NICE, London.

Spiller JA, Keen JC (2006) Hypoactive delirium: assessing the extent of the problem for inpatient specialist palliative care. *Palliat Med* **20**, 17–23.

Vahia I et al. (2007) Prevalence and impact of paratonia in Alzheimer disease in a multiracial sample. *Am J Geriatr Psychiat* **15**, 351–3.

Deciding on appropriate intervention

Elements of decision-making

One of the most complex but important areas one faces in caring for people with advanced dementia is to decide when and how far to intervene when things are not going well. Both a nihilistic attitude, with consequent refusal to ever investigate and treat aggressively, and a reluctance to acknowledge the consequences of the dementia, resulting in an unrelenting pursuit of improvement, can have devastating consequences for that person and their carers. Decisions have to be personalized and holistic. In this chapter we will review how to approach these decisions. Among other topics, we will deal with issues of feeding and hydration, and the management of intercurrent infections.

Decisions are almost always taken in situations of uncertainty, where we cannot be sure of the consequences of an intervention or of not intervening. This means that wrong decisions may sometimes have positive consequences, or that well-taken decisions may lead to the wrong outcome. It is a mistake to judge a decision solely by its outcome, rather than by the thoroughness and balance of the process by which it was reached. A bad decision can have a good outcome because of a chance happening, and a good decision can go badly. On the other hand, once a situation has reached an outcome, it is useful to go back over the decision-making process to consider whether all the important elements were considered and correctly judged. A decision that repeatedly leads to the wrong outcome is likely to have a flaw in the process by which it was reached.

In considering decisions about investigation and intervention, weigh up:
• The wishes of patients and relatives.
• The clinical state of the patient.
• Evidence base about outcomes.
• Ethical pros and cons.
• The legal situation.

In more detail, explore:
• *Currently or previously expressed wishes of the patient*, if they were competent when they made those decisions. These are legally binding if the conditions for an advance decision to refuse treatment under the MCA 2007 are fulfilled (📖 Chapter 18, The legal framework in the UK, pp. 313–322).
• *Acceptability to the patient*. Even if the patient has not in the past expressed a view on the treatment in question, one has to consider from what is known about them whether the proposed intervention or lack of intervention would be acceptable to them, e.g. some Hindu, Muslim, or Jewish patients may consider taking medication which contains beef or pork gelatin as an inert component unacceptable, and would be unlikely to consent to it if they were able to weigh up the information. An underused instrument is the Values History, where a document can be drawn up with the person affected if able to, or with relatives who represent the person's known attitudes and beliefs, to help decision-making when they

cannot express a view.[1] A specimen can be found at http://www.hospicefed.org/hospice_pages/valuesform.htm.

- *Views of carers and relatives:* these are not legally binding in the UK unless that person has designated LPA (📖 Chapter 18, Self-determination in dementia, pp. 309–312), but it is very strongly advisable to listen to carers' and relatives' views very closely, as guidance from the General Medical Council (GMC) and British Medical Association (BMA) state.[2] Never simply take expressed views at face value. Try to get a feel for what lies behind them, how the carer formed that opinion, the carer's understanding of the present and future of the patient's illness, their own fears and beliefs, their overall attitude to the person and their account of views expressed by the person in the past. When exploring views the individual communicated to them in the past, check out that these really are the patient's own views. You could ask them about the specific situations in which conversations were had, what specific words or expressions the person used, and in what context. However, keep in mind that carers often have a more holistic view than we do as professionals; listen to them and learn.

- *Burden of the condition without intervention.* Think through the consequences of not intervening. What symptoms would result? How would not intervening impact on quality of life, independence, prognosis?

- *Burden of intervention for that particular patient.* Will it involve hospital admission, and for how long—as a day case, for a few days, or weeks? Will distressing interventions, e.g. painful procedures or the passage of a NGT be involved, and will the patient be able to understand what is being done to them and why, or will it feel to them like an assault? How long will the intervention take? What aftercare will they get? Can one soften the impact on them, e.g. have family members who they know well available throughout, use a general anaesthetic, etc? What are the possible complications, how likely are they to happen to that patient, what long-term consequences will those complications have, and how will one handle them if they do arise? Do not just think in theory, but think in terms of real resources available locally. A centre that carries out an intervention hundreds of times a year is much more likely to carry it off with fewer problems than one which carries it out occasionally, for example.

- *Benefit of the proposed intervention.* What is the likelihood that the intervention will have a positive result? What positive result? What will be the impact of the intervention on the person's comfort, quality of life, or independence if it succeeds? How long is the benefit likely to last? Are the conditions in place to make the intervention succeed (e.g. an operation on a joint without good post-operative physiotherapy may reduce pain but not improve mobility).

- *Are there alternative, less burdensome, ways of achieving the same or comparable results?* If the risks to quality of life or outcome are considerable, a good enough result from a less intrusive intervention,

---

1 Doukas DJ, McCullough LB (1991) The values history. The evaluation of the patient's values and advance directives. *J Fam Pract* **32**, 145–53.

2 British Medical Association Ethics Department (2008) *End of life decisions: views of the BMA*, p. 6. British Medical Association, London.

rather than a perfect one from an aggressive procedure, may be more acceptable.

- *Prognosis*, How long is the patient likely to survive? How long is it before their condition changes to the extent that the benefits of the intervention will be nullified? How much of that prognosis will be spent in convalescing from the intervention? For example, if a patient is given palliative chemotherapy, how is that going to affect their quality of life in the short term, how long will it be till they recover from the effects of chemotherapy, and how long will the benefit last after they recover? Are they likely to deteriorate from another reason before they enjoy the full benefit?
- *What are the risks of intervention and non-intervention?* The benefits on intervention and non-intervention must also be balanced against the risks of either course.
- *What are the legal constraints and guidance under which you operate?* These vary with situations, but you should be well familiar with the ones that apply in your country and in the particular condition. But remember that legislation is passed with the intent of enabling good and effective care for those who cannot decide.
- *Then decide* to act or not to act!

Handling conflict situations

At times different individuals within a family disagree, or professionals' views may differ strongly from those of family. In such cases:

- Remember: most people are reasonable.
- Try and understand what drives the family's views (📖 Chapter 16).
- Listen closely, understand their fears, doubts, and motivations, and communicate this understanding to them by verbalizing their concerns and addressing each of them respectfully and thoroughly. Don't say 'I understand'; show you do by your behaviour.
- Try to get to the underlying reasons. They may have past experiences of illness, medication, or authority that affect the way they behave.
- Explain your understanding of their relative's situation and their future.
- Address the pros and cons of each option, and show your thought process.
- Take what they have expressed into serious consideration when taking decisions, and show how you did this when discussing the options.
- Avoid arguing; it only makes positions rigid.
- Empathize, but on key points of principle or practice, also be firm.
- Most people will respect your decision, even if they do not agree, if you show you have taken great care in reaching it.
- If there is serious ongoing conflict, arrange for a second opinion.
- Do not tolerate violence or bullying. While some aggression is to be expected in people under stress, there is a limit to what is acceptable that should not be crossed. If a patient or staff are being intimidated, lay down strict boundaries you expect to be respected. If violence takes place or is seriously threatened, involve the police.
- If crucial irreconcilable differences persist, you may need to apply to court.

In cases of doubt

There will always be situations where the alternatives are particularly difficult to weigh up, where, for example, all options have serious possible negative consequences, or where the cost–benefit analysis is open to differing interpretations. Avail yourself of these aids:

- Seek a second opinion from an uninvolved colleague who comes to the situation with fresh eyes. The right to a second opinion is enshrined in GMC and NHS guidance.
- Consult your medical defence organization: remember, however, that this will give you advice about what is legal, and tends to suggest the safest option, but you will still have to weigh up the ethical issues.
- Your trade union (e.g. the BMA or Royal College of Nursing (RCN)) may have an ethical advisor who you might discuss the situation with.
- Consult with a local medical ethicist, e.g. from a local university department.
- Take your situation to your institution's clinical ethics committee: more and more institutions now have these, and they can play an invaluable role in making difficult decisions. Membership comprises senior and junior clinical staff, medical ethicists and legal experts, and lay members. Meetings can be called at short notice to discuss specific situations. If urgent, some will use e-mail to discuss and advise. Regular meetings also examine complex live and recent cases, guidance being generated by the organization, etc. At other times, a meeting would take too long to organize in urgent situations, and virtual meetings through shared exchanges of views over e-mail, via conference calls, or through video conferencing enable a quicker response. Much advice regarding clinical ethics committees (including a directory) can be found on the UK Clinical Ethics Network website (http://www.ethics-network.org.uk/).
- In continuing situations of serious doubt or disagreement, take legal advice or apply to the courts for a decision.

Be aware of the law and guidance from regulatory organizations. For example, both a court and a regulator would take an extremely dim view of decisions taken without proper consultation with carers. However, never practice defensively, with your eye mainly on the possible legal consequences for you rather than the patient's best interests. Defensive medicine leads to precisely the kind of mistakes one is trying to avoid, because it unbalances a holistic view. Document your decision-making process in detail. No court or disciplinary body will condemn you for well-documented, thoughtfully made decisions which carefully weigh up the alternatives and consult broadly, even if the outcome turns out to be seriously negative for the patient.

Always remember the difference between law and ethics; in some people's minds ethics has become confused with the legal situation. The law aims to enforce a minimum standard of behaviour that is widely acceptable within that particular society to people with widely differing views or cultures. Ethics, on the other hand, aim to help individuals and organizations conduct themselves with the highest standard of integrity in personal, interpersonal, and community situations. Both legal and ethical perspectives have to be weighed up. The two inform and relate to each other closely, but they must not be confused.

Some ethical approaches

There are a number of commonly employed ethical approaches to weighing up situations. Some argue that actions are right or wrong in themselves (the *deontological* approach) and others judge actions mainly by the rightness and wrongness of their outcomes (the *consequentialist* approach). Consequences can be classified into beneficial and burdensome, and weighed up against one another. Both approaches have their attractions and limitations. Principles are universal but can be difficult to interpret and counterbalance in the complexity of certain life situations. Many 'principles' turn out to vary greatly from culture to culture. Consequences are a practical measure, but by definition they only become apparent after the event; and by what ethical criteria does one judge the outcomes? Consequentionalism can descend into a superficial and empty moral relativism just as much as a rigid principle-based approach can be dehumanizing and overbearing.

Principles-based approach

This is best exemplified by the work of Beauchamp and Childress (see Further reading). It applies four principles, by which to weigh up medical decisions. The principles are:

- Autonomy: people have a right to make their own choices, e.g. in accepting or refusing treatment.
- Beneficence (do good).
- Non-maleficence (do no harm).
- Justice: fairness and equality in distribution of scarce health resources.

Beauchamp and Childress suggest that priorities between these principles differ according to the situation. They also derive some context-dependent rules from these principles: honesty and truth telling; confidentiality; privacy; maintaining promises.

In many situations there will be conflict between the various principles. Beauchamp and Childress suggest that one must then justify departure from one principle by showing that another principle has a higher stringency in that situation. These departures are justifiable if: 'There is a realistic prospect of reaching the moral objective that appears to justify the infringement; the infringement must be necessary in the circumstances; the infringement should be the least possible, commensurate with the primary goal of the action; and the agent must seek to minimize the negative effects of the infringement.[3]

Many criticisms have been levelled at principle-based approaches. They have been described as an algorithm-based approach to ethics, which can be reductive, open to mechanistic application, and can analyse human situations and human actions in a disembodied fragmentary manner; they apply abstract theories to complex situations found in medical practice; they can be inflexible and unresponsive to particular circumstances. In particular, the work of Beauchamp and Childress has been criticized for trying to reconcile the deontological and consequentialist approaches,

---

3 Childress JF (1998) *A principle-based approach. In: A companion to bioethics* (ed. H. Kuhse, P. Singer), pp. 61–71. Blackwell, Malden, MA.

even though in many respects they point in very different directions. However, the model has proved adaptable and can allow analysis of complex situations. For some decades now, this model has been the predominant one in Western bioethical circles.

Casuistry

The main alternative to the principle-based approach is that of casuistry. This does not depart from absolute rules but gives a lot more attention to the circumstances of the situation to make practical judgments. It starts off with paradigmatic cases where the situation is clear cut and those involved in discussion can agree about the right and wrong ways of behaving. It then analyses the case in hand to discover the ways in which it departs or corresponds to the paradigm, and therefore how the conclusions drawn from the paradigm do or do not apply to the current situation. The right course of action can be worked out by confronting a situation to any number of paradigms which throw light on the situation.

Casuistry utilizes certain maxims as a shortcut for starting from first principles in every case. One commonly accepted maxim, for example, is that competent patients can choose or refuse treatment.

Clearly casuistry is open to abuse, allowing people to make judgments of convenience rather than rigour. But then any ethical analysis must assume that the person is doing their best to act ethically. Ethics is not law, and is not about enforcement but about behaving with integrity. Legal deliberations overlap but do not start from the same premises. Any system incorrectly applied is open to abuse. Equally, one may fail to discern properly similarities and differences between the cases one is considering. The strengths of casuistry are its flexibility, its responsiveness to particular situations, the fact that it starts from the human rather than from theory or principle, and the fact that consensus can be achieved even if the participants come from widely differing ethical or cultural backgrounds. The other problem with casuistry is it can end up in hair splitting, intellectual cleverness and nitpicking which misses the wood for the trees. The essential practicality and flexibility of casuistry is enshrined in common law and case law traditions which embrace this approach. In moral circles casuistry was for a long time treated by some as specious argument lacking in rigour, but in recent years it has regained respect and its responsiveness has been embraced by many.

Other ethical principles often invoked in advanced illness

A number of other ethical principles are often introduced into discussions about intervention in advanced illness. The main ones are:

Double effect

Some interventions may be ethical even if while achieving good they bring about foreseen but unintended harmful consequences. For example, a drug may be used to settle somebody's severe ongoing agitation even if it might result in the patient's earlier death. However, there are some very precise conditions for double effect to operate:
- The nature of the act itself is good or morally neutral: one cannot use poison to reduce agitation but only medication with a therapeutic effect.
- The good effect is the effect intended, e.g. the reduction in agitation not the death. The bad effect is foreseen but not intended. You know the person could die sooner but that is not why you are doing it.

- The good effect is not reached through the bad effect: for example death is not the means by which agitation is reduced.
- Circumstances must be sufficiently grave to justify causing the bad effect: the agitation must be very distressing and intractable.
- There is no safer way to achieve the good effect.
- The good that comes out is proportionately greater than the harm that results.
- The person taking the action does their best to reduce the harm resulting as much as possible.

Some criticize double effect as a form of intellectual dishonesty or sophistry; they argue that it is the outcome that counts, whatever the intention; and one may pretend one wanted one outcome while really desiring the other. Others respond that actions are not disembodied but acts of a human being, and that the process by which that human being arrives at decisions has an effect on them and their development as moral beings as well as on the recipient of these decisions. Even the law believes intention matters greatly: the most serious crime on the statute book, murder, is defined by the fact that death was intended, so to keep intention out of ethical reasoning is unreasonable.

Double effect is often invoked, but rarely operative in modern medical practice and in palliative care in particular. For example there is a common belief that morphine used for pain often kills patients quicker, but there is no evidence that this really happens unless the drug is used carelessly or in very rare situations where the patient has other very serious conditions which make them very vulnerable to it. Good drug availability (e.g. having opioids which are safe to use in renal failure) prevents most such situations.

Interestingly, it may well be used to allow the appropriate use of antipsychotics in dementia. In this situation we know that they are both effective for some as well as clearly harmful.[4]

Acts and omissions

Another distinction sometimes put forward is that between actively doing something negative (unethical) and refraining from doing something positive (acceptable), as in killing someone or letting them die by withdrawing life-support measures. Again, some fail to see a distinction between the two options as the outcomes are similar. Others argue that there are circumstances in which treatment can and should be withdrawn or withheld:

- When it is ineffective (cardiopulmonary resuscitation (CPR) in patients with widely disseminated cancer).
- When burdens and risks outweigh benefits.
- When the treatment does not advance the patient's medical good.
- When the treatment does not advance the patient's total good.
- When resources available do not allow treatment to be given.

They contend that the meaning of not starting or stopping treatment in these circumstances is totally different from administering life-shortening treatment.

4 Treloar A, Crugel M, Prasanna A, Solomons L, Fox C, Paton C, Katona C (2010) Ethical dilemmas: should antipsychotics ever be prescribed for people with dementia? *Br J Psychiat* **197**, 88–90.

Ordinary and extraordinary treatments

Interventions are extraordinary if they cause severe pain or suffering (including fear), if they incur a high risk of morbidity or mortality, if they are financially burdensome, or if they carry a low chance of success. While one should always accept (at least in some moral traditions) or give ordinary treatments, like feeding, there is no obligation to subject oneself or others to extraordinary treatments. Sometimes deciding not to give such treatments is important for preserving a person's dignity. Again, some find this distinction specious while for others it is deeply insightful.

Basic care

In UK law the MCA sets out the concept of basic care; care that cannot be refused and must be provided. This is at least analogous to the concept of ordinary and extraordinary means.

Applying ethical analysis in dementia

In decisions regarding patients with advanced dementia, the principle of autonomy is of limited applicability because the person cannot understand the consequences of the alternatives open to them and weigh them in the balance. The best approximation is finding out about past expressed wishes and working out what would be in line with the way the person lived their life and made their choices. While beneficence and non-maleficence are clearly laudable, often ethical problems in advanced dementia centre on uncertain outcomes, or on choosing between two potentially harmful outcomes in no-win situations; and what is good and what is harm may depend on one's view of life at its limits. This is not to imply that the principles model is not helpful here, but if applied by different people they might come to very different conclusions. The same applies to casuistic models. That is not surprising: in complex situations, right and wrong are rarely self-evident.

Is it then worth going through all the trouble? Emphatically yes, for several reasons:

• Working one's way through competing claims and exploring all the factors impinging on a situation makes it more likely one can reach a balanced view.

• It increases one's sensitivity to the various elements involved so that one can pick these up and respond better when one next meets them.

• It has an impact on the affected person and family and it has an impact on the person making the decisions and choices.

• Constant involvement with the ethical aspects of care, discussion with others, and reading around the subject sharpens our sensitivity and makes our responses more thought out and measured, more consistent and less based on the whim of the moment. It also allows us to become more nuanced in our judgments and decision-making, and more human. Above all, it personalizes decisions and makes us engage with that person and with that situation, it makes us get to know the person better and get a real feel of who they are, rather than resorting to production-line decision-making produced by over simple rules of thumb that may lead to grave injustices.

A case example: the pacemaker battery

C was a patient in a nursing home who suffered from AD and had had a dual chamber pacemaker inserted for complete heart block. She had had a stroke, needed two to transfer, and her speech was an incomprehensible mumble. She slept most of the day and showed no interest in her surroundings except at meal times, which, however, she did enjoy from her wheelchair. She kept her eyes shut most of the time but when talked to would eventually open her eyes and make brief eye contact. However, she was unable to follow simple instructions. The pacemaker battery was running low and the cardiologist reckoned it would need replacing in about 6 months, despite setting the pacemaker on VVI mode to eke out the longest possible lifetime from the battery.

The situation was discussed with C's daughter. She was very close to her mother, who had supported her through recent multiple losses in her own life. Her main concern was that the serenity her mother had found in the nursing home, where she was well cared for and loved, might be disrupted if she was admitted to a busy hospital ward, and she might never recover the same sense of peace. Her mother's previous experiences of hospital had been disruptive and difficult, and she had been unhappy there.

A letter going through the alternatives was drawn up and circulated to all professionals involved in her care and to the daughter. It described the symptoms she would have if she went into complete heart block again (after consultation with her cardiologist); the likelihood this would not respond to pharmacological treatment; the battery-changing procedure and what it would mean from her point of view (for example admission to the alien hospital environment, an uncomfortable procedure she could not understand, the use of sedation); her prognosis, including the condition she would be left in, her likely rate of deterioration and the chance of further strokes; what could be done to alleviate the symptoms of heart block (most probably deep sedation if she was distressed—it was unlikely to respond to pharmacological manipulation); her family's situation; and her family's wishes. The consultant also expressed his own feeling that changing the battery would be very distressing and that C should be allowed to die in peace if she developed complete heart block, but asked the other professionals for their opinions.

Some responded, and the responses were in agreement. The cardiologist offered to do the procedure as a day case, but even after considering this it was felt by clinicians, carers, and daughter to be too intrusive for no quality of life benefit. Emergency drugs were prescribed and obtained for the nursing home and a plan drawn up to be adopted should the battery fail. The GP was still in two minds over the situation. The matter was therefore presented to a virtual meeting of the hospice's clinical ethics committee. There was universal agreement from respondents (a medico-legal expert, an ethicist, and a number of palliative care professionals) that replacing the battery was likely to be detrimental to C's well-being. Some weeks later the battery did start to show signs of failure, and sedation was used to good effect when C became symptomatic. C recovered, and had no further episodes until she died comfortably a year and a half later, with no further episodes of severe bradycardia, well past the point where battery failure had been predicted. Afterwards it felt like it had been the right decision, not because the outcome was right, which might have happened as a matter of luck, but because the process involved weighed up the different aspects and involved all concerned, and came up with a practical plan. It did show the uncertainty of even expert expectations, which makes such decisions so complex.

Some specific clinical situations

This section will focus on specific clinical situations in which one has to make judgments about whether or not to intervene, and examine the evidence base to see what we know about outcomes. This is crucial in determining the balance between benefits and burdens, but is rarely examined in the depth required to inform real-life decision-making.

Feeding and hydration

The point at which feeding and hydration become problematic in dementia is a difficult one for patient, relatives, and professionals. The way to deal with this is to integrate the current evidence base with what is known of the patient's views, the views of the family, and ethical considerations.

This should be read in conjunction with 📖 Chapter 9, GI symptoms, pp. 139–155.

Nutrition and weight loss

- 30–40% of people with moderately severe to severe AD suffer clinically significant weight loss. Weight loss and malnutrition often start before diagnosis. They is more likely to be associated with difficulties in feeding than with hypermetabolic states such as cachexia (see 📖 Chapter 9, GI symptoms, pp. 139–155.
- In older people, weight loss of over 4% in a year is associated with increased morbidity and mortality.
- Reduced food intake often has behavioural roots early on in dementia, eventually giving way to physical difficulties in eating and swallowing.
- Studies looking at the effect of skilled assisted feeding are contradictory in outcome: some show it reduces weight loss, others do not.
- Neurogenic dysphagia first affects drinking, then swallowing solids. Swallowing can at first be helped by appropriate techniques (Tables 9.3 and 9.4) but eventually severe dysphagia or aspiration may ensue.
- What clearly also changes is the susceptibility to the harmful effects of aspiration, due to immunological problems and a higher infection burden in the mouth, rendering serious consequences much more likely.
- Many episodes of aspiration pneumonia arise from aspiration of saliva not food.
- Increasing feeding difficulties increase caregiver burden.
- It is very natural to see artificial feeding through gastrostomies or NGTs as the answer to these problems. However, the evidence for a beneficial effect of these interventions in late-stage dementia is lacking (see 📖 Chapter 13, Some specific clinical situations, pp. 246–252 for fuller discussion), and there is some evidence of increased serious risk and harm, including high mortality soon after insertion. In essence, perhaps somewhat counter-intuitively to those unfamiliar with the clinical condition of these patients, the evidence shows that gastrostomy is not life-prolonging in late dementia, a conclusion which has obvious ethical repercussions.
- Proponents of gastrostomy are concerned that patients may feel hungry or thirsty even if it does not prolong their life. Again, studies of people in whom the decision to forgo enteral feeding had been taken

showed few expressions of discomfort, and when these occurred they were related to non-nutritional symptoms.

- Patients who had PEG insertions often needed further hospitalizations to deal with problems arising from these devices, or physical or pharmacological restraint to keep them in place.
- Patients with dementia drink and eat less as illness progresses, and do not appear disturbed by this. Many think the sensations of thirst and hunger are blunted in late-stage disease, although there is no way of proving this.

Decision-making about artificial nutrition and hydration

- Analyse the patient's general condition, prognosis, and the underlying cause of the dysphagia before making decisions.
- What has been described above is the dysphagia that supervenes in many patients with AD as they reach the end of their lives, and there is no good evidence that enteric feeding then helps survival or comfort. However, it is important to recognize different situations and to treat each on its own merits.
- In most cases, persisting with gentle, skilled hand feeding and accepting that the risk of aspiration is probably inevitable is the most sensible and kindest option in advanced dementia.[5]
- The Law Lords in the UK, the Supreme Court in the USA and in Australia, among other countries, have defined artificial nutrition and hydration legally as a medical intervention. Its appropriateness needs to be decided on as for other interventions. These bodies were considering persistent vegetative state, where the import of stopping feeding and hydration is quite different. It is important not to get the two conditions confused.

Is hydration a special case?

- If there is no evidence that artificial feeding is beneficial in late disease, should artificial hydration also not be provided? Unfortunately the literature is very scant in this regard, as hydration and feeding are almost always considered together.[5]
- i.v. hydration is rarely appropriate at this stage. Cannulation needs skill; the need for reinsertion is frequent; there is a risk of thrombophlebitis and occasionally septicaemia; fluid overload could produce pulmonary oedema; and i.v. fluids will usually mean hospitalization, with its negative impact. Patients may frequently pull out an i.v. line which they may see as a foreign object that may harm them.
- Hypodermoclysis (s.c. fluid administration) is an alternative. Up to 2L of fluid per day can be given through one cannula, which can be disconnected for part of the day. Infection and fluid overload risks are lower, though overload is still possible (frailty, often low serum albumin). Questions one needs to address include whether it can be monitored safely in one's home or a nursing home, and what concrete gains the patient will actually receive. In palliative care few people at the end of life need parenteral fluids for comfort; the risks of pulmonary oedema, increased sweating and urination, skin damage

5 Royal College of Physicians and British Society of Gastroenterology (2010) *Oral feeding difficulties and dilemmas: a guide to practical care, particularly towards the end of life.* Royal College of Physicians, London.

and oedema often outweigh any benefit. If the mouth is kept moist few seem to suffer discomfort.[6] Blood tests at the end of life rarely reveal dehydration. Transfer to another institution for parenteral hydration is almost never in a patient's best interests at this stage.

- But if there is good evidence, in a specific circumstance, that fluids will reduce distress at the end of life, they ought not to be withheld.

Intercurrent infection

- People with dementia are more likely to have emergency hospital admission than controls. The main causes are syncope, bronchopneumonia, UTI, and dehydration. Infections also cause morbidity. Early detection and treatment, and advance care planning, could reduce admissions.
- Infections become commoner as patients become frailer.
- At what point does treatment stop adding life and merely prolong dying?

Lower respiratory tract infection (LRTI)
Risk

- For aspiration pneumonia see 📖 Chapter 9, Respiratory symptoms, pp. 156–159.
- Post-mortem series show that bronchopneumonia is the commonest cause of death in advanced dementia. It is a disease of frailty, often the consequence rather than the cause of deterioration.
- Bronchopneumonia tends to be less severe in those who are still functionally independent, leading to shorter hospitalizations.
- Patients on antipsychotics (atypical > conventional) are more prone to develop pneumonia, even after allowing for delirium.
- Pneumonia causes multiple losses in physical performance. These may or may not persist after recovery, even in advanced dementia. Patients hospitalized for their LRTI show a greater decline in ADLs.

Outcome

- As patients develop dysphagia, they become unable to take oral antibiotics.
- Pneumonia is common as death approaches. Two-thirds of a retrospective sample of nursing home residents developed an average of 1.5 episodes of pneumonia each in their last 6 months of life. In another series, a third to a half of nursing home residents who developed LRTI died within 6 months.
- Poor prognostic factors for LRTI include feeding dependency, reduced alertness, tachycardia, respiratory difficulty, tachypnoea, inadequate hydration, male gender, and pressure sores.
- A Dutch study showed that oral antibiotics for pneumonia in advanced dementia are associated with less discomfort, while parenteral hydration is associated with increased discomfort. The authors suggest that oral antibiotics may have a place in symptom control even at the end of life.
- People with pneumonia fed through a NGT have a higher mortality.
- US physicians are more likely to hospitalize people with severe dementia, give antibiotics, including i.v., and rehydrate patients than their Dutch counterparts. Symptom control measures were rare

---

6 General Medical Council (2010) *Treatment and care towards the end of life: good practice in decision making.* General Medical Council, London.

in both groups. Mortality was higher in the Dutch cohort, although another study found that mortality was similar and more related to baseline health than antibiotic use.
- Patients who were restrained while being treated for LRTI suffered more decline in their ADLs
- A study of nursing home residents in the US dying of dementia showed that just under half of them were given antibiotics in the last 2 weeks of life, and just under half of these antibiotics were given parenterally. LRTIs were the commonest reason for antibiotic administration.

UTIs

- UTIs are common in older people, especially in women, in men with urinary tract obstruction, and in those with catheters. Condom catheters carry a lower risk than indwelling catheters, and suprapubic catheters less risk than urethral. Intermittent catheterization carries a lower risk still but is unlikely to be practical in advanced dementia.
- UTIs are associated with an increased risk of delirium and falls, which is higher in people with dementia.
- Although they appear to often cause morbidity, UTIs appear to be less commonly associated with mortality than LRTIs in this population.

Decision-making with infections

- It is clear that pneumonia is at first treatable, but that the first episode in advanced illness may be a marker that the end stage is being reached.
- Pneumonia is both a consequence and a cause of deterioration.
- Treatment with oral antibiotic and symptom relief measures (see 📖 Chapter 9, Respiratory symptoms, pp. 156–159) is worthwhile for prognostic and symptom relief reasons. After treatment, patients may be able to return to a contented life.
- However, oral antibiotics eventually become impossible to take.
- Antibiotics also carry some risk themselves of adverse effects which may impact on quality of life (e.g. nausea, diarrhoea); of superinfection (e.g. *C. difficile*, 📖 Chapter 9, GI symptoms, pp. 139–155; thrush, 📖 Chapter 9, Oral symptoms, pp. 134–138); of accumulation in organ failure (e.g. nitrofurantoin in renal failure; erythromycin can cause reversible hearing loss in renal failure unless the dose is adjusted), etc.
- Administration of i.v. antibiotics would necessitate a move to hospital and would be invasive. In view of the risks associated with acute hospital admission for this population, one should think hard about whether admission is justified.
- A mobile i.v. administration team that could administer these drugs to patients at home and in nursing homes might cut down hospital admissions. However, the appropriateness of i.v. treatment would still have to be considered.
- It is still possible to treat pneumonia symptomatically and to maintain patients in comfort when it is no longer possible to treat the infection itself.
- Discuss all this early on with relatives and staff, possibly after the first infective episode, and try to agree a plan. Decide on parameters by which one would agree when infection should be treated with antibiotics, and when not. The decision will of course have to be taken

at the time, but sharing these criteria early on allows people to think about them and contribute more to decision-making, as well as to see the underlying process, and the rationale and deep consideration for the person affected that is employed in reaching these decisions.
• Similar considerations apply to UTIs.

Fractures and trauma

Risk

• A survey of 280 community-dwelling people with AD gave a risk of over 50 injuries per 100 person-years. Half of these were due to falls and about one in eight resulted in fractures. Soft tissue injury is common.
• People with AD have an increased risk of osteoporosis due to deficiencies of vitamins D and K, calcium and parathyroid hormone (PTH), low sunlight exposure, low dietary calcium, and inactivity.
• Frailty, medication, especially neuroleptics, slow response times, infections, visuospatial disorders, etc. make people prone to falls (📖 Chapter 11, Managing disability in dementia, p. 204).
• Most fractures result from direct trauma to the hip.
• People with dementia are more likely to suffer fracture as a result of falls than controls. They are less likely to take protective action in time due to the above factors. Some think poor soft tissue cover may be more important than bone strength in producing fractures.
• Their faster walking speed also increases falls risk.
• Physical restraints, e.g. cot sides, can make fracture more likely after falls.
• In specialist dementia units, hip protectors do not alter the incidence of falls but do result in significantly fewer hip fractures.

Outcome

• In the general older population, hip fractures have a 15–20% 1-year mortality. Mortality is highest in the weeks after fracture but takes a year to return to baseline levels.
• Fractures with more displacement, more fragments, or more soft tissue injury have a poorer prognosis for healing and rehabilitation. Intracapsular fractures are more prone to non-union and avascular necrosis of the hip, which is painful and interferes with mobilization.
• Dementia increases mortality after hip fracture, and increases post-operative mortality at 3 months about 2.5-fold. Delay before operation strongly affect post-operative mortality, by about 6% per extra day of delay.
• In a Spanish series, concurrent dementia at the time of fracture was a stronger predictor of 3-year mortality than concurrent cancer or heart failure.
• Peri-operative analgesia is often very inadequate. A well-known study showed that people with dementia were given a third of the total opioid dose given to non-demented patients over the peri-operative period, and around half of the (better pain-controlled) non-demented patients complained their analgesia was inadequate anyway. p.r.n. analgesia was rarely prescribed for either group. Untreated pain can contribute to delirium, whether it arises from an untreated fracture or untreated post-operative pain.

- Post-operative delirium results in a longer hospital stay, lower likelihood of recovery of pre-operative function, and higher mortality at 1 year.
- Post-operative delirium may also be the first event in frank dementia; whether it uncovers pre-existing dementia or precipitates it is unclear.
- In general, about 80% of those operated on for hip fracture will walk again; this falls to about 50% if aged >90. A small recent study found no difference in mortality or functional outcome between operatively and non-operatively treated hip fractures. However, a study of patients over 90 found no case of restored mobility in non-operatively treated patients.
- Rehabilitation after hip fracture is correlated to the severity of dementia.
- In Lincolnshire in the UK patients with dementia were found to have a 44% longer length of stay on orthopaedic wards than non-demented patients.

Decision-making with trauma and fractures
- Reduce the risk by addressing risk factors detailed above and in 📖 Chapter 11.
- Consider X-ray for fracture in all cases, but especially if frail, frequent falls, signs of fracture, high impact injury, advanced dementia, or poor ability to protect themselves.
- Remember pain expression may be reduced: examine in detail and give adequate analgesia (📖 Chapters 7 and 8).
- If a patient develops a fracture, consider the severity of the dementia, concurrent medical conditions, and likely prognosis in weighing up whether to transfer for surgical intervention.
- Most people should be treated operatively, as in the frail elderly this gives quicker, better pain relief and a better chance of mobilizing or of nursing in comfort.
- Peri-operative analgesia is often poor; discuss with the surgeon and ward staff, or take back early to your institution if possible.
- Nerve blocks are useful for peri-operative analgesia and reducing analgesic consumption. Skin traction can also reduce pain in hip fractures, but patients with dementia may find this hard to understand and maintain.
- In patients too frail to be treated operatively, hip traction or nerve blocks may give adequate analgesia—but assess often, especially in the first days after fracture, and give extra analgesia according to the degree of pain.

Remember the core message!

In deciding about investigation and treatment, weigh up patient and family preferences, legal requirements, ethical issues, and what is known about outcomes, and consult with others if you are still uncomfortable. Know the evidence base, as it may alter the balance of decision-making in ways which at first may seem counterintuitive.

Further reading

Beauchamp TL, Childress JF (2008) *Principles of biomedical ethics*, 6th edn, p. 432. Oxford University Press, Oxford.

General Medical Council (2002) *Withdrawing and withholding life-prolonging treatments*. General Medical Council, London.

General Medical Council (2010) *Treatment and care towards the end of life: good practice in decision making*. General Medical Council, London.

Jonsen AR, Toulmin S (1989) *The abuse of casuistry: a history of moral reasoning*. University of California Press, Berkeley.

Nuffield Council on Bioethics (2009) *Dementia: ethical issues*. Nuffield Council on Bioethics, London.

Royal College of Physicians and British Society of Gastroenterology (2010) *Oral feeding difficulties and dilemmas: a guide to practical care, particularly towards the end of life*. Royal College of Physicians, London.

The terminal phase

Introduction

Entering the dying phase in a terminal illness is the culmination of a process which began, often years before, with diagnosis. It is usually impossible to know how aware the person with far advanced dementia is of their impending death. But the carers and family will have gone through massive change, adaptation, and emotional turmoil over the years in anticipation of this moment. For some, death will bring a sense of relief, or of the satisfaction of having lived out their promise to look after a loved one. But at the end of a long and terminal illness, the final parting is still often associated with emptiness and profound loneliness and loss for those left behind. Managing the death in a dignified, caring, and competent way is of the greatest importance in helping carers and family feel that the life they cherished has come to an end in a fitting manner. It is also of course crucial for patients themselves that they are kept comfortable in this most vulnerable time. But managing the terminal phase well is also important preventively. Deaths perceived as badly handled are common precipitants of mental illness, and in palliative care one frequently meets relatives who, years after a death, are still struggling to put their life together again and have numerous questions arising out of the last days of life. Again, families which have been divided but come together when a loved one is dying will often form new, lasting, strong emotional bonds, but families which remain split at this point may well never heal the rifts.

Late illness awareness

There are times when a person with severe dementia had appeared unresponsive for days and then appeared aware just towards the end of life. Always presume awareness and talk with a patient as you would if they were aware. Doing so will enhance the dignity and respect which you show them.

Case example

Edna was dying at the end of a long illness with dementia. She had been looked after by her daughter with whom she had often fought during the previous months, despite her daughter's excellent attention. As she drifted away into semi-consciousness and became less responsive, her daughter was able to be with her a little longer. Finally, just hours before she died she looked at her daughter, appeared to recognize her and smiled. Huge comfort flowed from this awareness and recognition of her daughters care and presence.

The risk of medicalization of dying

Death is not primarily a medical event but a human event signifying the irretrievable closure of relationships central to people's lives. Medicine needs to play a facilitating role, and to be as unobtrusive as possible, allowing relationships to be centre stage. Paradoxically this is sometimes achieved by more medical intervention: if someone is very agitated, or in severe pain, or very breathless, the anguish this engenders in everybody makes corrective medical action the key to reclaiming the human, personal face of these precious last moments. But for much of the time medicine needs to be practiced competently but in a low key in the background.

- All unnecessary procedures and interventions should be stopped; only those that contribute to somebody's immediate well-being should be continued.
- Problems must be anticipated and prevented whenever possible.
- The means to correct problems that do occur must be immediately at hand.

Advance planning is key to a good death.

Be prepared

Preparation involves both anticipating potential medical problems and setting the scene to deal with social and emotional issues. This implies:

- Getting to know the patient and family as early on as possible, assessing strengths and risks.
- Discussing their fears and wishes around the death. It is useful to enquire about previous experiences of death.
- Finding out about preferred priorities for care and death. Be wary of a misplaced emphasis on place rather than on desired qualities of the care and death. The place chosen may be unavailable, or may not deliver the quality of care desired—things may have changed since the choice was made. Another place might better fulfil the type of care and death desired. All this should be discussed with families when decisions about preferred place of care are talked about. (see 📖 Chapter 13, Elements of decision-making, pp. 236–239).
- Ask the family about any religious and cultural concerns and rituals early on (📖 Chapter 19). This allows one to fulfil the patient's and family's wishes, but also demonstrates respect and amenability. Never assume from somebody's religious or cultural background—people are individuals. Always ask!
- Prescribe emergency drugs in anticipation.
- Have medication and equipment for any likely medical problems on site (📖 Chapter 14, Managing the last few days of life, pp. 261–266). The last thing a family needs in an emergency is medical staff wasting precious hours looking for medication while their loved one suffers.
- Plan staffing needs to move and manage the patient safely and comfortably.
- Procure equipment proactively (hoists, hospital beds, SDs).
- Have a plan, share it with the carers, and with the family if appropriate.

Recognizing approaching death

One cannot deliver good care of the dying unless one is able to recognize when death is near. This is not always easy, especially for those who rarely witness dying, as people will occasionally recover partially from what looks like a terminal event. It can be particularly difficult in advanced dementia, when patients are already very frail and have very restricted physical activity.

Signs of approaching death

Premonitory signs include (*often already present in advanced dementia):
- Withdrawal from active participation in social situations.*
- Increased weakness and lethargy; sleeping through most of the day.
- Reduced verbalization and communication.*
- Loss of interest in feeding or drinking.*
- Restlessness and agitation as one approaches unconsciousness (terminal restlessness; 📖 Chapter 14, Recognizing approaching death, pp. 256–260)
- Sometimes a falling off in urine production.

When the dying process is established further changes occur:
- Deteriorating level of consciousness.
- Sometimes newly developed incontinence of faeces and urine.
- Breathing pattern changes (📖 Chapter 14, Recognizing approaching death, pp. 256–260).
- Loss of control of cutaneous microcirculation.

Terminal restlessness
- Although widely recognized, the definition of this condition is imprecise. It has been defined usefully as 'agitated delirium in a dying patient, frequently associated with impaired consciousness and non-purposeful movement'.[1] It is believed to have a multifactorial aetiology: physical (pain, bladder distension, nicotine withdrawal) and emotional (delirium, anguish at declining faculties, fear of impending death).
- Conditions which may be mistaken for terminal restlessness include delirium and multifocal myoclonus (due to dementia itself, renal failure, opioid toxicity, and other less common causes).
- Terminal restlessness can be differentiated from delirium in a number of ways. Terminal restlessness occurs in the picture of a progressive deterioration and approaching death, whereas delirium can strike unexpectedly, although it too often builds up over time. Delirium is often reversible, whereas terminal restlessness is unlikely to be—but this is only obvious retrospectively. Investigation will often elucidate a cause for delirium, whereas terminal restlessness is part of a profound general decline. In terminal restlessness, the individual is globally intellectually impaired, while many people with delirium will still use comprehensible, if confused, language, and their thought processes may be possible to follow on their own terms even if they appear to us to be unjustified. For example, someone with delirium may suffer

---

1 Kehl KA (2004) Treatment of terminal restlessness: a review of the evidence. *J Pain Palliat Care Pharmacother* **18**, 5–30.

from a delusion that the staff are trying to harm them; if that premise is accepted, their behaviour becomes rational. On the other hand in terminal restlessness there is no logic or unifying belief—it is a global change. Terminal restlessness is often accompanied by anxiety, and restlessness is of course a feature; delirium on the other hand may be hypoactive (see 📖 Chapter 10, Delirium, pp. 174–177).

- Terminal restlessness is particularly taxing for patients and relatives to witness, and needs to be treated aggressively.
- Of course, one can only be sure that restlessness is terminal retrospectively, but by excluding reversible causes and putting it all in the context of the premonitory signs of dying, one can be reasonably certain of the diagnosis.
- It is as unethical to leave people who have no means of protecting themselves to suffer unnecessarily as it is to turn a reversible dip in someone's condition into an irreversible downward spiral by writing them off prematurely. Avoid the temptation to sit on the fence: gather the evidence as best you can, look at it conscientiously in its totality, and then act.
- In serious doubt, seek an opinion from a physician experienced in this field.
- Once someone passes from terminal restlessness to unconsciousness, a sense of peace usually descends, and one can truthfully inform the family that the worst is now over and that it is unlikely that any dramatic changes or new severe symptoms will occur until death (but see 📖 Chapter 14, Managing the last few days of life, pp. 261–266).

> Restlessness and agitation are always signs of physical or mental distress, and always need treating aggressively. Comfortable patients are never restless.

Changes in the final phase (Fig. 14.1)

- By understanding the changes that take place as someone is dying, one can get an idea of when death is more likely to occur. This helps professionals direct care and guide relatives as to what to expect.
- The rate at which people undergo these changes is very individual, and may depend, for example, on somebody's prior state of health, other illnesses they suffer from, and the physiological reserves they still have left.
- Rigid predictions are impossible, particularly in dementia, but tracking the rate of change allows one an informed guess as to how close the end is.

Level of consciousness

- Most chronically ill people die after a period of unconsciousness. Sudden death is unusual, although it is more likely in conditions such as severe breathlessness at rest, severe aspiration, or arrhythmias.
- Descent into unconsciousness is a process of diminishing reactivity to the environment. Interaction with the environment is at first spontaneous (e.g. spontaneous eye opening, verbal responses,

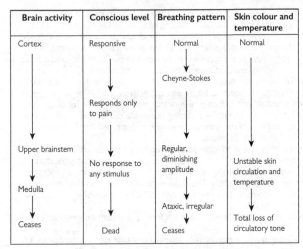

Fig. 14.1 Changes observed during the end stage of life

spontaneous movement), but then occurs only in response to progressively more extreme environmental intrusions into one's inner world: being called by name, being moved, being subjected to pain. A simplified form of the Glasgow Coma Scale (GCS) can be used mentally to monitor the level of consciousness. Deep unconsciousness implies no response to the environment even under extreme provocation (pain).

- Coma suggests extensive damage to both cerebral hemispheres, or damage to the ascending reticular activating system, arising in the brainstem.
- On average the transition from full consciousness to death takes 2–4 days in most people, but it can occur over hours or can take many days.

Breathing pattern

As a person becomes unconscious, their breathing pattern goes through a number of changes which can guide prognosis and appropriate intervention.

- *Spontaneous, regular breathing* of full consciousness gives way to
- *Cheyne–Stokes breathing*: regular, short periods of apnoea alternate with regular, short periods of hyperpnoea in a cyclical manner. As time goes by, the apnoeic periods become longer, occasionally to over 20s. Warn relatives about Cheyne–Stokes breathing beforehand, to prevent them thinking the patient is about to die during the apnoeic periods. Relatives also often experience the hyperpnoeic episodes as their loved one struggling to breathe, and explanation of the automatic nature of this is reassuring. Cheyne–Stokes breathing is supratentorial in origin, starts when a patient is still almost fully conscious, and continues until deep unconsciousness. Just as the gaps in breathing become longer and

longer over several hours, they eventually shorten until the breathing becomes regular again.

- *Regular breathing of deep unconsciousness*: also called central hyperventilation. It occurs when the driver for breathing is the higher brainstem. The breathing is regular, occasionally very rapid, which if distressing to relatives may require intervention (explain that this is not breathlessness but an automatic, brainstem-driven pattern; occasionally give a small dose of i.v. or s.c. midazolam or an opioid to slow down distressing respiration). The patient is by now deeply unconscious, unreactive to external stimuli, and totally unaware of him- or herself. Over hours, the breathing becomes progressively gentler, occasionally becoming so small in amplitude as to be almost undetectable. The lower brainstem is now in control.
- *Ataxic or agonal breathing* occurs in the last few minutes of life, when the breathing becomes totally irregular, unpredictable and gasping, sometimes accompanied by movement of the upper body as it struggles to take in its last breaths. Eventually breathing ceases altogether as the patient dies.

The earlier phases of these changes may be overridden by other breathing patterns, e.g. Kussmaul breathing if acidotic (rapid shallow breathing at first, later becoming deep and slow as acidosis becomes more severe).

Autonomic changes

Skin colour and temperature can become very unstable in deep unconsciousness; skin colour can change rapidly, or different parts of the body can have different appearances. The brainstem is losing its control over the sympathetic adrenergic tone of the cutaneous circulation.

Discussion with relatives

It is good practice to discuss these changes with relatives as soon as there are signs that the end is near. If relatives have been pre-warned of Cheyne–Stokes breathing, central hyperventilation, and skin colour changes they are often less anxious. They particularly appreciate an understanding of the patient's level of consciousness and awareness of them. In advanced dementia, awareness of loved ones may already be very diminished, but this may not be the case in people dying earlier in their illness. In particular, reassure relatives that:

- It is still possible to pick up discomfort in people who are unconscious, as their behaviour changes—they will grimace, or become restless, etc.
- Continuing existing analgesia means people will usually not be in pain. If pain still occurs, it can be easily and adequately controlled.
- Awareness of the environment is hard to judge, though by the time one is brainstem breathing and unreactive, lack of awareness can be assumed. However, it is useful to talk to and touch the dying person, and to only say things in their presence which one would have said if they were conscious.
- Medication for symptom control can now be used freely, if required, as the only aim from now on is maintaining comfort.

Many carers will have been very intimately involved in the care of the dying person, only to find themselves pushed aside as professionals take over. Ask carers how far they would like to be involved in care and leave clear caring roles for them if they wish, e.g. help with mouth care, washing, making beds.

Make sure any young children in the family are not ignored—they are easily forgotten in the general business and distress. Help the parents to support them, and be prepared to explain things to them in a manner suitable to their age.

Managing the last few days of life

Once the diagnosis of dying has been made, the situation needs to be managed to ensure the most comfortable outcome for the patient, maintaining their dignity at all times, and for the relatives. The basic principles are simple:

- Know what to expect (see 📖 Chapter 14, Recognizing approaching death, pp. 256–260 for common symptoms).
- Simplify medication to what is strictly necessary for controlling symptoms at the time. Anything else is burdensome.
- Anticipate problems and have the right medication and equipment in place.
- Have a plan for management and for crises, document it clearly, and share it with all relevant staff and where appropriate with the family.
- Communicate with the family at all stages, imparting information sensitively and geared to their needs at the time.
- Be guided by the family's and by the patient's own past expressed wishes, but take responsibility for any decisions yourself. Families are often in great turmoil; be sensitive as to how much they can and want to be involved in complex decision-making. Do not burden them unfairly. Explain, reply to their questions, explore their attitudes, understand their thinking, but then decide. You have the professional training, experience, and detachment to judge the best means to arrive at the end desired.
- Good care is personal, not formulaic. Visit, and listen.

Stop unnecessary medication

Many drugs will already have been stopped, particularly if the person with dementia has been having difficulty swallowing. Drugs to stop include:

- Diuretics.
- Antihypertensives.
- Cardiac medicines.
- Antidiabetic drugs.
- Antibiotics.
- Usually, steroids, unless essential for comfort, e.g. in some patients with brain tumours. In these rare cases they can be given via a SD, e.g. dexamethasone 8–16mg s.c. over 2 hours every day.

Stop all blood tests, artificial hydration (except in some rare cases where the patient is rapidly losing large volumes of fluid), and artificial nutrition.

Continue essential symptom control drugs

- Continue analgesia and other essential symptom control drugs.
- If the patient has been needing antipsychotic medications it may be risky to stop them now as they are symptom control drugs. Haloperidol can be added to SDs and also acts as an anti-emetic
- If the patient is unable to swallow, give drugs either by repeated injection (usually through a s.c. cannula left in place long term to avoid pricking the patient repeatedly) or through a SD.
- The s.c. route is preferred over i.v. (more difficult to place and maintain, can rarely be maintained at home, more prone to infection)

or i.m. route (needlessly painful, especially if cachectic). *The only occasion where i.v. or i.m. routes are justified in the dying patient is when he or she is in shock, as s.c. drug absorption would be erratic, or with rarely given drugs like phenobarbitone where undiluted s.c. injection can cause skin necrosis.*

- Rectal and buccal routes (ensuring the mouth is moist) may also be useful.
- Prescribe p.r.n. medication for crises. If safe, prescribe dose ranges so that experienced staff can calibrate what they give according to response. See Table 14.1 for some commonly needed p.r.n. drugs and common doses.
- Ensure a supply of drugs in the home. Few things are more inimical to good care than spending precious hours looking around for drugs in an emergency.

Common symptoms

Bubbliness ('the death rattle')

Some series put the frequency of bubbliness in dying patients as high as 60%. It is thought to arise from the oscillations of secretions in the throat (saliva that cannot be swallowed, sputum from the chest) with the inspiration/expiration cycle. It may distress relatives and staff; many patients appear unaware of it.

Management

- *Repositioning:* many nurses believe that sitting someone upright is more likely to reduce bubbliness than other positions, though sometimes the left lateral (recovery) position allows secretions to drain.
- *Suction:* rarely effective; uncomfortable; irritation from suction catheters may worsen secretions. Suctioning is only recommended where thick secretions occlude the throat and obstruct breathing, and even then its use should be limited. Deep suction is very distressing and not warranted.
- *Medication:* anticholinergics can reduce secretions (see Table 14.1). Generally, glycopyrronium or hyoscine butylbromide are to be preferred, as anticholinergic drugs which cross the BBB may worsen confusion and psychotic symptoms, particularly in dementia. Even with optimal management, a large minority of patients (40% in one audit) will remain bubbly. Giving larger doses of anticholinergics may not help in this situation.
- Explanation to relatives about why bubbliness happens and the fact that most patients do not seem to be aware is essential.

Pain

New pains in the terminal stages are uncommon, but old pains will not disappear. In addition, stiffness from lack of spontaneous movement, especially with extensive muscle loss and cachexia, may cause distress. Restlessness signifies discomfort, and pain has to be considered as a possibility. In semi-conscious patients it is sometimes possible to ask very simple questions but much of the time one has to judge whether to use a trial of painkillers if a dying patient appears to be in discomfort (see 📖 Chapters 7 and 8).

Table 14.1 Common emergency drugs used in the terminal phase

Indication	Analgesic	Common doses, route	Notes
Pain Breathlessness at rest Severe dry cough	Morphine sulphate	1–10mg s.c. p.r.n. (or 1/6th of 24h dose—this is a starting rule of thumb to help one titrate p.r.n. analgesia to response). Repeat after 30 minutes if needed. Common doses are 10–120mg s.c./24h via SD (more if needed)	Titrate dose to response—no upper limit. If using higher doses or alternative opioids, seek specialist palliative medicine advice
Colicky pain. Bubbliness	Hyoscine butylbromide	10–20mg s.c. p.r.n. Repeat after 30 minutes if needed. 20–120mg s.c./24h via SD	Colic: waves of pain and restlessness, with pallor, tachycardia, sweating, sickness. Does not cross BBB: no central effects.
Neuropathic pain. Anticonvulsant	Clonazepam	0.5mg s.c. stat. 1–4mg s.c./24h via SD	Compatibility issues common in SD—check. Consider specialist palliative care advice
Bubbliness. Colic	Glycopyrronium	0.2mg s.c. p.r.n. Repeat after 30 minutes if needed. 0.6–1.2mg s.c./24h via SD	Does not cross BBB: no central effects. Takes slightly longer to act than hyoscine, lasts longer
Bubbliness. Colic	Hyoscine hydrobromide ('Hyoscine')	0.4mg s.c. p.r.n. Repeat after 30 minutes if needed. 1.2–2.4mg s.c./24h via SD	Crosses BBB: sedative, anti-emetic, lowers seizure threshold, causes confusion
Sedation. Muscle relaxant. Anticonvulsant	Midazolam	2.5–5mg s.c. (or 1/6th of the 24h dose—see note on morphine). Repeat after 30 minutes if needed. Give 5–10mg s.c. or 5–10mg s.c./buccal p.r.n. for uncontrolled seizures. 10–40mg s.c./24h via SD	Short-acting benzodiazepine. Small doses usually enough for sedation. If prolonged seizures, larger doses may be given sc, im or buccally.

(Continued)

Table 14.1 Continued

Indication	Analgesic	Common doses, route	Notes
Anti-emetic	Cyclizine	50mg s.c. p.r.n. 150mg s.c./24h via SD	Good general purpose anti-emetic. Compatibility issues in SDs common—check.
Anti-emetic	Metoclopramide	10mg s.c. p.r.n. 30–90mg/24h s.c. via SD	AVOID if DLB or PD
Anti-emetic. Sedative (esp. psychotic symptoms, e.g. hallucinations)	Haloperidol	0.5mg s.c. 0.5–3mg/24h s.c. via SD	AVOID if DLB or PD
Anti-emetic. Sedation	Levomepromazine	3–6.25mg s.c. p.r.n. 6.25–12.5mg s.c./24h via SD. For heavy sedation, use 25–100mg/24h	AVOID if DLB or PD. May cause serious postural hypotension at higher doses

Management (see Chapter 8 for detailed guidance):
- Motorized beds enable easier changes of position and can be very useful for improving comfort and ease care.
- Pressure-relieving mattresses cut discomfort down significantly. Turning and repositioning on a regular basis is essential to reduce stiffness—joints and skin become uncomfortable if they are not moved. Moving stiff joints passively may help, although one has to judge the appropriateness of this in a dying patient. Do not underestimate simple things like ensuring smoothed sheets, well-positioned pillows, and clear catheters. Moving someone with an inadequate number of staff can be extremely uncomfortable; equipment such as hoists may also be needed, and an assessment of this is part of the preparation for the dying phase.
- When required analgesics should be given s.c. through a SD, or as stat doses, or via skin patches if the patient was previously on painkillers. TD patches take a long time to establish a stable serum level (12–16 hours for some, longer for other longer-lasting patches; see Chapter 8, Strong opioids, pp. 116–125), so they should not be introduced at this time but only used if put on a few days earlier.
- Use Appendix 5 to work out rough equivalent doses of medication.
- Morphine is often the ideal analgesic to give.
- Be sure not to undertreat pain.
- Most people with dementia require very low doses of analgesia, and the use of very low-dose opioids is very unlikely to be associated with serious risk.

- Avoid pethidine. It is too short-acting (2–3 hours) and may worsen confusion and agitation and increases the risk of seizures.
- For colic, e.g. bowel obstruction, constipation, use anticholinergics.
- If the patient had been on oral drugs for neuropathic pain (e.g. antidepressants, anticonvulsants), consider clonazepam in a SD. Obtain specialist palliative care advice in these complex situations.

Restlessness and agitation

Terminal restlessness (📖 Chapter 14, Recognizing approaching death, pp. 256–260) is ongoing in character over a few hours or days. Restlessness may also occur if there is discomfort, pain, fear or anxiety.

- Treat the cause, e.g. pain, urine retention (catheterize), loaded rectum (suppositories, enemas, or, if these are inappropriate, heavier sedation).
- Midazolam is a short-acting benzodiazepine suitable for short-term sedation. It can be given s.c. or buccally (Table 14.1).
- Midazolam or clonazepam can also be used if a patient has been on an anticonvulsant to prevent seizures, Fairly high doses would have to be used, e.g. midazolam 30mg/24 hours, which is almost certain to render the patient unconscious. This should be explained to relatives beforehand, along with the risk of seizures if an anticonvulsant is not used.
- Patients who have been on antipsychotics which they cannot now take could have haloperidol added to their SD if necessary and not contraindicated, e.g. DLB. If death is truly imminent, this is less of a contraindication. Alternatively, heavy sedation with benzodiazepines, e.g. midazolam, may be needed. Small doses of benzodiazepines do not have an affect on psychotic symptoms and the distress they cause.
- For people whose agitation does not settle with high doses of midazolam, consider levomepromazine or occasionally, phenobarbitone via a SD. In such cases, seek specialist palliative medicine advice.

Mouth care

- A dry mouth and coated tongue is a common problem at the end stage of life due to a combination of reasons: open mouth breathing, reduced hydration, the use of anticholinergic and other drugs etc.
- This can be extremely uncomfortable.
- Good nursing care with regular cleaning of the mouth with mouth sponges (up to every 2 hours), moistening with water, judicious spraying of saliva substitutes into the mouth, and the application of a very thin layer of petroleum jelly to the lips, not forgetting the corners of the mouth, can make a great difference. Relatives can be encouraged to participate in this.
- There is no evidence that artificial hydration at this stage of life reduces the dryness of the mouth or increases comfort.

Urinary problems

- Catheterize if in acute retention, as it can be intensely painful.
- Bypassing catheters with restlessness may signify bladder spasm, which responds to an anticholinergic or changing to a *smaller* catheter.
- Urinary incontinence will need a catheter, conveen, or padding. Choose the least intrusive means that will do the job.

The question of resuscitation

See ⬚ Chapter 20, Care at home, pp. 340–348.

Case study

Nancy, a 76-year-old woman with VaD, deteriorated at home over a 6-month period. She was now bedbound, needing total care from her daughter and carers. She no longer recognized her family and was unable to communicate. She was on sodium valproate 200mg b.d. to prevent seizures. Her pain from osteoarthritis was controlled with a 20mcg/h buprenorphine transdermal patch. End of life care drugs and a SD had been delivered to her home.

A call from the daughter informed the nurse that Nancy had become bubbly and unable to swallow medication. On visiting it was clear she was now unconscious, had audible chest secretions, and was twitching down the left side. A DN had given midazolam 2.5mg s.c. twice during the night for agitation, ?seizure, but this wore off after 3 hours.

A SD was set up with midazolam 20mg (for agitation and to replace the valproate) and gylcopyrronium 0.6mg in water for injection to run over 24 hours (see ⬚ Chapter 14, Mana-gement of syringe drivers, pp. 270–271). There was no need for analgesia in the driver as the buprenorphine patch was controlling her pain. As she was currently symptomatic, a stat dose of midazolam 2.5mg and glycopyrronium 0.2mg s.c was given for agitation, to stop twitching and to alleviate bubbly secretions

The rationale for changes was explained to the daughter.

Morphine sulphate 2.5mg p.r.n. was prescribed, should more pain occur. Regular assessment 4–8 hourly by DNs was kept up. Medication was assessed daily, and stat doses given were discussed to decide if they needed to be added to her regular medication from the following day.

NB: If the patient is symptomatic, always give stat doses of medication, as it takes time for the medication administered via a SD to become effective.

The Liverpool Care Pathway for the dying patient[2]

The Liverpool Care Pathway (LCP) provides a template of care for the very last few days of life, incorporating the above principles into a document so that key features are not missed, and allows audit to improve quality of care. Its implementation is a cornerstone of the National End of Life Care Programme. It can be used in hospitals, in the community, in hospices and in care homes.

However, the LCP was never envisaged as a standalone document, but rather as a tool in a wider and deeper context of improving care of the dying. Therefore, to implement the LCP a number of steps are highly recommended:

• Gaining specialist palliative care support and executive endorsement for the implementation of the LCP in that environment.
• Registration and training of the coordinator with the LCP central team in Liverpool (Marie Curie Palliative Care Institute Liverpool, MCPCIL). This allows the coordinator to receive support and benefit from previous experience in implementing the LCP in other contexts.
• Setting up a local steering group, and producing local documentation.
• Carrying out a base review of the documentation of dying in a number of patients (20 is recommended).
• Running an education programme before initial pilot site implementation.
• When the pathway is implemented, maintaining competencies by reflective practice and post-pathway analysis.
• Ongoing education and training of staff.
• Eventually, ensuring that all those carrying out care of the dying are trained to do this and that the LCP is used as part of the clinical governance setup locally.

The use of the LCP without adequate preparation and supervision can lead to misinterpretation and poor care. The premise of the LCP is that imminent dying has been diagnosed, and yet this can be at times very difficult. There are no easy criteria by which dying can be definitely diagnosed or ruled out; it needs experience, judgment, and the ability to see the whole picture. MCPCIL recommends that people are only put on the LCP when the multidisciplinary team is in agreement that they are indeed entering their very last few days of life. As with other instruments, misuse can lead to harm, e.g. when the appropriateness of the LCP for a patient who has survived longer than anticipated is not reviewed.

The LCP provides guidance on:
• Comfort measures.
• Anticipatory prescribing of medicines.
• Discontinuation of inappropriate interventions, and reviewing treatment.
• Psychological and spiritual care.

2 Liverpool Care Pathway for the Dying Patient: http://www.mcpcil.org.uk/liverpool-care-pathway/index.htm

- Care of the family (both before and after the death of the patient).
- Implementing the LCP implies a multidisciplinary approach to end of life care.

Clinicians also need to consider the administration of and need for ongoing fluids. These are not necessary if the patient is imminently dying but need careful consideration if there is doubt about the diagnosis of imminent death.

After death has occurred

- Confirm death if required, and complete the death certificate. Include dementia as the cause or contributory cause of death.
- Explain to the family and leave clear written instructions about the procedures needed, e.g. for registering death.
- Offer to meet family members again if they have outstanding questions about events surrounding the illness and death.
- Offer information about local bereavement services.
- Screen family members for bereavement risk. Advise those at risk to seek specialist bereavement support, and inform the GP with their permission.
- Be mindful of potentially suicidal relatives: inform the GP and psychiatric services if high risk. You must do this even if they withhold consent.

See 📖 Chapter 15 for more information on bereavement.

Management of syringe drivers (SDs)

What is a SD?

A SD is a small portable battery-operated pump which slowly delivers drugs to the patient by continuous s.c. infusion over a set period of time. It is commonly used in palliative care when the oral route is no longer possible. There are several different pumps in use and practice varies from area to area. Please consult your own local policy and guidelines.

NB: It is imperative that the rationale for using the SD is explained to family, carers, and at times health care professionals who may be unfamiliar with their use and perceive this as a last resort in trying to control symptoms.

Why use a SD?

- For control of persistent nausea and vomiting.
- Intestinal obstruction.
- Severe dysphagia.
- When the patient is too weak to swallow.
- Unconscious patient.
- Poor absorption of drugs (rare).
- Poor patient compliance.

What are the advantages?

- A 24-hour infusion achieves constant plasma concentration, avoiding peaks and troughs in symptom control.
- Multiple symptoms can be controlled with a combination of drugs.
- Avoids the use of intermittent injections.

What are the disadvantages?

- Local skin reactions:
  - Inflammation/swelling or bleeding at the cannula site, especially with certain drugs at higher concentrations (cyclizine, levomepromazine).
- Mechanical problems:
  - Battery not working, infusion lines can become disconnected or kinked.
- Loss of flexibility if only changed every 24 hours.
- Compatibility problems with some drug combinations.
- Training for staff.

NB: For detailed compatibility of drugs in SDs see Dickman et al.[1]

If using a SD

- Remember to consult local policy. There are now a number of different SDs in use (e.g. Graseby, McKinley), so that detailed instructions cannot be given that would apply to all.
- Never set up a SD unless you feel fully competent.
- Explain to the patient and family about the use of the SD in advance and show them the equipment.
- Consent the patient (if they have capacity).
- Educate patient and carer
  - How it works/what to check.
  - What to do if they are worried (who to contact).

- Provide reassurance about giving the same drug doses by another route.
- Discuss with patient and family rationale for medication changes or increases.

On-going care of the patient with a SD

- Ensure that all drug regimes are correctly written up by a doctor or suitably qualified non-medical prescriber. Patients' symptoms should be assessed 4 hourly. If symptomatic a stat dose of s.c. medication will be needed.
- Check infusion site and look for:
  - Redness
  - Oedema
  - Bleeding
  - Moisture beneath dressing around cannula site.
- Re-site cannula if necessary.
- If the drug is irritant to the skin the following may help:
  - Dilute the solution as much as is practicable
  - The SD can be changed every 12 hours to allow further dilution if needed.
  - Hydrocortisone 1% cream can be applied to the skin around the cannula site.
  - Dexamethasone 1mg can be added to SD.
  - Rotate the site more frequently (non-irritant site can last for ≥7 days).
  - Change cannula from steel butterfly to Teflon cannula.
- Check that the pump is still working.
- Check the rate is set correctly and the correct amount has been infused in the last 4 hours.
- Note solution in syringe, e.g. precipitation/crystallization.
- If the alarm sounds:
  - Check that the tubing is not kinked, cannula/tubing is not blocked, if crystallized, replace tubing and increase amount of diluents (the SD will need to be completely redone).
  - The SD may be empty.
  - Malfunction of driver (change to new pump).

Reference

1 Dickman A, Littlewood C, Varge J (2005) *The syringe driver. continuous subcutaneous infusions in palliative care*, 2nd edn. Oxford University Press, Oxford.

Chapter 15

Bereavement

Introduction

'The cost of commitment'
Dr Colin Murray Parkes

Looking after the terminally ill does not end with their death. Because the family (in its broadest sense) is the unit of care, palliative care also involves itself with care of the bereaved.

Anyone in palliative care will have seen many people who are themselves dying who suffer a bereavement; they will be struck by how often the pain of this overshadows the pain of cancer, for example, and the distress of their own impending demise. Bereavement is an extraordinarily powerful experience.

People with dementia frequently suffer bereavements themselves. Sometimes they will remember this and suffer a sense of profound shock and bewilderment. At other times losing the company of a loved one may not be recalled or understood, but the absence of that person may still have strong emotional effects. In either case it can affect their behaviour and care profoundly. Our understanding of this process is in its infancy.

Carers and family members of someone with dementia suffer from severe grief both while the illness progressively removes the person's abilities and also when the person with dementia dies. The relationship of carers with the deceased will often have been particularly long and intimate, not just from their past life, but from a very intense involvement in their illness, so the feelings may be acute. The sense of emptiness may be coupled with relief that the suffering of the person who has died is over, and often with a sense of a load lifted from one's shoulders if one has been the main carer. Many skills learned from being a carer suddenly have no outlet, and one's role is no longer clearly defined. Personal memories become very private, as the other person who embodied them, despite themselves having no recall of them, is now gone forever. All the time previously tied up with the care of the person who has died is suddenly freed up. The carer may find that their total absorption in care, often for years, means that they have left behind many of their commitments and relationships outside the home, making the void particularly stark. However, there is often a strong sense that no one can fill the place of the person who has died. One's world becomes a lot lonelier, and a large part of it which used to be shared with someone important suddenly becomes only one's own, which no one else will ever quite understand. For many, bereavement brings intense sadness and disorientation.

Theories of grief and bereavement

Stage-based models of bereavement

- Various models of bereavement have evolved over the past 50 years.
- Early models (Kübler-Ross, Parkes, Worden) tended to be stage-based, seeing the bereaved person go through a number of stages to resolution. The authors never intended their stages to be conceived rigidly, but inevitably this often happened, as people with less experience and nuanced thinking fitted those they were 'helping' into artificial schemas.
- No model of grieving will explain what everyone goes through. Models need to be used to develop one's understanding, not to become straitjackets into which people's experience is made to fit. Good theory can help one proceed in a sensible way in an unfamiliar situation. Theory is not a substitute for sensitivity, but should be an aid to it.

Kübler-Ross

- In 1969, Elisabeth Kübler-Ross, in her book *On death and dying*, described five stages of adapting to terminal illness (denial, anger, bargaining, depression, and acceptance) which were later applied to bereavement.
- The importance of this model now is its hold on public perception. People will often say they are going through an angry phase or have reached acceptance. Kübler Ross always intended her stages to be seen as individual, and recognized that people could oscillate from one stage to another and back intermittently, or miss certain stages altogether. Her work provided one of the first coherent and useful theoretical underpinnings of grief, and raised it back into popular consciousness, but its picture is now recognized as simplistic.

Colin Murray Parkes

- Colin Murray Parkes, a psychiatrist at the Royal London Hospital and St Christopher's Hospice in London, probably did more than anyone to establish the study of bereavement on a scientific and theoretical basis.
- In his book *Bereavement* (1972), Parkes proposed a model of grief based on a change in the nature of attachment to the person who had died. In his model, the bereaved person goes through a number of stages:
  - *Shock and numbness*. The first few days after death are characterized by a sense of unreality, depersonalization, and emotional anaesthesia.
  - *Yearning and searching*. The bereaved person has intense longing for the missing loved one, and looks for them everywhere. People often describe seeing someone in the street who they are sure is the person who died, only to realize that it is someone who looks similar. They may have intense feelings of the presence of the dead person.
  - *Disorganization and despair*. The realization that the loss is irrevocable throws the bereaved into an intense awareness of this void that cannot be filled. The pain is very acute, and very strong feelings are sparked off by minor day-to-day events. The bereaved

person's concentration suffers, they become forgetful, and may neglect themselves or others, as everything seems trivial next to the aching loss.

- *Reorganization.* The loss is eventually assimilated, with a reframing of the place of the person who has died. The feeling of loss never goes, and acute feelings can still be sparked off by memories, anniversaries, or everyday events, but in general, the bereaved picks up the threads of a life that is now reconfigured in a newly coherent way despite the loss.

- Parkes' other major contributions include his definition of normal and abnormal grief and an elucidation of some of the factors which increase one's risk of maladaptive grief.

- Abnormal grief is defined as grief which is unusually prolonged and accompanied by depressive or anxiety disorders or other health conditions.

- There has been a reaction against this conception of bereavement because it can lead to the medicalization of grieving at the expense of social factors. However, there is no doubt that some grief is associated with serious physical and mental illness. By identifying those more likely to develop major problems, one can target appropriate help and preventive work.

Table 15.1 Risk factors for complicated bereavement

Type of death: traumatic, sudden or unexpected death, multiple deaths
Uncertain death: absence of body of deceased
Relationship with the person who died: dependence, conflict
Concurrent major life stressors, e.g. loss of role or income
Ill-health of the survivor, especially if dependent on the deceased for care
Economic or social insecurity and hardship
Multiple previous losses
Perceived social isolation
Unsupportive families
Past depression, anxiety, or other serious mental health problems
Post-traumatic stress disorder
Drug or substance abuse
Pessimistic orientation
Younger age at bereavement
Male sex

William Worden

Worden, a psychologist at Harvard, in *Grief counselling and grief therapy* (1983) presented a number of tasks of grief. Grieving people need to:

- Accept the reality of the loss.
- Work through the pain of grief.
- Adjust to a different environment.
- Relocate the deceased and move on in life.
- Grief counselling has corresponding functions:
- To increase the reality of the loss.
- To help the counselled person deal with expressed and latent affect.
- To help the bereaved person overcome the impediments to adjustment to loss.
- To encourage the bereaved to say goodbye and become able to reinvest themselves in life.

However grief is not unitary, with one purpose and direction, and this model, while useful, again is limited in its reach.

More recent models of grief

- More recent models of grief have shed the stage-based approach, pointing out that there are many different ways in which individuals grieve, and that one's grieving pattern can alter over time. The idea of a single orientation, goal, or direction in grieving has been superseded.
- Such models emphasize the differences in the grieving process at different stages of life, between different people, and in different cultures and the need to personalize our understanding of grief.
- Men and women often grieve differently, although most people have mixtures of both coping styles. Women tend to have wider social networks, express emotion more openly, and seek and obtain more emotional support. Men, on the other hand, tend to deal with loss in a more problem-orientated, cognitive, and often private way. This has implications for bereavement and bereavement support. In the past, there was a tendency to provide support which explored the emotional while brushing aside a practical orientation as a distraction from the grief work that had to be done. There is a growing recognition that support needs to be delivered in the style of the person needing support. 'Male' problem-solving behaviour often works with other losses, but the permanence of loss in bereavement may mean that what has usually been an effective way of working through loss no longer works well. One is then left facing a devastating situation with no tried and tested model for approaching it. Equally, though, there is little evidence that emotionally orientated behaviour alone helps one cope with loss of a spouse.
- There is now a stronger realization that bereavement work needs to have both an emotional and a cognitive orientation. Margaret and Wolfgang Stroebe pointed out how people who are grieving tend to oscillate back and forth between times of profound grieving, where they feel intensely any or all the feelings of loss, anger, etc. (bereavement orientation), to times of restoration orientation, focusing on the rebuilding of the self.

- Men are also more likely to react to bereavement through self-harming behaviours, such as heavy drinking. In many partnerships, women play an important part in their spouse's positive health behaviours, and the loss of this also increases risk of bereaved men's health suffering.
- Attachment theory looks at styles of attachment developed through life experiences, especially during childhood, and how the coping styles these engender tend to be reproduced when facing the insecurity of loss in later life. Some people are insecure, anxious, and clingy; others are afraid of rejection, so avoid closeness; others still become deeply depressed, anxious, or disorganized, and may be at high risk of self-harm. More secure individuals still develop these traits, but are able to return more easily to a sense of stability and security.
- This has led to a surge of interest in resilience in the face of life's traumas. Can one develop supportive styles which foster resilience?
- Resilience and recovery are distinct. In recovery, the disruption in one's life is high after the loss but slowly comes back to a low level. In resilient individuals, there is less disruption from much earlier on, and they are still able to function in their relationships or at work despite the loss.
- The relationships lost by resilient individuals appear to be similar to those of people who are less able to cope, suggesting that resilience is a quality of the person, not the type of loss. Low self-esteem, dependency on the partner, and sudden death are linked to low resilience. Some researchers have found that resilient individuals have a more complex emotional experience, suggesting that resilience does not result from denial or rigidity but from being able to include and adapt. Resilient individuals do not bury the sense of loss but are able to continue functioning while grieving. 'It's hard, but I can cope'.
- Other theories are based on the effect bereavement has on one's narrative of life, the story one tells oneself about the meaning and direction of one's life. This has been called one's assumptive world—one could call this one's personal theory of oneself. Bereavement suddenly shatters the plot one has constructed over many years and brings this assumptive world into conflict with the world as newly perceived—insecure, painful, unpredictable, and meaningless. Narrative theory looks at ways in which the bereaved can be assisted to rebuild a new narrative of their lives which includes the loss.

There are clearly two broad models of bereavement and bereavement care.

- The more 'medical' model looks at risk factors and recovery. This runs the risk of pathologizing normal human experience, squeezing people into boxes so they fit classifications, and elevating the role of the expert without whom it is difficult for people to work through their problems. Equally, it is now clear that risk factors (e.g. multiple past losses) put some individuals at risk while in others they build resilience and experience in handling crises. Risk factors are clearly not the full story.
- On the other side is a more personalized, fluid orientation emphasizing resilience and the personal reconstruction of a coherent narrative to make sense of the deep losses one has gone through. There can be something trite about resilience theory—the idea that resilient people

do better after loss is a rather circular one. It is clear that we need to move towards long-term social changes that build resilience. But it is not yet as clear how one can promote resilience in the short term in people who have little of it and are facing massive loss. The key probably lies in harnessing existing skills, relationships, and creativity, but that can be very difficult in individuals beset by deep depression and feelings of panic whose trust in the future has been shattered. More exploration of factors that promote resilience and evidence of how these can be nurtured in acute situations is proceeding. What is certain is that, by restituting an emphasis on social factors in helping people manage grief and bereavement, and by again making grief a normal event rather than an illness, such stances have restored a very important balance.

- The 'medicalized' approach emphasizes risk and vulnerability factors; the 'personalised' approach stresses characteristics that are likely to promote adjustment. It is likely that the two approaches will in future be seen to be complementary rather than opposing, although there are clearly elements in each which are incompatible. Bereavement is not an illness, but it can have very detrimental mental and physical consequences.

Bereavement in people with dementia

'*Understanding the concept of death is not a prerequisite for experiencing the emotions associated with grieving*'
Dodd (2005)

- People with dementia may experience the loss of someone close to them. Equally, old bereavements may seem to them as if they had just happened and cause distress anew.

- The clarity with which people can grasp and contextualize the information varies with the type and stage of dementia. For example orientation to time: some case reports describe people with dementia whose spouse died, who rapidly developed delusions that it was their parent who had died.

- Staff of residential care facilities and family members often shy away from talking about the bereavement because of a fear of distressing the person or because they feel they lack the skills to do it. They may also minimize reactions to the death or misinterpret behavioural changes.

- The literature on the experience of bereavement in people with dementia is limited. Much can be learned from the more extensive literature on bereavement in people with learning difficulties. However, there are clear differences. People with dementia tend to be older and to have had more experience of death and its rituals than people with intellectual disability, and hence may have a more embedded understanding of the meaning of death. The memories of people with learning disabilities are often better.

- It has been suggested that people with intellectual disability might be more susceptible to complicated grief, because they face more associated secondary losses (loss of a carer in a dependent individual, financial insecurity, placement in care at short notice), barriers to communicating about the loss, and difficulty finding meaning in the loss. There is no clear evidence that this is so.

- There is no prospective long-term study of grief in people with dementia. In learning disability, grief is associated with increased psychological disorder, but most of it also common to other grieving individuals. Whether grief increases psychopathology in this context is unclear, although evidence suggests that people with intellectual disability often suffer more prolonged grieving. It is not known whether bereavement increases BPSD in dementia.

- In an Irish study, people with intellectual disability had more complicated grief symptoms if they had taken part in more rituals after the death (seeing the body, attending the funeral). This seems counterintuitive, as it is believed that in people with no cognitive impairment, rituals aid adjustment. However, the authors point out that this might have been the first time the person with intellectual disability attended a funeral, so this experience would heighten the sense of strangeness rather than provide comfort in familiarity. A ritual is not a ritual when it is strange and new. There is no published evidence on whether involvement in rituals has an impact on people with dementia, although participation in rituals from their past does seem to be very evocative in other contexts.

- People with dementia may forget that the deceased person had died and persistently ask for them and enquire when they are coming to visit. This can be very painful for grieving family members, and the distress of the person with dementia every time they are told the news again is fresh and raw
- The decision as to when and what to tell the person with dementia is a difficult one. They have a right to know but also to be protected from things they cannot handle. Every choice should be personalized. However, the question is not if they should know but when and how.
- It is remarkable how often the loss is remembered when so little else seems to be. It is as if the emotional impact sears it deeper in the memory.

Case study

Marg, aged 96 with advanced AD, and her sister Dot, 92, left their family home to move into a nursing home when care for Marg became too much. Marg repeatedly asked her sister if they could go home, to sit by the fire with their mother and sisters. This upset them both, as Dot had to tell Marg several times a day that her mother and sisters died years ago. Both were usually in tears, with Marg becoming quite agitated at times. The carer saw their distress and explained that Marg's short-term memory was poor and that this was the reason for the repetitive questions and that her memory was back to when her mother and sisters were alive. She suggested, to alleviate the distress, so that Dot was not reliving the event as new, to respond by saying that they would see their sister and mother shortly. Reorientation to distressing events in the advanced stages can be futile and harmful.

Handling bereavement in people with dementia

- Convey information about the death clearly, simply and without euphemisms. These can confuse even cognitively intact people, and people with dementia think very concretely.
- Provide the information within a supportive context. Take time to answer questions, ensure there are family members, friends, or particularly close members of staff to provide continued support.
- Provide concrete objects which remind them of the lost person. These may make them feel closer to the dead person, and may also help anchor and jog memory. These could be pictures, belongings, or furniture that the person with dementia will have associated with the deceased.
- Frequent reality orientation may be useful, by bringing the person into the conversation and the fact that they have died. It would seem particularly important that family members talk to the person with dementia about the dead person and include them in the grieving process. However, it is equally important not to bring this up all the time, and to change tack if the news is clearly very distressing as if new every time it is mentioned. It is useful to reinforce the fact that

someone has died so it is remembered, but not to keep imparting this as a new fact again and again.
- Carers often are not aware how long grieving can take—months or years—and may expect people to 'pull themselves together' after a few weeks.
- The caring team must also support family members through this process. On top of their own grief they have the grief of someone whose understanding is fragmented and whose reactions may be repeatedly overwhelming.
- A small RCT suggested that bereavement counselling provides significant improvement in mental health in people with intellectual disability, and that volunteer bereavement counsellors quickly learn how to adapt their style to these situations. No similar studies have been done in dementia. One would expect the results to vary widely according to the stage of dementia.

Bereavement in carers of people with dementia

- Carers of people with dementia will often have invested enormous physical and emotional energy in caring, and when the person they cared for dies, they may be exhausted, alone, and with little support.
- Their previously clear caring role, which may have been burdensome but provided a strong sense of being very needed by someone they loved, disappears, and the skills they developed over years of caring suddenly have no outlet. Above this is the loss of someone with whom a life was shared through thick and thin.
- Grieving for a person with dementia starts while they are still alive, as they lose more and more of the qualities which defined their relationships. This anticipatory grief involves a loss of the shared past as the person's memory fades; a taking over of roles by the spouse or other family member; a loss of the shared present as fewer and fewer habitual activities are shared; and at times shock at unaccustomed behaviour such as agitation or violence. Towards the end of life, many people with dementia become very limited, unable to talk or feed or move independently. Carers also suffer loss of their own freedom, of many social relationships, and of their planned future. Caring for someone with dementia involves a long period of incremental loss.
- Some studies have shown more sadness, guilt, regret, and frustration in spouses of people with dementia in care homes, and more anger in spouses of people cared for at home. A perception of good care in care homes was associated with better adjustment after death.
- A recent study found that risk of pre-death grief was higher in relatives who had lived with the person before nursing home admission, who were less satisfied with care provided in the home, who had more depressive symptoms, or where the person with dementia was younger.
- Anticipatory grief is high in the early stages of illness, then settles to a more stable level, but again rises towards the last months of life.
- More severe anticipatory grief has been linked to less grief after the death, although the evidence on this is mixed, some even suggesting a short-term improvement just after death followed by intense grieving in the longer term.
- A US study by Meuser and Marwit comparing experiences of spouse and adult children caregivers showed that in the early stages of illness, children of people with dementia were much more likely to be involved in collusive denial with their parent, whereas spouses tended to be more open and accepting of the dementia and its implications for the person with the illness and for them. In the mid-stages of disease, children's realization of their parents' illness was accompanied by intense emotion, with anger, jealousy at healthy older people, and guilt about a wish their parent would die. Emotions so far suppressed often erupted. In spouses, progression was accompanied by a more linear increase in sadness and in empathy and compassion. They rarely shared the sense of unwanted burden experienced by children carers. Nursing home placement, usually at the advanced stage of illness, was accompanied by a release from a sense of burden and a mellowing and

increased empathy and sadness in children; but in spouses it intensified the feelings of guilt. In spouses, grieving increases in parallel with the progression of the illness, while in children the middle stages are usually the worst. At the end stage spouses also experience a greater sense of their own loss as, for example, they become decoupled from their spouse. The authors suggest gentle education of children-carers about the illness at early stages and attention to anger management techniques in the middle stages; while support groups and help towards independent living may benefit spouses.

- A care-giving role is not only a source of burden and stress. A comparison of former carers and former non-caring relatives showed better long-term well-being in the carer group. For many, the caring role is a fulfilment of a promise made decades earlier, and is carried with pride and satisfaction despite the innumerable difficulties.

- Evidence regarding carers after the death of a family member is more limited. Depression levels in carers fall after death, especially if the person with dementia had not been placed in a care home. Those in whom emotional distress was high before death appear to suffer even more distress afterwards, whereas stability before death is associated with continuing stability afterwards. Role overload has negative prognostic implications, while good psychosocial support and self-esteem are protective.

- Grief and depression are distinct entities. Psychotherapy and antidepressants reduce depression in bereaved dementia caregivers without reducing grief. 16–25% of bereaved carers are depressed months to a year after the death, with depression while caregiving, lower income, greater caregiver burden, less family support, and adverse health behaviours increasing depression risk.

- A combination of brief individual and family counselling intervention, participation in support groups, and ad hoc counselling fairly early in the course of dementia results in less depression both before and for up to a year after death. This intervention was found to significantly increase the number of resilient carers.

Providing bereavement support

- So far the bereavement support of carers of people with dementia has been haphazard, and most carers are left without support once the person dies. A more proactive stance is warranted, as is more research to understand the particular issues affecting this group.
- Bereavement is a normal process, and most bereaved people do not need professional support. There is evidence that intervention focused on problematic bereavements achieves useful outcomes, but unselected intervention does not.
- If possible, starting well before the person with dementia dies, assess carers for risk factors and explore their coping styles. By getting to know carers this can be achieved informally.
- After death, official procedures, e.g. death certificates, have to be sorted out, and the family needs to contact a funeral director. Relatives find written information about what they need to do, e.g. how to register the death, very helpful, as the newly bereaved may retain little complex information. Ask whether they have questions about the death or illness, and offer to see them again at a later date should any issues crop up.
- In the initial periods, the best support is to be there and listen. Respond to the content and emotional tone, but let the bereaved person talk freely.
- As far as possible, utilize the bereaved's own network of resources, if necessary supporting them to carry out this role. While for the first few days after death help is often abundant, after the funeral this may fizzle away leaving the bereaved person alone. Time by oneself is important to take in what has happened, but prolonged isolation is not good. Friends and family, primary care, voluntary organizations, self-help, and church groups can all provide practical and emotional support.
- Normalize reactions in bereavement that people might find strange, such as the tendency to see or hear the voice of the person who has died. The bereaved need to be reassured that this is normal and does not mean they are not coping or are going mad.
- Assist people to realize that there is no map for getting through grief—we all struggle, as the experience is different for each of us. At times one is lost and does not know whether one is doing the right thing, and that is not because one is doing it wrong. However, this is also a time when people discover personal resources they never knew they had, and support must be geared to enable people to tap these resources.
- If you have concerns that a bereaved person is finding the situation overwhelming, consider referral to a local bereavement support service. GPs, hospices, and Primary Care Trusts (PCTs) may have contact details for these. However, not all bereavement services operate in similar ways, and you should satisfy yourself that the kind of support provided is well thought out.
- When serious psychological issues occur, e.g. major depression, severe anxiety, or alcoholism, refer to a psychologist or psychiatrist. Consider risk factors and coping styles in deciding.

- In people who are depressed, always ask about thoughts of self-harm and suicide. Confidentiality does not apply when there is a serious risk of self harm: discuss urgently with the GP or psychiatric team.

Further reading

Dodd P, Guerin S, McEvoy J, Buckley S, Tyrrell J, Hillery J (2008) A study of complicated grief symptoms in people with intellectual disabilities. *J Intellect Disabil Res* **52**, 415–25.

Meuser TM, Marwit SJ (2001) A comprehensive, stage-sensitive model of grief in dementia caregiving. *Gerontologist* **41**, 658–70.

Stroebe M, Schut H, Stroebe W (2007) Health outcomes of bereavement. *Lancet* **370**, 1960–73.

Chapter 16

Communication

Introduction

Good communication is at the heart of good dementia care. Patients with dementia communicate less easily, understand less easily, and respond to advice and support less easily. Communication with family and friends is also crucial, as is the ability to discuss and explain bad news. Sharing information with other professionals is an essential part of good clinical care and there are simple rules to enable this to be done well and effectively.

Effect of dementia on the quality of communication

- Dementia causes inability to both communicate and to understand. These abilities are lost relatively early on in the course of the illness.
- This makes dementia somewhat different from most other conditions where palliative care is provided.
- Dementia also causes a reduced ability to integrate, understand, and process information. Therefore what is said is not only quickly forgotten but may also be responded to in a different way. For example, a good and sensible explanation about the need to take blood or dress an ulcer may not overcome the reluctance of the patient to accept a brief period of pain or discomfort.
- Complex suggestions which are less easily understood may appear more threatening and be resisted vigorously.
- Dementia will often reduce the ability of the person to express themselves. Patients may be unable to make their requests known to staff, or may simply lack the skills or authority to make staff listen to their requests.
- There is also a high incidence of dysphasia in dementia, even in the early stages, which often leads to intense frustration on the part of both dementia sufferers and their carers.
- Difficulties with facial expression and the ability to gesticulate as a part of normal conversation further reduces the ability of the person with dementia to express themselves.
- Finally, frailty itself may reduce a person's ability to communicate and may also reduce the likelihood of care staff listening to what is said.

Maintained ability to communicate but without capacity

A minority of people with dementia may be able to argue persuasively and coherently the case for what they want, when they are entirely unable to understand the reasons why it is not possible. This can present a huge challenge; a verbal and persuasive individual may make a strong case, built entirely upon misunderstanding, for an outcome or intervention which is simply dangerous or unworkable. A common example will be a person who is desperate to go home but unable to understand that at home they will be at risk, alone, and deeply distressed. The rationale for the right care might well be explained but that explanation will be forgotten within minutes.

Often, in such circumstances, as a result of the clarity with which the wish is expressed, professionals may fail to recognize that the patient lacks capacity. As always, where the patient lacks capacity, solutions must be provided in their best interests. But the persuasiveness and passion with which the patient makes their case is always a substantial challenge both emotionally and practically for care workers even when the lack of capacity is clearly noted. Indeed it will sometimes be the case that the desire to respect autonomy in such people will lead to attempts to put in place inappropriate and risky solutions. Even worse, those who see that the person lacks capacity and must be treated in their best interests to avert substantial risks may then be regarded poorly for providing that necessary protection.

Techniques for communicating with people with dementia

- Treat any treatable medical conditions or sensory impairments as this may improve capacity and understanding.
- Pain demands attention[1] and is likely to do this much more in those made already highly distractible by their dementia. Simple analgesics, etc. might help in such circumstances.
- Other physical conditions may reduce the ability to communicate If the dementia causes a fluctuating capacity or understanding, assess the person at the better times.
- Taking a bit more time to have the conversation will produce substantial dividends for many people with dementia. Explain in simple terms and simple language. Maintaining eye contact and waiting for 10–15 seconds will often produce a response when at first there is none. It takes time to absorb and process things in dementia.
- Location matters. If possible see the person at home, or in a quiet place away from the hurly burly of the ward.
- Hold the conversation in a relaxed way in a quiet and calm setting. People who have difficulty understanding will be far more fearful if they are feeling pressured or threatened.
- Sit at the same level as the patient or lower.
- Have the important discussions when someone who the person with dementia trusts is present. A friend or relative may nod or smile approvingly when sensible things are said, supporting the individual
- Explain in simple language and try to educate the person about the decision to be taken: careful setting out of what is known can be effective even in advanced dementia.
- Sometimes, forms of distraction can be used to enable care to be provided. For example, to get someone washed, dressed, or fed, singing a little song, cracking a joke, or talking about something quite irrelevant will be enough to relax that person so that they can accept the care they require.
- There is further discussion of ways of improving communication in the BMA guidance on assessment of capacity.[2]

1 Eccleston C, Crombez G (1999) Pain demands attention: a cognitive-affective model of the interruptive function of pain. *Psychol Bull* **125**, 356–66.
2 British Medical Association (1995) *Assessment of mental capacity, guidance for doctors and lawyers*. British Medical Association, London.

Giving bad news

- There is always a reluctance to give bad news to patients or those who love them. But clinicians have discovered the importance of discussing serious illness such as cancer and its likely outcome with patients. There is now widespread agreement that it is right to tell people they have dementia at an early stage of their illness and thus to allow them to have the right discussions at the right time as a result of that intervention.
- Sharing bad news:
  - Reduces the sense of isolation and unrealistic fears resulting from knowing something is wrong but not knowing what it is.
  - Enables patients and carers to face the future together rather than separately and in isolation.
  - Allows people to plan for the future and make decisions about what they want of their future care.
  - Builds a relationship of trust with professionals, as patients and carers know they are being treated with respect.
  - Treats patients as adults.
- Families will often keep their concerns from the patient and avoid discussion with them. The secret concern about dementia becomes a dire and distressing one which cannot be broached. As a result, the person with dementia becomes excluded from conversations about the most important thing in the family.
- Often enough there will be a discussion with relatives about the diagnosis but not with the patient.
- Sometimes, early on in dementia, patients do become distressed and angry as a result of a conversation about dementia. But it is almost always the case that having had an open conversation about the reality of dementia with both patient and family present, the dire and distressing secret is acknowledged and there is usually a sense of relief and better care can be provided.
- Enabling a conversation about the reality of dementia in front of the patient can hugely reduce the ongoing distress and challenges faced by the family.
- It is important not to deny the reality that dementia will get worse and progress. It is often helpful to point out that dementia is a terminal condition. This does provide the opportunity to plan to some degree for the future and in some respects this is a relief for both patient and family as they then know that the illness is time-limited.
- It is dangerous to give a prognosis in terms of life expectancy. People with dementia may die of other illnesses and the dementia may cause far less trouble than might be feared, or it might be much more aggressive and rapid. The timing of death is even harder to predict in dementia than it is in other conditions for which palliative care is provided.
- The bad news must be complemented by a good description of the help and support and ongoing review on offer.
- When challenging behaviour and wandering may be at their height, relatives are often deeply afraid that things will merely get worse and worse until the patient dies. In fact, wandering and challenging behaviour almost always settle as the illness progresses.

- Appropriate medication should be discussed and the patient and relatives should be reassured that distress can be effectively reduced.
- The time of imparting bad news is a good opportunity to introduce discussions on advance illness planning, financial planning, lasting powers of attorney, and advance statements; this again gives the opportunity to make positive use of bad news.

Issues of giving bad news in someone with severe memory problems

- It can be argued that giving bad news to someone with severe memory problems, especially if the news is acutely distressing, is pointless as they will only forget within a few minutes.
- It is important to share the bad news at least once along with the family and others who need to know. The ethics of shielding patients from a difficult truth is dubious.
- It is important to be clear and direct and not use euphemisms, as the potential for sowing confusion is great. Bad news is made easier by giving good support, not by fudging the discussion. Bad news is bound to distress.
- On the other hand families and carers are often left with the need to continue imparting bad news day in day out. For example, many people with dementia will repeatedly ask to go home. In these circumstances a long discussion as to why that is not possible, or explanation that the home so carefully built, maintained, and loved has been sold is distressing and unnecessary on a daily basis. Families can be reasonably advised to reply in rather simpler terms such as 'that will not be possible today I'm afraid'. For the person with severe memory problems that leaves open the possibility of the future while closing off the possibility of danger and distress within the memory span of today. Such simple but honest sidesteps may substantially reduce some of the distress when questions are repeatedly asked.

Giving bad news

Before you start
- Check your facts: about the illness, the patient, and the relatives.
- Quiet location, no interruptions.
- Sit down at the same level.

Find out what the patient or relative knows or suspects
- What is their understanding of their condition?
- What do they think is happening now?
- Listen to: factual content of the replies; style: educational level, personality, emotional content (verbal and non-verbal clues).

How much do they want to know?
- Ask them!

Share medical information
- Match their language and style—but be yourself.
- Give a warning shot: 'I'm afraid the news is not very good', 'Things are a bit more serious than that'.
- Use simple language: keep things simple, avoid jargon at all costs. Patients can often only take in one main message if it is very serious.
- Check understanding—ask the patient questions that relay back what you are saying to them.
- Reinforce the message: say it in a number of different ways.
- Repeat it in the same words: slogans help patients remember.

Elicit their agenda
- Your plan must reflect what matters most to them as well as what you feel is important at this point.

Respond to the feelings
- Acknowledge and accept them: 'You must feel devastated', 'This has thrown your life into great uncertainty'.

Acknowledge the patient's own problem list
- They need to know that the problems they have expressed are being responded to, not just what you assume their problems to be.

Be realistic about what you can and cannot do, but come up with a joint action plan
- Having a plan gives people a sense of direction and reduces the sense of helplessness. Be realistic but also emphasize the positive.

Utilize the patient's own resources
- Family, friends, patient's own strengths, etc.

Summarize the main points of the meeting
- Go over the plan in brief again, ask if there are any other questions, and if necessary book another meeting.

Based partly on ideas developed in: Buchman R (1992) *How to break bad news: a guide for health care professionals.* Johns Hopkins University Press, Baltimore, MD.

Communication with families

- Families consistently prove to be the best advocates, best carers, and best advisers for patients with dementia and it is important that they are involved in both care and decision-making. Families also know the patient far better than professionals ever can, and can be a very rich and useful source of information. They may be able to put odd behaviour into a context that makes its meaning clear; they might pick up nuances and small changes that you would miss. They have their own distress and their own reactions, and sometimes their own agendas; but in most cases, families can be harnessed as great sources of help to the patient.
- They may not like to ask questions or criticize for fear that their loved ones will get less good care.
- In a very real sense, families are affected by the illness, often just as much as the patient is. It is their illness too, although not in a pathological sense, but certainly if illness is seen in a more social context. They are therefore as entitled to support as the patient is. Facing major loss can sometimes lead to long-term health consequences, including mental health; a good supportive environment will reduce the risk.
- Great care must be taken to talk with and hear the concerns of families.
- Be open welcoming and willing to talk with families.
- Tell families how to contact you and raise concerns if they are worried.
- Copy letters to families so that they know what is going on.
- Involve families in major decisions around treatment and placement.
- Always explain the reasons for and purpose of treatment.

Difficult families

- Some families prove to be very challenging. Difficult families are not a homogeneous group.
- When health services get it wrong and the patient is being harmed families should be expected to be unhappy. 54% of complaints to the health ombudsman in the UK related to end of life care and key causes of complaints are:
  - Poor support for basic comfort.
  - Family and patient privacy.
  - Poor spiritual, cultural and psychological care.
  - Poor communication limiting a patient's sense of empowerment and their ability to make an informed decision about their care.
- Often the decision to move from 'curing' to 'caring' was not clearly communicated, leading to needless and painful interventions that diminished the patient's quality of life, and referrals to specialist palliative care teams were sometimes made too late, or not at all.
- So it really is incumbent upon those providing palliative care for people with dementia to understand that this is a difficult and uncertain task and to be willing to recognize when the care plan is not going as well as it should.
- Many families are simply not good at expressing themselves to professionals. They do not know how to have an effective discussion with health workers, or feel intimidated, especially at consultant ward rounds.

This group of people requires special care, time, and sympathy. Some people communicate better with other members of staff, e.g. HCAs, so it is vital the multiprofessional team communicates well within itself.

- Interpreters should be provided for families whose first language is not that of the doctors. Relying on family members for translation is poor practice:
  - They will often filter what is communicated, either because it conflicts with their own views or, more commonly, because they are not used to discussing bad news directly and openly, and may misguidedly shield the recipient.
  - When bad news is being communicated simultaneously to patient and family, the interpreter does not have the option of taking in the news and being upset and reacting to it as they would normally, as they have to communicate the news on to someone else while they are still themselves reeling from it.
  - Professional interpreters can be much more precise in their language.
  - Professional interpreters can also explain cultural nuances to the professionals that might have a major bearing on what is being communicated, or how it is being received.
- Advocates and community leaders or pastors may also be of help in supporting this group of people. It is important to ensure they understand the issues and that they play an enabling rather than a controlling or restrictive role reflecting what they think should happen. Sharing information with them would of course require the consent of the patient or their representative.
- Some families bring to the patient's illness some of the deep conflicts and/or difficulties of earlier life.
  - The children of the patient may have been abused, separated, or have difficulty as a result of a long-standing wound within the family.
  - The family may have been divided by a deep, distressing argument.
  - Others will have become separated by distance as a result of migration.
- Some patients will have reacted to such difficulties by taking sides in a family, or by doing their very best to heal rifts but without succeeding.
- Sometimes the patient has been the 'strong' one and in these circumstances families may find it very difficult to accept that the patient has dementia or that the patient is dying.
- Such situations may reduce the family member's ability to understand and empathize with the sick person.
- Some relatives may conclude that the patient is unwell because they are getting the wrong care and support.
- In some circumstances, as a result of the deep conflicts, the distress that they feel cannot be expressed in sympathy and empathy with the patient. The anger and aggression may become directed towards staff.
- A one-to-one or family meeting with a skilled facilitator can be very helpful in looking at these conflicts and attempting to find a way forward that can be beneficial for all.
- Some relatives have their own difficulties: personality disorders, mental illnesses, and other grave intercurrent crises. A sympathetic and caring approach with good communication will normally ameliorate

the majority of these difficulties. Communicating with other health or social care professionals looking after them, with their permission, can be of great help in providing joint support for someone who is especially vulnerable and facing a very major upheaval in their lives.

The hazards of using family as interpreters

One of the authors was looking after a Kosovan refugee in a hospice; he had lung cancer but had not been told the diagnosis. A professional interpreter was brought in, but unfortunately the agency sent someone who could only speak Serbo-Croat rather than Albanian. Although some communication was possible, it was limited. The next day, the author casually dropped in to say hello to the patient and see how he was. The patient's 9-year-old son, who spoke excellent English, was there, and was volunteered as interpreter. At one point, and with little warning, the patient asked what was wrong with him, and how long he had left to live. It felt to the author that he could not equivocate or postpone an answer without causing even more distress to son and father, and he had to use the 9-year-old boy to tell his own father that he had lung cancer, and that he only had weeks left. This was immensely distressing for everyone, and the boy was crying even before he had begun to translate. The boy and the father both needed to know the facts, to help them to prepare for a difficult future, but they needed to be told in their own time, in their own way and apart from each other. Using the boy to tell the father was very regrettable and plainly wrong, but to this day the author is unsure of how else he could have handled the situation when he was unexpectedly put on the spot.

Consultation skills

- Take time.
- Sit down and try to adopt a posture so that you do not look down upon the patient.
- Adopt a 'listening poise': do not sit straight on and stare at the patient, tilt your head a little and be attentive.
- Ask open questions (not ones with yes/no answers).
- Ask specifically about fears, worries, and hopes.
- Ask if there is anything the patient or relatives are unhappy about and reassure them it will not be held against them.
- Be willing to discuss issues of dying and end of life.
- Do not think that if they cry that means you did it wrong; distress is often a key to discussing the really important issues.
- Recapitulate and summarize.
- Do not expect to finish everything in one go; two or three consultations may be better and needed.
- Always be sympathetic.

How to conduct a family meeting

Family meetings can be useful for sharing information, planning for the future, or resolving conflict. However, badly handled meetings can damage relationships and the caregiving process. Some hints on managing family meetings are given below (based partly on the work of Monroe and Oliviere, 2008):

- The caring team need to discuss and clarify their objectives between themselves in advance.
- Tensions and differences of opinion between team members need to be addressed before the meeting as any conflict within the team will be quickly picked up, can be distressing for families, and sometimes exploited by some family members to further their agendas.
- The patient should, if competent, give their permission for such meetings, even if they do not wish to be present. This preserves trust.
- A lot of thought should be given as to which professionals should be invited to attend a family meeting. Too many people will make it feel too formal, and families might find it difficult to express their real views.
- A good balance between numbers of professionals and family members needs to be kept if the meeting is not to feel intimidating.
- Clear boundaries are essential for people to feel safe in the meeting.
- Start with introductions and setting out the time available for the meeting. Start on time and end on time.
- Find out what the family would like to get out of the meeting at the beginning, and merge it with the team's agenda.
- Use an open style and promote open communication with open questions.
- Acknowledge uncertainty and acknowledge feelings simply.
- Acknowledge conflicts and allow differences. Try and get people to understand each others' points of view. Encourage compromise.
- Reinforce similarities and strengths.
- Reframe problems so people have an agreed understanding of them.

- Be concrete about the resources available and exactly how care will be delivered by services and family. Clear agreed plans reduce conflict later.
- End in a safe place. Give a warning shot a few minutes before that the end is close and any other issues need to be brought up now.
- Summarize decisions, acknowledge the emotional tone of the meeting, validate the family's contribution.
- Finish on emotionally neutral, shared territory.
- Offer opportunities for follow-up.

Promoting family resilience

Carers and families face huge stresses, and professional input can help them face them more effectively and in ways which do not damage them and foster their own development. Over the last few years, building resilience has been a big topic in palliative care. Factors affecting family resilience are now better understood.[3] Caregiver resilience can be promoted in a number of ways.

Communication with children

In the distress that occurs when facing a major loss, children are often forgotten as adults struggle hard to cope. Yet it has been shown that children suffer long-term consequences if they are not supported through loss. It is impossible not to communicate with children; they will pick up altered behaviour, changing moods, and hushed conversations. Therefore it is better to have open and honest communication which allows them the support they need. Some points are worth remembering:

- What is said, how, and when depends on the age and development of the child. Children at different ages have different conceptions of ill-health and death, and the concepts and language should be appropriate to that child
- The best support is usually provided by parents, and professionals need to support them to provide their children with help.
- Children need simple, age-appropriate explanations of what is happening and what will happen next.
- They need reassurance that they have not caused the problem (young children are prone to magical thinking, believing that their thoughts or wishes can have major consequences).
- They need to talk about the here and now; time moves much slower for young children in particular, and discussions many months in anticipation of a change may be premature.
- They need reassurance about the practical aspects of their own lives and care: who will look after them, what will change and what will not.
- They need to share their feelings with an adult they trust. This may occur fleetingly but is just as important.
- They often need reassurance that an illness is not catching and neither they nor their parents or siblings are going to succumb to the same illness in the near future.
- Parents should be encouraged to alert the school about what is happening.

3 Zaider T, Kissane D (2007) Resilient families. In: Monroe B, Oliviere D (ed.) *Resilience in palliative care*, pp. 67–81. Oxford University Press, Oxford.

- Children need to have ongoing contact with the ill person, and to participate in that person's care in their own way of they can.
- They need to be considered an integral and essential part of the family, not just someone to be protected form a difficult situation.

Professional input may be required, both during an illness and in bereavement. Brief interventions are often highly effective.

Promoting and enhancing resilience in carers

Physical resilience:
- Moving and handling training.
- Exercise programmes such as walking for health or swimming.
- Self-care such as healthy eating, responsible drinking of alcohol.
- Opportunities to attend health screening and dental checks.
- Preventive medicine such as influenza immunization.

Mental resilience:
- Mastery.
- Perceived control.
- Self-efficacy.
- Optimism.

Social resilience—aims to maintain and improve social situation and relationships:
- Social network.
- Perceived social support.
- Engagement with desired leisure activities.
- Opportunities for intellectual stimulation and education.

Financial resilience—aims to maintain and improve social situation and relationships:
- Financial management.
- Access to benefits and social welfare.
- Employment.
- Pensions.

Spiritual/existential resilience—aims to provide meaning in caring role
- Finding meaning and purpose in life.
- For some people, engagement with religion or faith.
- Anticipatory grief and acknowledging loss.

Reproduced from Payne S (2007) Resilient carers and caregivers. In: Monroe B, Oliviere D (eds.) *Resilience in palliative care.* Oxford, Oxford University Press, p.94, with permission.

Communication and the protection of vulnerable adults

- People with dementia are particularly vulnerable, and health and social care professionals have a duty to protect and promote their safety. As part of this, they must be able to identify and take firm action in instances of abuse, be it physical, financial, or mental, either from other professionals or from family members or other acquaintances.
- *Any suspected instances of serious abuse must be recorded and reported to one's line manager and thence to the institution's designated safeguarding coordinator. Try to obtain consent from the person reporting abuse, but if serious abuse is suspected, confidentiality becomes secondary to the need to protect the vulnerable. In these cases, expert advice should be sought, but the duty to respect confidentiality may be waived.*[4, 5, 6]
- Abuse may be a criminal offence which needs to be reported to the police and social services through the appropriate channels for a full investigation.
- It is important to protect the vulnerable person from abuse but also to support the abusing carer. Elderly people are sometimes abused by carers at the limit of their endurance because they have had no support in facing a very difficult situation. While criminal activity needs to be dealt with appropriately, it is essential to provide good ongoing support to enable a caring environment to be created for the benefit of both carer and person cared for.

Removing the next of kin from the decision-making process

- Sometimes as a result of all the difficulties it becomes clear that the next of kin is either
  - insisting upon clinical decisions which are harmful to the patient or
  - acutely distressing the patient by their presence.
- In exceptional circumstances it becomes necessary to remove certain relatives including the next of kin from the decision-making process. Where no LPA has been appointed, under the MCA the duty of professionals is to consult with relatives rather than seek consent. In that circumstance, treatment is provided in the best interests of the patient without the agreement of the objecting person. Where a LPA does exist it will be necessary to demonstrate that the attorney is not acting in the best interests of the patient and to proceed without their agreement while contacting the Court of Protection to remove their authority. Clinicians should seek legal advice in such circumstances.

Excluding people from visiting

- Very exceptionally, it may be necessary to exclude people from visiting, either because the person has been violent or behaved inappropriately

4 Department of Health, Home Office (2003) *No secrets: guidance on developing and implement-ing multi-agency policies and procedures to protect vulnerable adults from abuse.*. http://www.doh.gov.uk/pdfs/nosecrets.pdf

5 http://www.dh.gov.uk/en/Policyandguidance/Healthandsocialcaretopics/Socialcare/Vulnerableadults/index.htm)

6 http://www.elderabuse.org.uk/

in other ways towards staff or because the person causes deep distress to the patient with dementia or acts in a manner which is considered harmful to the patient. An example of this would be someone who is supplying illegal drugs to a patient who is frankly psychotic.

• The other reason for excluding someone from visiting would be that the patient themselves does not wish to be visited. Generally in advanced dementia the patient will be unable to make such a choice but it might be made by the next of kin or a LPA. Further advice on these matters should be sought from the Code of Practice of the MCA.

Getting a second opinion or switching consultant

A second opinion or change of consultant can be helpful for all if trust in the consultant has broken down to such an extent that it is almost impossible to provide the care required. Such a switch can give the opportunity for a fresh start and will often occur in the context of a very distressed patient or family beginning to recognize that things are changing and that the hoped for return to health or the previous status quo will not be achieved. Such switches need not occur within the context of blame, and can sometimes benefit patients and families hugely as well as allowing clinicians a solution to a difficult situation for them.

Sharing confidential information more widely

- It is accepted that within and among health professionals confidential information will be shared between health care workers on a need to know basis.
- In advanced dementia care, the number of those who need to know what to do so as to provide the best possible care is far larger than that within which medical confidentiality is normally confined. Without spreading information appropriately to such non-health care workers the care of the patient is likely to be compromised.
- An essential part of excellent palliative care is effective communication with all those who need to know what is required. *The palliative care of dementia differs from other forms of palliative care because the patients themselves are really not going to be able to retain, carry, and convey information about their needs. This provides some difficulty with medical confidentiality. But the MCA allows and requires appropriate sharing of information in the patient's best interests.*
- People with advanced dementia are unable to consent to the sharing of information with health and social care workers. A substantial component of good quality care is provided by people who are not health workers.
- If information is not shared, the care of the patient will suffer.
- Another very useful method is to use shared care notes which are written in by all professionals.

Sharing letters with patients and families
- The practice of sharing letters with patients as their right was introduced by the UK Government in 2000.
- It has been demonstrated that in dementia care sharing letters with patients and relatives enables better awareness of the treatment that is planned and better engagement with patient and relatives.[7] Clinical experience has shown that writing to relatives and letting them know that some of the more controversial treatments (such as antipsychotic medication) are being used appears to reduce the level of complaints significantly.
- When information is in writing, families have far more chance to read, review, and integrate that information than they would do otherwise. Sharing letters can enable challenges to and questions about what is done in terms of treatment to be made more effectively and more appropriately.

Sensory disabilities
Deafness, blindness, and other sensory disabilities occur frequently in dementia and must not be forgotten. A lost hearing aid, or ears blocked with wax is more disabling for those with dementia than it is for those without, although it is likely to be less frequently considered as patients

---

7 Treloar A, Adamis D (2005) Sharing letters with patients and their carers: problems and outcomes in elderly and dementia care. *Psychiat Bull* **29**, 330–3.

themselves will not complain about the difficulty. Sight problems make falls and getting lost and disorientated more likely. Aggressive management of sensory disability, providing appropriate lighting, and transforming the buildings where people are cared for to make it easier for them to navigate around, can go a long way to improving communication for patients with dementia (see 📖 Chapter 11).

References

Christ GH (2000) *Healing children's grief: surviving a parent's death from cancer.* Oxford University Press, Oxford.

Department of Health, Home Office (2003) No secrets: guidance on developing and implementing multi-agency policies and procedures to protect vulnerable adults from abuse. http://www.doh.gov.uk/pdfs/nosecrets.pdf

Department of Justice Code of Practice (2007) *Mental Capacity Act.* Her Majesty's Stationery Office, London.

Dyregrov, A (2008) *Grief in children: a handbook for adults,* 2nd edn. Jessica Kingsley, London.

Elson P (2006) Do older adults presenting with memory complaints wish to be told if later diagnosed with Alzheimer's disease? *Int J Geriatr Psychiat* **21**, 419–25.

Fahy M, Wald C, Walker Z, Livingstone G (2003) Secrets and lies: the dilemma of disclosing the diagnosis to an adult with dementia. *Age Ageing* **32**, 439–41.

Healthcare Commission (April 2008) *Spotlight on complaints – a report on second-stage complaints about the NHS in England.* Healthcare Commission, London.

Monroe B, Oliviere D (2008) Communicating with family carers. In: Hudson P, Payne S (ed.) *Family carers in palliative care: a guide for health and social care professionals,* pp. 1–20. Oxford University Press, Oxford.

Monroe B, Kraus F (2004) *Brief interventions with bereaved children.* Oxford University Press, Oxford.

Ouimet MA et al. (2004) Disclosure of Alzheimer's disease. Senior citizens' opinions. *Can Fam Physician* 50, 1671–7.

Zaider T, Kissane D (2007) Resilient families. In Monroe B, Oliviere D (ed.) *Resilience in palliative care,* pp. 67–81. Oxford University Press, Oxford.

Person-centred dementia care

Introduction

Person-centred care is first and foremost a philosophy of care. It emphasizes the importance of caring for the whole person with dementia, a person with agency and human needs. It is a philosophy which argues that we need to care for a person as a living, human being. It emphasizes these aspects because it argues that someone with dementia is at risk of being no longer viewed by others as a person. It is concerned with supporting all aspects of the person's experience of living with dementia—cognitive, emotional psychological, physical, and spiritual. We can no longer say there is nothing that can be done to support people to live well with dementia. Perhaps the most pressing concern is to put what we know into practice.

The person-centred approach to caring for people with dementia is a philosophy of care which argues that how and whether we care for the person with dementia will affect their personhood and well-being. This approach:
• Was pioneered by the late Professor Tom Kitwood.
• Has a robust evidence base attesting to its effectiveness.
• Is enshrined in guidelines on best practice by NICE/SCIE (Social Care Institute for Excellence) guidelines on dementia and is implicit in the National Dementia Strategy for England.

Kitwood drew on ideas from social psychology and counselling to provide an alternative view of dementia and dementia care. His approach was based on Rom Harre's social psychology of self, and also drew on Carl Roger's client-centred therapy where the therapist's 'unconditional positive regard' was considered an essential ingredient to the therapeutic encounter.

There have been, and continue to be, other related psychosocial approaches in dementia care, including:
• Validation therapy (Feil).
• Resolution therapy (Goudie and Stokes).
• Integrity promoting care (Brane and colleagues).
• Individualized care (Rader and Tornquist).
• Person-focused care (Cheston and Bender).
• Emotion-oriented care (Finnema).
• Most recently, relationship-centred care (Nolan and colleagues).

This short chapter gives an overview of the key concepts in person-centred care as described by Kitwood, including dementia as a dialectic process; personhood; agency; psychological needs; subjective experience; and moral worth.

Dementia as a dialectical process

Kitwood began by recognizing that there were psychological and social influences on a person's behaviour, and therefore psychological and social approaches which would promote their well-being.

- The traditional biomedical paradigm of dementia attributed much of what a person did, or failed to do, to their neurological disease.
- As the neurological disease could not be changed, it was assumed that little that could be done to improve life for a person with dementia. In short, people with dementia were viewed as being beyond therapeutic potential.
- As dementia could not be cured, people with dementia were seen as failures.

Kitwood looked beyond the medical illness and concerned himself with the human experience of the condition. He argued that non-biological factors such as psychological and social factors had as great an influence on the person's cognition and well-being as biological factors. He was not alone in thinking this. Around the same time, in the US Karen Lyman (1989) wrote a seminal paper entitled 'Bringing the social back in: a critique of the bio-medicalisation of dementia', while Jaber Gubrium challenged us to consider the social construction of AD (1986).

Personhood

Kitwood viewed the greatest threat to a person with dementia as being at risk of no longer being seen as fully human. He asserted the importance of the person with dementia being seen as:

- A PERSON with dementia, rather than
- A person with DEMENTIA

In Kitwood's relational approach to personhood a person is a person among others. What other people do can enhance or diminish that person's standing as an individual. Kitwood describes behaviours which increased the sense of person as 'personal enhancers' or 'positive person work' and these he listed as including:

- Validating the person's experience.
- Celebrating the person.
- Holding the person's emotions.

Actions that diminish the sense of person (or 'personal detractors') constitute a 'malignant social psychology' and include:

- Ignoring the person.
- Outpacing the person
- Banishing the person.

Such malignancy was never considered to be intentional on the part of families or care staff but resulted from accepting dominant cultural beliefs and practices. From Kitwood's perspective, distressed behaviours were seen as legitimate responses to assaults on personhood, rather than as an inevitable part of the disease process.

So from this person-centred perspective there is huge therapeutic potential in dementia care and it lies within the interpersonal and social dimension of people's lives. It is through human interaction and engagement that the sense of person and feelings of well-being are attained and maintained. By changing the nature of the interaction we can directly affect the individual's personhood and well-being. The patient's social environment is crucial. The aim of person-centred dementia care is to enhance the sense of person and to improve well-being.

Agency

People with dementia far from being passive victims continue to be active agents who seek meaning in their world and act upon the meaning they make. We now have a wealth of evidence demonstrating that people with dementia actively strive to make sense of the world and their place in it and that this continues up to the final stages of dementia. For example, in advanced dementia relational bonds continue to support many family members and carers. The relationship is rarely a unidirectional one.

Psychological needs

Person centred care holds that a person's emotional well-being is as, if not more, important than their cognitive functioning. In Kitwood's view:

- A person's well-being is intimately connected to the extent to which their psychological needs are met.
- People with dementia have an overarching need for love and interconnectedness.
- People with dementia have needs for attachment (the need for secure bonds with carers).
- People with dementia have needs for comfort (the need for relief of pain, closeness, and tenderness).
- People with dementia have the need to be known by others (identity).
- People with dementia need occupation (the need to be involved in the process of life).
- People with dementia have the need to have their social standing as persons recognized (belonging).

Since Kitwood, many have seen challenging behaviour as a part of the person's attempts to meet their needs. Cohen-Mansfield and Stokes have described many of the 'behavioural symptoms' as attempts by the person to have their needs met. Challenging behaviour may often be driven by need. The need-driven dementia-compromised behaviour paradigm is a formalization of that view. Person-centred care aims to reduce challenging behaviour by meeting the person's emotional, psychological, and social needs.

Subjective experience

A central part of person-centred care is to take the person's perspective and try to understand how they are feeling, what the world looks like from their perspective. He suggested this be ascertained by methods including

- Traditional interview and observation.
- Other methods of role play and the arts.

Kitwood, with his colleague Bredin, developed Dementia Care Mapping as an observational framework for measuring the quality of care from the perspective of the person with dementia. Such information can be gathered on a regular basis and fed back to staff to stimulate the development of more person-centred action plans. Ongoing feedback and review enables continuous quality improvement in dementia care and is recommended by the Audit Commission and NICE/SCIE (2006) guidelines.

The importance paid to the person's perspective has grown enormously since Kitwood first championed this idea. Person-centred care is now recognized as being essential to both day-to-day care and to the development of appropriate service development and evaluation. Indeed, although this was rare in the early 1990s, collectives of people with dementia, whether meeting in person (e.g. the Scottish Dementia Working Group) or as virtual groups (e.g. the Dementia Advocacy and Support Network International (DASNI), http://www.dasninternational.org/) are now relatively commonplace.

Moral worth

The person-centred approach has been credited with reinstating the person as a valued human and social being with moral worth and human rights. This is true regardless of degree of cognitive impairment. A key need was for the intrinsic value of people with dementia to become enshrined in public policy and to eradicate stigma and discrimination. That value must now remain enshrined in public policy. In England the Department of Health's National Dementia Strategy (2009) emphasizes the importance of eradicating the stigma associated with dementia. Kitwood formalized a value base that people have moral worth and entitlement to social standing, regardless of their degree of cognitive impairment. Beyond that, one of his last papers was concerned with the moral development required for care work, which continues to be a real and important challenge.

Further reading

A fuller discussion of person-centred care along with a full reference base is available in:

Downs M (2009) Person-centred care as supportive care. In: Hughes J, Lloyd-Williams M, Sachs G (ed.) *Supportive care for the person with dementia*, pp. 235–44. Oxford University Press, Oxford.

Chapter 18

Choice, capacity, care, and the law

Self-determination in dementia

For each individual there is a desire to promote choice, involvement, and consent as far as possible, but it is also right that those who lack capacity can access the best and most appropriate care. Good dementia care will engage the individual in decision-making as far as possible, but also enable good decisions to be made and the best clinical care to be provided throughout the their illness to all those who cannot consent.

How does one promote self-determination of the person with advancing dementia?

- In dementia, progressive loss of memory occurs alongside progressive loss of the ability to understand, weigh up, and balance decisions. The eventual inability to express oneself verbally may mean that even when a preference can be chosen, it cannot always be communicated.
- Once someone has a disability, people will often ask carers what the disabled person wants rather than asking the person directly. Such behaviour may stem from the extra time needed to find out from individuals themselves, or from an assumption that they will no longer know. We will often not ask people with dementia what they want or think, rather we will decide what we think they want.
- In fact very many choices can still be expressed late on into an illness. Most people with dementia will continue to try and reject things that are painful or distressing. Late on in dementia people may well prefer a savoury thick soup to a raspberry flavoured diet supplement, and while both may have the same nutritional efficacy, the attentive carer can easily work out the person's preference. Similarly, preferences can be determined for choices such as drinks, music, and activities, as well as where the person is happiest sitting, etc.
- The choices made by those who are sick are often not the same as those made when healthy, and it is important to continue to try and work out what people want when they are ill. Someone who previously rejected active treatments may well say they want antibiotics when offered in advanced dementia, and there is then a real need to allow a current expressed wish to trump a previously made rejection of care. Continued attempts to discuss decisions are important.
- Several techniques can be employed to make this easier:
  - Offer choices in simple language at convenient and varied times.
  - Offer choices when the person with dementia is at their most relaxed.
  - Carefully explain in terms that can be easily understood.
  - Accept non-verbal communications: a nod, smile, or hand gesture (especially where aphasia is significant).
  - Discuss issues when a family member of friend is present: they often have extra skills in communicating with the individual.

Advance care planning

- Advance care planning provides opportunities early on during dementia to think through the possible choices that will affect people with disease progression when they may no longer be able to make or express their own decisions.

Such attempts are always fraught with hazard and uncertainty. Our fears for the future rarely turn out to be the actual problems we eventually face. The experience of birth plans in obstetric units has been one of considerable fluidity of decisions by perfectly competent women once faced with the realities of childbirth. Even though they are well thought through in a relatively predictable condition, at the time of need, advance decisions are set aside by the competent, as they conflict with current choice. If such fluidity is seen in birth plans, it will also occur in dementia, where planning has to encompass an understanding of the uncertainty of prognostication.

- People with dementia often bring to their illness hopes, fears, and wishes for later illness. Most of all perhaps, people wish to ensure their comfort and dignity in what will become a terminal illness.
- Given that fear in the person affected by dementia and in their carers will be a very strong driver for decisions, it is imperative that time is taken to discuss fears. Some useful themes to discuss include:
  - Preserving health and enhancing memory is useful and right at early stages.
  - Some of the challenges faced early on (such as depression, wandering, etc.) often settle later.
  - The aim of care is to maintain and maximize function and independence for as long as possible.
  - Distress is a key issue that health care workers should seek to alleviate.
  - Expert help is available when needed.
  - Relatives, friends or carers can be engaged as advocates to discuss and plan care when the individual is unable to do this.
- Detailed discussion usually leads to a sense of trust that, despite the illness being long and disabling, care will be ongoing and that distressing symptoms will be alleviated. Clinicians have to negotiate a difficult tension: many people with dementia fear the future and find it hard to trust ongoing care, but on the other hand making very categorical and firm decisions for the future may also put them at risk of enhanced suffering.
- Advance care planning is still unusual in the UK, although surveys of care home managers, for example, have shown widespread endorsement of the practice.
- In the USA, the Patient Self-Determination Act (1990) requires many health care providers to give information to patients about advance health planning before admission to their health care institution.
- In the UK, Advance Care Planning utilizes a number of tools. In England and Wales, these include advance statements of preferences and wishes, advance decisions to refuse treatment (ADRTs), and nomination of someone with LPA to stand in for the patient should they become incapable of making legal decisions. In Scotland advance directives do not hold the same legal status (📖 Chapter 18, The legal framework in the UK, pp. 313–322), but facilities for someone else to have power of attorney also exist.
- Appreciating this requires an outline of the legal framework for advance care planning in the UK (📖 Chapter 18, The legal framework in the UK, pp. 313–322).

Advance statements of wishes and preferences

Having established the person's own thoughts, fears, and hopes, further discussion should include

- Ongoing discussion about support, care packages, medical care, ways of assisting living, access to care, etc.
- The availability of treatment to reduce and alleviate distress.
- Discussion about future transition from the more disease-modifying early approach, to a palliative end of life approach.
- Discussing wishes about future care.

This open and broad discussion should allow people to ask questions but will also allow those who do not wish to know, not to know.

- Dying and chronic illness is a social not a medical event. Planning should look at who should be involved in care, what input, support, and resources are wanted, religious needs, planning for future care in a home or at home, etc. Decisions must be reviewed in the light of how things turn out. Choices should be stated in terms of the underlying desires and values, rather than in very rigid terms of place, because if circumstances change (say a care home gets a new manager and care deteriorates) one would want to allow carers with professionals to make the choice that will still best deliver the person's wishes (see 📖 Chapter 13, Elements of decision-making, pp. 236–239).
- Some commonly expressed decisions are often problematic later. Perhaps the most frequent is the statement 'never put me in a home'. While not a medical decision and thus not eligible for an ADRT, a person may well make such a statement in strong terms. The fear of poor care in such homes as well as a general fear of 'becoming like them' is enough to make most people never want to live in a care home. And yet, at times, home care breaks down and quality of life as well as activities, comfort, and dignity may be greater in a well run care home.
- Other decisions that may be expressed are those around money and who should manage it; around resuscitation of patients who suffer a cardiac arrest; strong statements for adequate relief of distress in advanced dementia; and refusal of some active treatments such as antibiotics or complex surgery.
- Very firm requests or prohibitions may bring with them unintended adverse consequences. A discussion of broad wishes and hope is useful.
- Preferred Priorities of Care (PPC) documentation may be very helpful here.[1] PPC has been developed in the UK to aid decision-making both in terms of where care is to be provided and to suggest what style of care is wanted, who is wanted to be around in advanced disease, and how this is to be implemented. Originally designed to be set out while people have capacity, the documentation has now been enhanced to allow decisions to be made in the best interests of those who lack capacity.
- Issues such as artificial feeding and management of repeated infections may be explored at this stage. Benefits and risks must be laid out to allow qualified answers which permit intervention in certain situations but not in others (📖 Chapter 13).

1 http://www.endoflifecareforadults.nhs.uk/eolc/eolc/current/CS310.htm

- Good, open discussions build confidence and instil a sense of being known and heard. The extent to which advance care planning currently changes things for the better has yet to be demonstrated. The current literature shows that take-up is still very low and that it rarely brings about much change. This may improve as its use becomes more widespread.

The legal framework in the UK

Treating those who lack capacity

The MCA (2005), amended in 2007, reflects the Adults with Incapacity Act (2000) in Scotland, although there are important differences. Similar legislation occurs throughout the world. Both Acts sought to develop the decision-making framework for those who lack capacity. In Northern Ireland a law covering both incapacity and mental health care is expected by 2013.

Good dementia care will engage the individual in decision-making, promoting choice, involvement, and consent, but also protect the right to the best and most appropriate care for all those who cannot consent.

The MCA defines mental capacity and sets out the rights and duties of those who provide care to people lacking capacity.

Treatment without consent

- Section 5 of the MCA (Acts in connection with care or treatment) absolves clinicians or carers of liability when acting in the best interests of a person who lacks capacity. In other words even though something is not consented to, it is to be done as if consent was given.
- Nothing in this section lets clinicians off retribution resulting from negligence and what is done is subject to any ADRT.

Best interests decisions

The MCA sets out that when capacity is lost, decisions must be made in the best interest of the patient. With a person lacking capacity one would work out the best options that one would offer to the patient if they had the ability to choose. A decision is then made in their best interests. In arriving at a decision the following must be considered (quotes from the MCA):

- The decision must not be based 'upon age or appearance, or a condition or an aspect of the [patient's] behaviour', and must consider 'all the relevant circumstances' and think through 'whether it is likely that the person will at some time [regain] capacity in relation to the matter in question'.
- If it appears likely that the patient will regain capacity, decision-making should be deferred to then, if possible and reasonable.
- The clinician or carer must not be motivated by a desire to bring about the patients' death.
- The clinician or carer must then consider, so far as is reasonably possible to ascertain:
  - The person's past and present wishes and feelings (in particular, any relevant written statement made by him when he had capacity).
  - Their beliefs and values.
  - Other factors that the person affected by the incapacity would be likely to consider.
- The clinician or carer must take into account,
  - Anyone named by the person as someone to be consulted on the matter in question or on matters of that kind.
  - Anyone engaged in caring for the person or interested in his welfare.

- Any one (recipient) of LPA granted by the person.
- Any deputy appointed for the person by the court.

Guiding principles set out by the MCA

- A person must be assumed to have capacity unless it is established that he lacks capacity.
- A person is not to be treated as unable to make a decision unless all practicable steps to help him to do so have been taken without success.
- A person is not to be treated as unable to make a decision merely because he makes an unwise decision.
- An act done, or decision made, under this Act for or on behalf of a person who lacks capacity must be done, or made, in his best interests.
- The Act cannot be achieved in a way that is less restrictive of the person's rights and freedom of action.

The injunction to use the least restrictive option has to be seen in the context of the well-being of the patient, and it must not be invoked to justify sub-optimal care.

Determining capacity in clinical practice

Mental capacity is defined in the MCA as the ability to understand the information relevant to the decision, retain that information, use or weigh that information as part of the process of making the decision, and communicate the decision (whether by talking, using sign language, or any other means).

In dementia it is rare for incapacity to be caused by the inability to communicate a decision, but common for people with dementia to be unable to understand information, unable to believe and retain the information and unable to weigh it in the balance. A common scenario would be that a person with dementia has forgotten that they had difficulties at home and does not believe they cannot cope there.

Others will not understand the need for treatment, or have a delusional understanding of treatment or the persons providing it. Although not all psychosis causes incapacity, hallucinations and delusions commonly cause fear, etc. This requires treatment to which the patient is unable to consent, as they are unable to understand that what they are experiencing is not real.

Good practice in Capacity Assessments demands that the clinician:
- Explain in simple language the treatment, its purpose and why it is proposed.
- Explain the main benefits, risks, and alternatives.
- Record what has been explained and record the reasons why the patient is held to lack, or possess, capacity. It is important to present the evidence in the notes, as if the issue ever came to court, one would be required to show on what basis the conclusion had been reached.

Case example

A consultant carried out a capacity assessment of a man with a neuro-degenerative disease who wanted to change his will. A few months after the person's death the consultant received a letter from one of his sons' solicitors asking how the conclusion that he did have capacity had been reached. The consultant was able to attach a copy of part of the notes which detailed how each of the tests of capacity had been met by this man. The solicitor never contacted the consultant again and the case was dropped.

- Capacity is not an all or nothing phenomenon, and a person may have full capacity, limited capacity which can be enhanced with information and support, or no capacity. Different decisions require different levels of capacity. Capacity fluctuates and is situation specific.
- Incapacity generally leads to the use of the MCA, but the Mental Health Act (MHA) may be used in a few circumstances to allow psychiatric treatment (📖 Chapter 18, The legal framework in the UK, pp. 313–322). The MHA does not authorize physical treatments: these are all provided under the MCA. Common law applies in the rare circumstance where restraint is required to prevent harm to others.
- It may at times constitute neglect to not treat those who lack capacity but resist.
- Under the similar Scottish Adults with Incapacity Act (2000), a person lacks capacity if they cannot understand, make, act on, or communicate decisions, or retain the memory of those decisions. In these cases the law requires that all decisions are taken for the patient's benefit; that decisions are only taken if the benefit cannot reasonably be achieved without them; that the least restrictive option is followed; that consideration is taken of the person's past expressed wishes (including advance directives), that relevant others are consulted, and that the person is helped to use existing skills and if possible develop new ones.

ADRTs

- In England and Wales and many other jurisdictions, ADRTs made while an individual retains capacity are legally binding if they are validly made and apply to the treatment specified. A professional who disregards an ADRT without good reason to question its validity, is liable to prosecution.
- ADRTs may be written or verbal.
- ADRTs can refuse life-sustaining treatment, but only if they are in writing and witnessed.
- ADRTs can promote appropriate care which avoids burdensome treatment and accepts natural death. They can increase the control of an individual in advanced dementia.
- There are risks as well as benefits to ADRTs. The difficulty in spelling out choices a long time beforehand in very different circumstances has been alluded to.
- ADRTs that refuse all active treatments in advance dementia may unintentionally disadvantage a person. In the UK they are illegal, as the

circumstances for a refusal to apply have to be stated very specifically. For example:
- A person with dementia who is physically reasonably well develops an easily treatable UTI. The distress caused by a broad advance refusal to take antibiotics was probably never anticipated when the refusal was made.
- An untreated broken hip could leave one with severe pain and distress that is hard to manage.
- A directive to accept only analgesics in advanced dementia might cause problems if one develops seizures or vomiting.
- Refusal of certain forms of nursing care might leave the patient neglected, poorly cared for, and suffering.
- Discussion about an ADRT should be with a health or social care professional who can ensure that the treatment refusals are appropriate and will not compromise the patient's care at the end of life.
- It is sensible to be mindful at the same time of guidance on decisions about CPR.[2]
- It is good practice to review ADRTs regularly, e.g. annually, but this is not a legal requirement.
- If the person is competent, they can revoke their ADRTs at any time verbally or in writing, though adding in a refusal of life-sustaining treatment must be in writing.
- If subsequent to making an ADRT the individual appoints a LPA (🕮 Chapter 18, The legal framework in the UK, pp. 313–322) that covers decisions contained in the ADRT, then the ADRT is replaced by the LPA.
- *Health professionals are duty bound to ensure that an ADRT is valid, especially if it appeared to cause the individual harm. The MCA sets out reasons why an ADRT might be invalid.*
- In Scotland, advance directives replace ADRTs. They are not legally enforceable under the Adults with Incapacity Act (2000). Instead, Scottish law requires that past wishes (of which advance directives are one statement) must be taken into consideration. Advance directives can, however, be legally binding under common law. The same situation currently applies in Northern Ireland.

LPAs for health and welfare

In the UK and in many other jurisdictions it is possible to transfer decision-making powers to a representative or advocate. In England and Wales a LPA may be set up. This legal process requires specific forms and procedures (for an information pack see http://www.direct.gov.uk/en/Governmentcitizensandrights/Mentalcapacityandthelaw/Mentalcapacityandplanningahead/DG_194840). A LPA enables formal decision-making powers to be given, in advance, to someone whom the patient trusts. The LPA can make decisions on health, consent to or refuse operations and treatment, decide where someone should live, etc.
- For financial matters an Enduring Power of Attorney (EPA) can be set up. The EPA can sign cheques, dispose of money, property, shares, etc., and gain full control over the financial affairs of the individual.

2 BMA/RC/RCN (British Medical Association, Resuscitation Council, Royal College of Nursing) (2007) *Joint statement on cardiopulmonary resuscitation.* http://www.bma.org.uk/ethics/cardiopulmonary_resuscitation/CPRDecisions07.jsp

Validity and applicability of an ADRT

An advance decision is not valid if the patient:
- has withdrawn the decision at a time when he had capacity to do so
- has, under a LPA created after the advance decision was made, conferred authority on the donee (or, if more than one, any of them) to give or refuse consent to the treatment to which the advance decision relates, or
- has done anything else clearly inconsistent with the advance decision remaining his fixed decision.

An advance decision is not applicable to the treatment in question if:
- at the material time the patient has capacity to give or refuse consent to it
- that treatment is not the treatment specified in the advance decision
- any circumstances specified in the advance decision are absent, or
- there are reasonable grounds for believing that circumstances exist which the patient did not anticipate at the time of the advance decision and which would have affected his decision had he anticipated them.

An advance decision is not applicable to life-sustaining treatment unless:
- the decision is verified by a statement by the patient to the effect that it is to apply to that treatment even if life is at risk, and
- the decision is in writing signed and witnessed.

Case examples

Jason stated years ago that if he is frail and dying he only wants reasonable care and comfort. He now has advanced dementia and a severe pneumonia. He has been suffering a lot recently and is now very ill. It is decided that it is in accordance with his wishes he be kept comfortable and not treated with antibiotics. His advance refusal is helpful and is used to confirm the treatment path.

Jane wrote an advance refusal 4 years ago, stating that if ever she developed dementia she would refuse all active treatments including antibiotics. She now has moderate dementia and while she has lost the ability to decide about the need for treatment she is still able to live a fairly normal life at home with family. She has diabetes and a UTI. The advance refusal states that she may not be given antibiotics or diabetic medication, but it is concluded that she did not anticipate this circumstance and that stopping medication now would be seriously harmful and cause considerable suffering. Analgesics do not appear to be a suitable alternative for treating the pain of the UTI.

- By signing a LPA or EPA it is established that when capacity for a decision is lost, the decision will be made by the appointed attorney as if that decision it was made by the individual.

- The LPA is required to make decisions in the patient's best interests and in line with the person's wishes were he or she still able to express them.
- LPAs can be extremely useful in freeing up resources and enabling the best care. Because the decision-making capacity remains with a competent person in real time there are some substantial advantages of LPAs over ADRTs.
- However, there are risks. Financial abuse by EPAs is frequent: 15% of cases brought to the Court of Protection in England involve misuse of powers of attorney. Similar problems may arise with LPAs. A LPA can be removed by a court or prosecuted if it is suspected that decisions are being made in the attorney's own interest or based on his or her rather than the patient's presumed wishes.
- In Scotland, financial matters can be delegated to someone with Continuing Power of Attorney, and decisions regarding health and care choices to someone with Welfare Power of Attorney.

Deprivation of Liberty Safeguards (DOLS)

- In England and Wales the MCA was amended by the MHA (2007) to introduce new safeguards for those who lack mental capacity and who are deprived of their liberty. For the purposes of the Act deprivation of liberty includes being kept in a hospital or care home and not allowed to leave as well as interventions which restrict the access of visitors to the person involved. There must be a clear intention that the patient will not be allowed to leave or that visitors are restricted.
- The safeguards cover deprivation, but not restriction of liberty. Therefore if a patient tries to leave but accepts staying after persuasion, safeguards may not be necessary. But if they persist in trying to leave and are repeatedly stopped, they are deprived of their liberty.
- In such circumstances an order authorizing deprivation of liberty is obtained from either the Local Authority or from the local health authority (PCT). The order requires several assessments including a medical assessment by a doctor specially approved under the MHA, a mental capacity assessment, and a best interests assessment to ensure that the deprivation of liberty is reasonable and appropriate.
- The legislation aims to balance undue restriction of freedom with the potential for harm should patients choose a harmful option with little awareness of consequences. See the Code of Practice for more details.

Case example

Charles is really quite confused and insists upon leaving the unit; if he does so it is thought that he will come to harm. He tries to leave the ward and so the door is locked. Having been kept there he tries again and again to leave. He does not see why he should stay and wants to get back to work at the school from which he retired many years ago. He is well enough now to set off down the road and catch the bus, but if he does he will very likely be lost and come to serious harm. It is decided to keep him in the ward and stop him from leaving. He is deprived of his liberty, and therefore an assessment for a DOLS order to be put in place is requested. This is sent to the local health authority (in a care home it would be social services) and assessment is initiated.

How good are proxies at expressing an incompetent person's wishes?

The MCA and similar legislation rely on the assumption that a surrogate or proxy nominated by the patient will accurately reflect the patient's wishes. Is this assumption upheld in empirical studies?

- A meta-analysis by Shalowitz and colleagues in 2006 examined this issue. They reviewed 16 studies presenting 151 hypothetical scenarios to over 2500 patient–surrogate pairs, and analysed almost 20,000 responses.
- What they found was surprising. Overall, surrogates only predicted patients' preferences accurately in 68% of cases. Surrogates were least accurate in scenarios where the patient had developed dementia or stroke. Accuracy was not affected by the closeness of relationship of surrogate to patient. Training and discussion between patient and surrogate beforehand actually slightly reduced surrogate accuracy.

These disturbing findings have made some look for other ways of decision-making in situations of loss of capacity. One proposal has been to agree a consensus which sets limits to how far proxy decisions can depart from community values. This has clearly worrying repercussions. Another is to consider the whole tenor and value-system embraced in a person's life and to make decisions in line with that. The difficulty with this is who decides and how.

The MHA (1983 and 2007) and the Mental Health (Care and Treatment) (Scotland) Act 2003

- The MHA sets out the criteria that have to be met before compulsory detention for assessment and treatment of people with mental disorder can be applied, for their own safety and the protection of others.
- Under Section 2, a patient can be detained for assessment for 28 days if the application is signed by two medical practitioners, one of whom is approved in terms of the MHA, and an approved mental health professional (e.g. psychiatric social worker or nurse). The second medical practitioner should either have known the patient previously or be another MHA-approved practitioner. Assessment orders are not renewable.
- In emergencies, an application can be made by an approved mental health professional or the patient's closest relative, and signed by a medical practitioner who is familiar with the patient. Emergency detentions can last up to 72 hours, after which the patient is allowed to go or is detained as above.
- After assessment, an application for a treatment order under Section 3 of the MHA can be made which lasts for up to 6 months, and is renewable.
- Patients detained under the MHA can be given treatment against their will in many but not all cases.
- Capacitous refusal of treatment and ADRTs are overridden if treatment is required under the MHA, with the exception of electroconvulsive therapy, which can be refused. However, this to can be overridden in an emergency.

- Detention can only be applied to treat mental and not physical illness.
- Patients can under certain circumstances be treated compulsorily in the community under a Community Treatment Order.
- In Scotland, detention of a person who retains capacity but is a risk to self or others is not permissible under the Mental Health (Care and Treatment) Act 2003, unlike in England and Wales. An emergency detention order may be made by any registered medical practitioner without requiring the involvement of a mental health professional (known as a Mental Health Officer), although there is a presumption that such orders will be used very sparingly. However, detention under the Act against a person's will cannot be initiated by the person's welfare guardian. Compulsory detention or treatment after 28 days in Scotland must be authorized by a Mental Health Tribunal, much sooner than in England and Wales. Responsibility for producing medical reports to extend compulsory detention or treatment does not reside only with doctors but can also be undertaken by others, such as clinical psychologists, social workers, and mental health nurses. Some have questioned the legality of this under European human rights legislation.

National Assistance Act (NAA) (1947, 1951)

- There is one other piece of legislation which is occasionally used in the UK to protect vulnerable people from risks they may not recognize. This is Section 47 of the NAA 1948 and the Amendment Act of 1951.
- This allows a doctor, who need not be a psychiatrist, to transfer an older and infirm patient who is a risk to himself or others, without his consent, to hospital or other suitable care.
- A number of conditions are stipulated, but the wording is vague and open to various interpretations:
  - The person must be suffering from grave chronic disease (and?) or be aged, infirm, or physically incapacitated, and (or?) is living in insanitary conditions.
  - The person is unable to devote proper care and attention to himself, nor is he receiving proper care from others.
  - His removal from home is necessary, either in his own interests or for preventing injury to the health of, or serious nuisance to, other persons. (Serious nuisance could mean, for example, a serious infection or infestation risk due to poor hygiene.)
- The law requires 7 days' notice to be given to the person involved before an application is made, except in emergencies certified by the appropriate official (in practice, a public health doctor).
- The Act provides for the removal and detention of the person in question but not for their medical treatment without their consent. That is only allowed by invoking a compulsory treatment order under the MHA, which of course only holds for mental health treatment.
- An application has to be made to the local council for a public health doctor to sign the request. The request is then made to a magistrate's court to transfer the person involved to another care setting. Such

an order would allow detention for 3 months, but may be extended
further by reapplying for a court order.
- The compatibility of Section 47 of the NAA with human rights
legislation cannot be assumed. The Department of Health advises legal
advice to be sought in every case.
- Use of this Act is considered draconian—there is no requirement for
a court to hear the patient or his/her representative; in emergencies,
no notice need be given; and an appeal is only allowed after 6 weeks.
This is far more restrictive even than the MHA. Disquiet about the
wide remit and paucity of protection provided by this Act has been
expressed by lawyers, public health officials, and others involved in its
operation. It appears to be very open to legal challenge, and should
only be invoked in truly exceptional circumstances.

Determining capacity in clinical practice: an example

Case scenario

Charles is a 75-year-old retired head-teacher with dementia who had
seen his mother die in a nursing home. She had been placed there by
the hospital even though he thought that she could have been better
looked after at home. She seemed distressed and he had found it a very
difficult experience. As a result he always said that he did not wish to go
into a home or receive sedatives. He eventually reached a stage where,
although very verbally able to express his views, he had no understanding
of his current difficulties. He had been struggling at home with no food,
and lonely at night. He was unsteady on his feet and had fallen repeatedly, though he did not recall this. He hallucinated, and was tormented
by voices. It was felt that he would not be safe at home.

- The questions to be asked in Charles' case are complex. There is an
advance refusal of nursing care, probably based upon his mother's
experience and a desire to avoid that. Now, however, he has been
suffering a lot at home and may be happier in a care home. His refusal
probably did not anticipate his current circumstances and is probably
not binding (technically it is not binding anyway as nursing home care is
not strictly medical care).
- Antipsychotics, though potentially harmful, are probably the correct
treatment for his psychosis. His inability to weigh up the alternatives
and their respective consequences makes his refusal invalid.
- But if he lacks capacity, that does not mean he must be put into a
home. A care package at home with good support might work; given
that he was a head teacher he might even be able to afford 24 hour
care himself. That might well obviate the problems of his being alone at
night and falling, etc.
- So, especially in the case of those who cannot choose for themselves,
those caring for the person with dementia must make a detailed
assessment of the best clinical care options, their impact, and balance
those options in terms of their effect and the previous hopes and
attitudes of the person involved. This is the process of a best interests

decision—all best interests decisions are contingent upon identifying the best clinical option.

Further reading

Chapman S (2008) *The Mental Capacity Act in practice*. National Council for Palliative Care, London.

National End of Life Care Programme and National Council for Palliative Care (2008) *Advance decisions to refuse treatment: a guide for health and social care professionals*. NELCP and NCPC, London.

Department of Health (2008) Mental Capacity Act 2005: deprivation of liberty safeguards. Code of Practice to supplement the main Mental Capacity Act 2005 Code of Practice. http://www.dh.gov.uk/prod_consum_dh/groups/dh_digitalassets/@dh/@en/documents/digitalasset/dh_087309.pdf

Department for Constitutional Affairs (2007) Mental Capacity Act 2005 Code of Practice. http://webarchive.nationalarchives.gov.uk/+/http://www.justice.gov.uk/docs/mca-cp.pdf

Restraint

- At times restraint is a necessary component of good dementia care. Section 6 of the MCA sets out that restraint should be used to avoid harm to an individual and requires that the restraint should be proportionate to the harm avoided.
- But all caregivers need to be aware of the dangers of restraint.
- As well as being essential for good care, restraint may increase risk. For example, cot-sides on beds may increase injury risk as patients climb over them. Restraint may worsen incontinence, functional status, mobility, and pressure ulcers.
- Physical restraint may make some patients more angry and suspicious, and worsen the behaviour it is meant to control. And there is a grave risk to the self-esteem and dignity of the person with dementia. Restraint must therefore be used only after careful thought, and with great skill.
- It may be applied by unskilled people who may not fully understand its consequences, or without adequate staffing.
- Restraint comes in several forms:
  - Being locked into a unit (where DOLS may apply).
  - Being physically restrained to enable personal care (Section 6 of the MCA).
  - Being physically restrained to prevent harm to others (common law).
  - Being medicated forcibly either by injection or by the use of covert medication (Section 6 of the MCA).
  - Being treated under the MHA when that applies.
- Carers have a duty to provide good care for people with dementia who do not understand the risks they are exposed to. If this cannot be done with skilled persuasion and a careful approach this will sometimes mean restraint.
- The failure to provide appropriate restraint may be lethal and can constitute severe neglect. Under the MCA (England and Wales), Section 6 states that restraint may (or should) be used if harm will accrue to the patient if they are not treated. Harm will include the persistence of treatable distress.

Case example

Charles, a verbally able former head teacher, is convinced that he is fine at home and does not need to be in care. But several episodes of care at home have failed and he is being kept in hospital. There he is happy, and it is hoped to send him home to live with his family soon. But now he has a pneumonia and needs fluids and antibiotics. He removes the drip and refuses the medicines.

With restraint he can be treated and without restraint he will suffer and may die. At this stage of his illness treatment is judged appropriate. He is sedated and restrained, treatment is provided, and he improves.

Covert medication

Covert medication may be an essential part of the attempt to give good and appropriate care to people with dementia who do not understand why treatment is needed. But the issue has been seen as so difficult that nursing staff have been suspended for administering medication covertly. With discussion and debate, it is considered reasonable to medicate covertly in exceptional circumstances where harm will otherwise accrue to the patient. Guidelines by the UK Nursing and Midwifery Council[3] as well as the Royal College of Psychiatrists[4] suggest a framework for this practice.

- The key principles here are that:
  - In those who cannot validly consent to or refuse medication clinicians have a duty to provide good clinical care.
  - Resistance to taking medicine occurs in people who lack capacity and is in no way the same as a valid refusal.
  - If patients will suffer harm as a result of non-treatment then in exceptional circumstance, when all else has been tried, it may be reasonable to give medicine covertly.
- A recent survey in a UK tertiary centre found that 12% of older inpatients were being given medication covertly. They were all detained, mostly had dementia, and lacked capacity.
- Covert medication can be considered a form of restraint. Medicines administered secretly in food ought also to be considered a form of restraint.
- Some conditions need to be met before administering covert medication can be considered justified:
  - The patient must lack capacity in this matter.
  - Not giving medication is likely to cause serious mental or physical harm to the patient.
  - Non-drug alternatives have been excluded.
  - Attempts to give medication openly have failed.
  - The issue has been discussed in a multidisciplinary team, if at all possible formally in a best interests meeting.
  - Inform, and as far as possible get the consent of, the family.
  - The reasons for incapacity, and the reasons for giving medication, are clearly noted in the case notes.
  - The decision should be kept under review.

Case example

Charles, the retired head teacher from our previous case, has improved a little but remains very confused and spits out his medication as he hates the taste. He is taking thyroxine as well as anticonvulsant medication but does not understand what the pills are for. Missing both will make him ill. Neither can be given by injection. The medicines will safely mix with food and thus can be given easily. Without covert medication his care will be difficult and he may suffer serious harm. His family supports the use of covert medication. Careful consideration of the issue aims to reduce the risk of these measures being abusive.

3 Nursing and Midwifery Council (2007) *Covert administration of medicines: disguising medicine in food and drink.* http://www.nmc-uk.org/Nurses-and-midwives/Advice-by-topic/A/Advice/Covert-administration-of-medicines/
4 Royal College of Psychiatrists (2004) College statement on covert administration of medicines. *The Psychiatrist* **28**, 385–6.

Spiritual care

Introduction

Any serious illness is a life-changing experience, not just for the sufferer but also for those who love them. Dementia affects the personality in a totally pervasive way, which makes many fear it deeply. It changes relationships profoundly and permanently, and it can reduce previously very independent or able people to utter dependency. For the carers, and for outsiders, this raises disturbing and challenging big questions. What does it really mean to be human when so much we define ourselves by in day-to-day life can be lost to an illness like this? What happens to love—can one still feel it when one forgets shared moments, when one might even no longer recognize the people one loved and lived for? Is it fair to see someone who may have given so much to others ending up like this? What then can one expect of life? Is there a continuity in this person's identity with their past, or is it all fragmented? How do they experience life, stripped of so much we use to make sense of ours?

For people with dementia, there are often times of bewilderment, sometimes fear and threat and aggression, sometimes profound isolation and deep depression, sometimes total helplessness. Equally, however, both the carers and the person with dementia can discover a simplification of their lives and relationships to what is at the core, and among the traumas and anxieties of forgetting and loss can be found moments or even lasting states of deep joy and togetherness. Both these extremes are the realm of the spiritual, which is hard to define but easy to recognize. Yet the expression and communication of the spiritual in someone who is losing their language, internal and external, is difficult to conceptualize. This chapter will consider this. It will also discuss the elements of different belief systems and cultural identity, and how these should interface with day-to-day care.

In doing this, it is essential to remember that memory loss is patchy or late in appearance in some dementias, so one must not assume but check with the person and carers and try and work out for oneself how far this is a problem. One needs an idea of what else is impaired, and what is preserved, as well as what that person particularly appreciates.

People with dementia also suffer from other advanced illnesses, so that their dementia may be at a relatively early stage while their other illness is reaching the end stage. Spiritual care, more than even any other aspect of care, needs to be personalized and responsive to the person's state of being.

How we express our spiritual being

- While our actions and relationships are external and observable, we also have an interior life which drives what we do and choose, and helps us make sense of our experience. It is the thread that runs through our lives and gives us continuity and coherence. This prevents our lives from being a series of unconnected random events.
- Our inner being is shaped by what we learn from our parents, what we imbibe from our culture, our formal learning and knowledge, our experience of life, the people we meet, the adversities and joys we live through.
- This inner self ascribes meaning to what we experience, and helps us choose what we do and how we do it. It determines our passions and our dislikes, provides the lens through which we view our life, and gives us a sense that life has direction and purpose.
- It is challenged and altered when we face difficult situations that do not fit our previous views of the world, or times of great joy that can be equally momentous.
- Although shaped greatly by culture and knowledge, even for two people who apparently share the same outlook and the same beliefs about life, a person's inner life will always be different from anyone else's, it will always be personal, and it is ever-changing as one is exposed to new things.

This inner life can be described as the life of the spirit. We express our spiritual life in a number of ways:

- Through customs and rituals, which can often express states of being in situations where words would only do it very superficially.
- Through religion and prayer.
- Through our creativity, in making or responding to works of art, literature, and music.
- Through intimacy with the people we love.
- Through our solitude.

Yet, although the spiritual life is internal and in many ways beyond language, and is usually expressed symbolically (ritual, art, prayer), in order to describe it and analyse it, we use words. This can lead to the erroneous belief that it requires an articulate language to express it or even to experience it. Such a notion would effectively exclude people with advanced dementia from the spiritual realm. Our society has been termed 'hypercognitive', glorifying knowledge and understanding above all else, at times making it appear as the only dimension which marks us out as human. Dementia challenges that conception and provides an alternative reading of our humanity. The life of people with dementia is immediate, responding to their environment in the here and now, and it is emotional and relational rather than cognitive.

Religion and spirituality

As we have described, spirituality can be lived and expressed through religion or through other means. While it is possible to have a spiritual life without adhering to a religion, it is not possible to have a good religious life without being spiritual.

- In some Western countries, only a minority of the population are practising members of a religious group. However, older generations are currently more likely to be religious than younger.
- For some, religion has become an object of anger or ridicule and is blamed for divisiveness or thought control. For others, their religious belief is the source, means of expression, and aim of their spiritual life. It is important (though not always easy) to support people through their own world view rather than one's own. It is the product of their life experience.
- As more of the population of many Western countries becomes less religious, one casualty is the language of spirituality, which has grown and been expressed over hundreds of years through religion, religious rituals, and in religious terms. Caring staff may have no language in which to access or describe the spiritual. For many people their world is a day-to-day affair. This may affect their ability to detect and respond to spiritual concerns, and to discuss them in the caring team.
- It is essential to treat the person's and carers' spiritual beliefs with great respect—they are not a preference (like a favourite football team) but an outlook on life. This outlook is the key to their reading of the events they have lived through and what they have learned in their lives, and a lack of respect for it is a lack of respect for that person's lived past and present.
- Religion is sometimes presented as a list of customs and practices, and it is felt that as long as one adheres to these, one is respecting the person's religious belief. This dangerously misses the point: religion is about a world view and attitude not about practices, though practices may reflect this world view. Practices carried out without any notion of their significance are sterile and misleading. Many practices said to be religious are actually local traditional customs, and people of a similar faith in another area might have entirely different practices.
- No two people, even of very orthodox beliefs, practise their religion in quite the same way. It is essential always to ask the person or carers what is particularly important for them, and never to assume.
- It is easy to extrapolate erroneously from one religion to another. For example, the significance of the priest or minister in many Christian denominations is totally different from that of an imam or a rabbi for Muslims or Jews; some Christian denominations, such as Quakers, have no ministers. The participation of a minister may have great importance for some Christians at times of crisis, but the role of the imam or rabbi may be much more peripheral.

Major issues in spiritual care for people with dementia

A spirituality of dementia frequently needs to address particular issues:
- Bewilderment and confusion in the earlier stages of the illness, particularly as one's cognition becomes affected.
- When present, insight and awareness into early cognitive decline, and of the future devastating course of the illness, which can be frightening and demoralizing.
- Fear of the future and of future dependence and a perceived loss of dignity, especially while insight is preserved.
- Feelings of guilt about the effect on carers and loved ones.
- Distant memories, good or bad, in mild or moderate dementia.
- Immediate distress, disorientation, and confusion later on in the illness.
- Relived experiences from the past, e.g. of relationships which suddenly seem much more real (like the person with dementia worrying that their mother is not present) or of traumatic situations, e.g. flashbacks in people who have been in concentration camps as prisoners of war.
- Later, the person with dementia's poor understanding which may breed suspicion of care and carers and a strong sense of being under threat.
- In very advanced dementia, very major limitations in verbal communication and understanding of even simple concepts.

Tools for delivering spiritual care

Spiritual care for people with advanced dementia has to:
- Be a spirituality of the immediate, not of the past or the future. This is the case even when the past is being relived: it is the immediate, very real experience one is dealing with, not memories.
- Utilize symbols, ritual, sensory input, and simple human contact as cognition deteriorates. These replace understanding and cognition with evocative echoes of potent distant memories which persist for much longer, a sense of atmosphere, of immediate sensory input, and human relationship. In later dementia, cognitive capacity is broken down but the capacity for emotional attachment remains (📖 Chapter 4).

Symbols and rituals

Symbols, rituals, and experiences from a person's past can possess resonances for that person which go beyond words. Just as a smell can make us relive an experience with great vividness, we can recall the past through symbols in ways that are more powerful for being less literal.
- The power of symbols persists beyond verbal fluency, especially if symbols are well embedded in one's past.
- In dementia, where so much appears strange and unfamiliar to the affected person, rituals can be potent sources of comfort and reassurance.
- Explore with the person with dementia or their family which symbols hold great meaning for them. These may be personal or religious (e.g. a cross for a Christian, a menorah for Jews, statues of Hindu gods, sacred art, or holy pictures). Placing them in the person's environment or utilizing them in certain activities or interactions may be a way of supporting spiritual activity.
- However, it is vital to remember that people with dementia think very concretely, and verbal symbolic language may confuse them, especially after the initial stages. On the other hand the symbolic language of rituals they have participated in very often in the past is unlikely to disturb them.
- Rituals from one's past hold great power to evoke. In this context, a ritual is only a ritual if someone has engaged in it before to the extent that it holds symbolic meaning for them.
- For many Christian denominations, participation in the sacraments (as understood variously in Roman Catholic, Eastern Orthodox, and various Protestant traditions), especially the Eucharist, is a particularly potent experience.

Similarly, commemoration of significant religious festivals may trigger a sense of participation and involvement which is rare in day-to-day life. Examples include Easter and Christmas for Christians; Eid-ul-Adha for Muslims; Passover and Yom Kippur for Jews; and Diwali for Hindus. Institutions which care for people with dementia should strive to commemorate such meaningful days for their residents whenever relevant to them. Even more, they should give space and encouragement to families to commemorate such festivals in their traditional ways, as this will chime with the person with dementia far more strongly than a different, less familiar, celebration.

Music is employed in many religious systems as part of prayer or worship. Familiar hymns and religious songs are another useful tool in the spiritual care of people with dementia. Music is equally useful in secular spirituality. It is the experience of many carers that music can calm an agitated and distracted person with dementia and hold them in rapt attention. Both listening to music and making music, especially singing, can have this effect (📖 Chapter 23, Music therapy, pp. 388–390).

Do you think he has a soul?', I once asked the Sisters. They were outraged by my question but could see why I asked it. 'Watch Jimmie in the chapel', they said, 'and judge for yourself'.

I did, and I was moved... because I saw here an intensity and steadiness of attention and concentration that I had never seen before in him or conceived him capable of. I watched him kneel and take the Sacrament on his tongue, and could not doubt the fullness and totality of Communion, the perfect alignment of his spirit with the spirit of the Mass.... There was no forgetting, no Korsakov's then,... for he was no longer at the mercy of a faulty and fallible mechanism... but was absorbed in an act, an act of his whole being, which carried feeling and meaning in an organic continuity and unity, a continuity and unity so seamless it could not permit any break.

From: Sacks O (1985) *The man who mistook his wife for a hat*, p. 36. Picador, London,

Past experiences

- Particularly in early and moderate dementia, reminiscence, with a carer or in groups, can be very effective.
- Photographs and items from the past can bring it to life. These can be used during meetings or be placed around the house to absorb the interest of the person with dementia on their travels.
- All too often the rooms of people with dementia are institutional, impersonal, clinical, and uninviting. Creating a room that has resonances of one's past (furniture, soft furnishings, photographs, objects of significance, but also the style of the room) can provide opportunities for all sorts of reminiscences, conscious or not, and relived moments and sensations from one's history.
- It is important to include materials of significance to the generation of the residents and if possible to reproduce some of the traditional feel of homes from their past.
- Surroundings must also be built appropriately for people with dementia to reduce the sense of disorientation and communication techniques used also have to be appropriate—see 📖 Chapters 11 and 16.
- Group work can be valuable, but groups need to be clearly led, with the leader taking the initiative in leading throughout. The group may appear confused and uncoordinated to the casual watcher, as different participants may be doing their own thing at various times. Yet there is no doubt that the social experience of group participation is greatly valued and uses a number of the more persistent skills in dementia. To achieve a good result, everyone needs a chance to participate, the speed of the group must be adapted to that of the participants, and each person in the group must be acknowledged personally by physical

contact (e.g. handshakes at the beginning and at the end) and by addressing them by name as they contribute.

Sensory input

- Sensory input in the here and now, above all human touch but also fragrances (aromatherapy, gardens) and colours, textures, and sounds that resonate with that individual can reach out to the person with dementia who may be less accessible in other ways.
- The creative arts can play a large part in enabling contact with the spiritual. Painting, making music, and clay modelling can make time stand still and also provide a very tactile means of expression. Such activities need to be designed so that they can be engaged in and abandoned easily when concentration wanes.

Human contact, interaction and presence

- Simple companionship is very meaningful for someone who may find the world a lonely and bewildering place.
- Companionship can involve simple shared activity. A quiet presence and a being with, often without words, but with a strong awareness of each other's presence, can also reach the person with dementia, even in the later stages when verbal fluency is disrupted.
- The carer needs to be open to receiving from as well as giving to the person with dementia. This can be a long and painful process, but it restores the person to a place where they are not mere recipients of care but share in human interaction. Many family carers eventually find something sustaining in their interactions with the ill person.

Prayer and readings

- For people with a religious background, prayer can hold great significance.
- Reading to the person from their scriptures can be calming and reassuring as well as deeply meaningful. Readings should be short and simple, but their power does not always come from the text being fully understood; they may still be very evocative for those who miss the meaning but recognize them from their past.
- Praying with a person with dementia in the manner to which they are accustomed can be of great help to them. It gives them a sense of companionship at a meaningful level. It can be especially poignant when they themselves are losing their verbal fluency but someone else can still provide the words for them.
- Many religions have widely recognized short repetitive prayers, sometimes with prayer beads to aid the process. Mantras in Buddhism, the rosary for Catholics, and the Jesus prayer for Orthodox Christians are examples of simple repetitive prayers that may remain accessible to many religious people with dementia. Some Muslims use the misbaha (Islamic prayer beads), to recite the 99 names of Allah, but others find this repulsive. Always ask!
- It is clearly always essential to make sure that what one is doing has meaning for that particular person, and any imposition of unwanted or even resented prayers is an act of violence on that person. However, by talking to them and their families and being sensitive to their

reactions, and by asking every time, one can avoid this. Prayer provides an important dimension in the already restricted lives of people with dementia. This path needs to be trodden with great delicacy, but it must not be avoided.

- Take enough time in prayer; if we spend only a short while in prayer with sick people they may not have time to really become part of it. Do not rush.

End of life practices

- Different faiths have end of life practices which adherents may wish to follow. As always, check whenever possible.
- See Table 19.1.

On the night she died, Margaret had been unresponsive all day, eaten nothing, said nothing, and just lain quietly in bed. Her family and friends gathered round to pray the Rosary. Towards the end of this (after about 15 minutes) Margaret raised her arm and made a 'Sign of the Cross'. It was the last sign of awareness she showed. She died that night.

Further reading

Neuberger J (2004) *Caring for people of different faiths*, 3rd edn. Radcliffe Medical Press, Oxford.

Table 19.1 Brief guide to faiths and faith resources

Faith (and faith resources)	Diet	Sacred festivals	Washing	Modesty	Care while dying	Care after death
Buddhism: Religious leader: Buddhist monk, lay teacher or lama for Tibetan Buddhism. More information: http://www.buddhanet.net/	Often vegetarian. May avoid alcohol or mind-altering drugs	Buddhist New Year Jan, Feb or April, depending on country of origin. Puja days (days of festival/prayer linked to lunar cycle) Vesak (Buddha day) May.	No special needs	Variable needs. Asians may prefer same gender doctor/nurse	Important to die consciously with a clear mind. May refuse painkillers/sedatives. Prefer to know they are dying. May wish a Buddhist monk to be present but not many other visitors	Believe consciousness remains in the body for 8–12 hours. May not wish the body touched too soon. Chanting from the Abhidhamma (Theravada) or Tibetan Book of the Dead (Tibetan). Rituals and practice vary—check with family. Cremation common
Christianity: Religious leader: priest, vicar or elder. More information: http://geneva.rutgers.edu/src/christianity/	No special needs. Some abstain from a favourite food during Lent. Sometimes abstain from meat on Fridays or fast before communion	Holy day is Sunday (Saturday for Seventh Day Adventists). Advent (1–24 Dec). Christmas (25 Dec). Lent (40 days up to Easter) Easter (March/April calc. by lunar cycle). Whitsun or Pentecost (50 days after Easter)	No special needs (check for cultural preference)	No special needs	Sacrament of the sick/last rites may be important for Roman Catholics and some Anglicans. Prayers and communion may be welcomed. Other practices vary—check with patient, family, and faith community	Body treated with respect and dignity. Support from clergy as required. May wish to pray. No formal problems with post-mortem. Usually church funeral followed by burial or cremation. Requiem mass for Catholics

Hinduism: Religious leader: Brahmin priest or pandit. More information: http://www.hinduism. co.za/	Often vegetarian. Ban on beef. Fasting common	Divali (Festival of Lights) Oct/Nov calc. by lunar cycle. Sankrantis 12 solar festivals. Vasant Panchami spring festival Navaratri (9 nights) and Dassera (Mother Goddess) Holi (March). Many others celebrating Hindu gods	Wash daily in running water. Wash hands and mouth with water before/after food. Total privacy for bedbaths. Wash private parts with running water after excretion	Women often require female doctor/nurse. Men may request male nurse for personal care	Prefer to die at home. Atonement ceremony with Brahmin priest at home, may be followed by blessing and tying of sacred thread around the wrist (do not remove these threads). Family/extended family brings gifts for patient to touch for distribution to the needy. Sacred leaves and Ganges water may be placed in the mouth before death. May wish to die on the floor (close to Mother Earth).	Body left covered. Consult the family before touching the body. Family usually do Last Rites, washing patient with sacred water. Postmortem only for legal requirement. All organs to be returned. Funeral preferred within 24 hours. Always cremation. Eldest son is chief mourner, women may stay at home.

(continued)

Table 19.1 Continued

Faith (and faith resources)	Diet	Sacred festivals	Washing	Modesty	Care while dying	Care after death
Islam: Religious leader: Imam or maulana. More information: http://www.islam.com/	Ban on pork and alcohol. Ban on non-Halal meat, often vegetarian. Fast between sunrise and sunset at Ramadan (partial/ total exceptions for elderly or ill)	Muslim holy day is Friday Jum'a-tul-Mubarak (Friday prayer). Ramadan lasts 1 month (variable calc. by lunar cycle). Eid-ul-Fitr: end of Ramadan. Eid-al-Adha (April) Muharram Eid Milad-un-Nabi Shab-i-Miraj Lailat-ul-Qadr	Wash daily in running water. Wash before prayers. Women wash completely after menstruation. Wash private parts with running water after excretion	Crucial for men and women. Women clothed head to foot day and night. Women need female doctors/ nurses	May wish to face Mecca (SE in the UK). Family may recite the Koran. Family will probably wish to stay with the patient and may wish an imam to be present. Children often actively excluded from death and after-death rituals/ceremonies	Do not wash the body, cut nails or hair. Non-Muslim should not touch body. Wear gloves if vital to touch. Mosque or family will handle ritual washing of the body and prayers. Post-mortem only if legal requirement. Organs to be buried with the body. Burial (never cremation), within 24 hours performed only by men
Judaism: Religious leader: Rabbi. More information: http://www.torah.org/	'Kosher' diet. No pork or shellfish. Kosher meat. No mixing of meat and milk (even in food preparation)	Jewish Sabbath sundown on Friday until sundown on Saturday. Pesach (Passover) April. Shavuot June (49 days after Pesach). Hashanah (Jewish New Year) Sept/ Oct. Yom Kippur (Atonement)	No special needs	No special needs, generally. Ultra-Orthodox Jews may wish to keep hair and limbs covered. Men may regard physical contact from female staff as immodest	Dying patient is not left alone, family will usually want to be present at death. Prayers recited by relatives. May require Rabbi (ask family)	Allow time lapse before touching body and touch as little as possible. Arms extended by sides with hands open. Do not wash the body. Ritual purification by Holy Assembly. Post-mortem only for legal requirement. Burial within 24 hours apart from Sabbath. Cremation forbidden

Sikhism: Religious leader: Sikh community. More information: http://www.sikhs.org/topics.htm	Often vegetarian. Ban on Halal meat and alcohol. May avoid beef and/or pork.	Baisakhi (April). Gurpurab (10 per year; celebrating the 10 gurus of the Khalsa Panth). Prakash Utsav (festival of light). Holla Mohalla (festival of colour and happiness)	Wash daily in running water. Wash hands and mouth with water before/after food. Wash private parts with running water after excretion	Female doctor/ nurse for female patients if possible. The Kaccha (undershorts) is a sacred garment. Consult closely with patient if it needs removing	Family may wish to sing or say prayers. The 5 Ks are personal sacred objects, not to be removed: Kesh, uncut hair; Kanga, wooden comb fixing the hair; Kara, metal wristb and on the right wrist; Kaccha, undershorts; Kirpan, dagger	Body may be laid on the floor. Continue special regard for 5 Ks. Family may wish to wash the body. Viewing important. No formal problems with post-mortem. Always cremated as soon as possible (within 24 hours)

Reproduced from http://www.gp-palliativecare.co.uk/?c=clinical&a=guide_faiths. © Dr Eileen Palmer 2004, used with permission.

Chapter 20

Provision of appropriate care

Place of care in advanced dementia

People with advanced dementia can be cared for at home, in a care home, or in hospital. This chapter looks at how palliative care is provided in these various settings, and looks at how care needs can be organized and the risks managed. 📖 Chapter 5 contains an overview of palliative care provision in various settings, but does not focus on dementia.

Transitions across care settings

Problems are particularly liable to occur around transitions of care from one setting to another. It has been demonstrated that moving stable residents between care homes as a result of their closure, is associated with a mortality within 6 months of up to 30% The unfamiliarity of the person with the environment and of staff with the person's behaviour is at its greatest at this point. Moving patients with staff may reduce but not remove the risk, as can communication between settings.

The risks of confusion, disorientation, wandering, and aggression as well as the inability of staff to read and interpret behaviour correctly and to reassure the patient are all at their highest.

Where are people with dementia cared for?

Overall, in the UK, 63.5% of people with dementia live at home and almost all the rest in care homes. That said, few are specifically supported to live at home until they die and most move on to institutional care as their disease progresses. The number who live in institutional care increases with:
- Age (Table 20.1).
- Dementia severity.
- Lack of informal caregivers.
- BPSD (📖 Chapter 10, BPSD, pp. 171–173).

Table 20.1 Place of care of people with dementia with age (estimated)

Age	Percentage in institutional care
65–74	26.6
75–84	27.8
85–89	40.9
90+	60.8

Based on: Knapp M, Prince M (2007) *Dementia UK: a report into the prevalence and cost of dementia prepared by the Personal Social Services Research Unit (PSSRU) at the London School of Economics and the Institute of Psychiatry at King's College, for the Alzheimer's Society: the Full Report.* Alzheimer's Society, London.

References

Williams J, Netten A (2003) *PSSRU Personal Social Services Research Unit. guidelines for the closure of care homes for older people: prevalence and content of local government protocols.* Available at: http://www.pssru.ac.uk/pdf/dp1861_2.pdf

Care at home

- The majority of people with dementia are looked after at home. They depend, especially at more advanced stages, on informal carers, usually family members and more often female.
- Carers of people with dementia are most often spouses, and therefore may be old and unwell themselves. Women live longer, and traditionally have a caring role, and the brunt of care often falls on them. Daughters are the next commonest group of informal carers after spouses. See 📖 Chapter 22.
- There are concerns about the future viability of informal care on this scale, due to demographic changes, smaller families, increased geographical mobility, and changes in employment and social expectations.
- Improving home care rates in advanced dementia requires an understanding of the advantages and risks associated with care at home and how they can be managed, and of factors precipitating a move to institutional care.

Advantages of care at home

These include:

- Often, the presence of family carers who love and care for the person with dementia. This provides a continuity of relationships but also more personal care and often great efforts to optimize comfort.
- Familiarity with the environment and routine, reducing the risk of confusion, falls, disorientation, and wandering.
- Memories and associations which allow the person with dementia to relive moments of their past experience, often in the presence of carers who can understand this.
- Home care is less expensive, although at the last stage of dementia nursing home care may be cheaper.
- Distress may be better identified by family carers at home, and therefore treatments may be more appropriate.

Risks of care at home

- Isolation and lack of professional input with consequent substandard care
- Carer exhaustion, which may be extreme and lead to physical or mental health breakdown or the risk of elder abuse.
- The environment is not designed for caring for people with dementia, and may provide a number of physical hazards. This is often offset by familiarity.
- Patients who are alone for significant stretches of time are particularly vulnerable.

Many surveys have shown that, when asked, most people would prefer to die at home with their loved ones. Community palliative care teams have enabled many people with end-stage illnesses to fulfil this wish. These opportunities have been much less available to those with advanced dementia, for reasons outlined in 📖 Chapter 5. But both palliative care and community mental health teams have shown that this can be done for dementia.

Case example

Grace, in her 70s, developed multi-infarct dementia. She became very agitated and went into a nursing home. Within 2 weeks she had lost weight, was bruised, distressed, and was moved to a dementia assessment ward. It was difficult to see what could be done to alleviate her distress or to care for her. Judicious use of antipsychotics, antidepressants, and benzodiazepines had some benefit. She settled enough to go into a dementia specialist nursing home. She continued to lose weight, and remained distressed until her husband could not bear to see her in such a way. He asked if he could take her home. The nurses and consultant thought this a bad idea. Her husband insisted, and after discussion it was agreed that this could be tried. Grace lived at home for 8 years. She gained weight and was happy in the care of her husband along with a small but loyal group of supportive carers. For a lady who had been in need of full nursing care including feeding, it was extraordinary to see her on trips out to shopping centres and her beloved golf club. Grace's dementia stabilized for quite some time and did not progress.

What is needed to make home care work?

Home care can only work if:

- The patient's needs are met adequately (📖 Chapters 7–11, 13, 14, 16, 17, 19).
- The carers' needs are met adequately (📖 Chapter 22).
- Good planning is put in place, anticipating changes in the person's condition, care circumstances (e.g. carer's illness), and emergencies.
- The basis is a holistic, multi-axial assessment and approach, combining ongoing symptom review, good nursing care, equipment, social care, family interventions, respite, and good information. At the centre comes regular review, usually by an expert nurse with access to specialist medical support.
- Open and honest communication and education of patient and families is very important to achieve this.
- Challenging behaviour (📖 Chapter 10, Agitation and aggression, pp. 193–195) greatly increases carer burden, cost of care, and makes institutionalization more likely.

An appropriate model of care for dementia

The model of care for dementia has to take account of its fundamental differences from other, more acute illnesses in which palliative care has traditionally intervened. In dementia:

- The illness is slower to progress, and at times change may be hard to see.
- The period with severe disability may last much longer.
- The end stage is less clearly delineated.
- People affected have limited understanding of what is happening to them and limited ability to intervene themselves.
- The burden on carers is heavy and particularly long-drawn-out.
- The balance of health care and social care needs is shifted: few health problems are especially acute (although these can occur), but social needs are great.

- Behavioural problems, not particularly amenable to medication, may predominate in the middle period, and physical symptoms in the end stages.
- Recognition of symptoms in verbally uncommunicative people and even eventually to conceptualize their problems is not straightforward.
- The mix of skills needed to provide good care is different.
- The combination of mental and physical needs means that many problems may fall between two stools, not being sufficiently appreciated by staff familiar only with one type of need.

A model of care has to be able to provide care for a large number of people over a long period. It must lead to better coordination of care and if possible improve the skills of professionals and informal carers already looking after people with dementia.

Two models of care in south London

The Croydon model
In Croydon from 2006 to 2010, St Christopher's Hospice ran a project providing palliative care for people with dementia. Over 200 people were referred to this project in the first 4 years. Two-thirds were in care homes and one-third in their own home. The project revolved around a full-time palliative care trained clinical nurse specialist who worked closely with mental health, primary care, and care home teams. She assessed patients who were referred according to GSF criteria or the surprise question (📖 Chapter 4, Identifying the need for palliative care, pp. 63–65). Her role was providing ongoing assessment and symptom control advice, coordination of care between the various professionals, support for family carers, mentoring and formal education of professional carers, and triage so that those with more complex problems get specialist help. She had consultant palliative care support. She played a major part in improving communication with families and in referring patients to other agencies when it would help.

With this model of care, care of patients and communication with families and practice of care improved considerably. Staff became more able to pick up problems and to start to deal with them, and know when and who to call for assistance. And just under 90% of patients under the project died in their own place of care, without hospital transfer.

Hope for home
The Greenwich Advanced Dementia Service has looked after over 100 patients. It sets out to provide those who have severe dementia with ongoing care at home with their families until they die. The service is a small unfunded one that has been very highly regarded by carers and other professionals. Over the last 3 years, 75% of those cared for died at home. The others most often had very short hospital admissions as a result of a sudden unexpected and distressing change. But many more (distressing) hospital admissions have been saved and better quality care achieved, and there are substantial savings to both health and social care budgets. Most patients continue to require ongoing psychiatric care, and may require opiates and analgesia (usually in low doses) at the end of life.

The key principle is a combination of a psychiatric assertive outreach model (regular ongoing visiting) with palliative care and advanced physical care skills and availability.

Good medical care and ongoing assessment

Comprehensive assessment of needs must incorporate an assessment of:
- Medical diagnosis and need.
- Medical and psychiatric history.
- Personal background, family, housing, financial, and welfare situation.
- Functional ability and need for care support.
- Need for and provision of appliances and assistive technology.
- Previous expressed wishes regarding care.
- Full examination of mental and physical state.
- Assessment of carers and their needs and strengths.
- Care planning.
- Agreement on how to deliver care.
- Follow-up arrangements for ongoing support and regular review.

Requirements for successful home care

An informed family

- Without information about the illness, prognosis, the possible shape and appropriate response to potential crises, and assistance and support available, families will find it much harder to feel safe about providing care (📖 Chapters 16, 21, and 22).
- Information is best imparted person to person by the key worker or other professionals. This can be supplemented by written materials and online information, but these are rarely enough by themselves. Effective information needs to be personalized, based on an understanding of the specific circumstances; transmitting this understanding helps to make people feel safe.
- Care issues such as feeding need to be incorporated into the discussion and the family may need specific training n these areas.

Information sharing among professionals: QOF and GSF

- Professionals involved in caring for someone with dementia need to share information effectively and in a timely manner. This is done through copying each other into correspondence, phone, or email contacts, and regular face to face meetings.
- The information shared needs to be relevant to the participants—the Data Protection Act (1998) prohibits sharing of information that carers do not need to know, but equally lack of relevant information can be dangerous. Once they have received information, all professionals are ethically and legally bound by a duty of confidentiality, sharing it only on a need to know basis.
- A patient register for people with dementia or terminal illness was held in 90% of all practices in the UK in 2010 under the Quality and Outcomes Framework (QOF). This should be kept updated and forms the basis of primary care work in this area. In 2010, 20 QOF points were awarded for keeping a register of and reviewing dementia patients, and 6 for palliative care patients.
- The GSF aims to optimize generalist care for the terminally ill (📖 Chapter 4, Identifying the need for palliative care, pp. 63–65) (http://www.goldstandardsframework.nhs.uk/) through:
  - Providing diagnostic criteria for recognizing such patients.

- Keeping a register of terminally ill patients.
- Fostering good communication with patients and their family.
- Requiring regular multiprofessional discussions about each patient.
- Providing a framework for advance care planning (📖 Chapter 20, Care at home, pp. 340–348), including anticipatory prescribing.
- Informing on-call medical staff about these patients and having a plan for out of hours care.

- Each locality and each practice signed up to GSF has its own coordinator.
- GSF has been endorsed by the National End of Life Care Programme of the Department of Health, NICE, the Royal College of General Practitioners and the RCN.

Equipment and home adaptations

- Equipment provision can make the difference between successful care at home and needing to go into a care home.
- An occupational therapist can carry out a home assessment for any adaptations necessary, e.g. double banisters, wall rail.
- Rooms may also need to be reallocated to keep someone at home—e.g. bringing the bed downstairs if there is no upstairs bathroom, if the patient wanders and may fall down stairs, or to keep the patient integrated in family life. This may entail considerable sacrifice from carers.
- Equipment may include incontinence aids, a commode, toilet raiser, shower wet room, shower bath aids, shower stool, zimmer frame or walking stick, wheelchair, hospital bed, pressure-relieving mattress, reclining chair, hoist.
- Assessment for equipment is usually done by occupational therapists. Suitably trained physiotherapists and nurses can do limited assessments.
- Equipment is usually obtained from the local PCT or social services equipment store. Many facilities will respond urgently to requests for palliative care patients, whose lifetime is short.

DNs, long-term condition matrons, carers, and GP visits

- DN visits can be arranged if there is a procedure to be performed regularly, e.g. dressing change or refilling SDs; if there is a condition requiring skilled supervision, e.g. wound care or poor diabetic control; or if there are complex nursing needs, e.g. PEG tube.
- Carers can visit several times a day to get the patient out of and into bed, for toileting, washing, cleaning, shopping and cooking, or giving a meal. See 📖 Chapter 24, Health and social care, pp. 392–394 regarding entitlement to continuing care.
- Frequent GP or specialist nurse visits, say every 2–4 weeks, greatly reduce the strain on carers, who feel well supported. This together with DN visits enables early detection of problems and intervention.
- A GP must have seen someone alive within 2 weeks of their death in order to issue a death certificate—otherwise it may become a coroner's case with an unnecessary post-mortem. GPs would therefore be advised to visit patients close to death in a timely manner.

Involvement of other professionals and agencies

Good home care requires judicious referral to other professionals and agencies when this will improve care, while resisting the temptation to refer to more and more agencies in the vain hope that it will improve care without a clear overarching plan of the contribution of each to the whole. Involvement of too many people with unclear roles is confusing for patient, family, and professionals alike, increases the risk that 'what is everybody's business is nobody's business' and things fail to get done, and may add an extra strain on carers who have to wait on professionals for no clear gain.

- Having a key care coordinator is very useful to family and professionals. This may be a DN, GP, or in areas fortunate enough to have them, an Admiral Nurse. They are the key link to steer the family through the complexities of advanced dementia care, linking with other professionals as needed.
- Admiral Nurses or other dementia nurses/ community psychiatric nurses may be essential to good care of complex dementias.

On-call arrangements

- Crises can occur 24 hours a day, and are more anxiety-provoking out of working hours, especially at night.
- It is always important to have details of out of hours services that carers and family can access for advice or visits. The service needs to have at least some information about the patient and their current state. The family needs to have contact details available, an idea of what these services can offer, and if possible an alternative should the first contact be unavailable.
- Some families end up with multiple possible contacts, each with special circumstances in which they should be called, and possibly different working hours or procedures. This is confusing; a single point of call which then redirects calls as needed is the ideal.
- Having emergency medication prescribed and available at home makes responses from on-call services much quicker and more fruitful.
- On-call deputizing doctors' services and DNs are available almost everywhere, though some DN services do not provide 24-hour cover.
- Specialist mental health for old age and palliative care facilities may be available to give advice 24 hours a day in some localities. Some will give advice to patients and families already under their care, but will also advise professionals regarding patients not on their books.

Keeping it simple

- The greatest aid to success in many areas of life is to adopt a simple but robust system.
- Regularly review medication to eliminate anything that is not absolutely necessary for comfort (see 📖 Chapter 14, Managing the last few days of life, pp. 261–266).
- Medication may be given in liquid form. It may be mixed with food, but pharmacy advice must be obtained to make sure the medication is stable in these circumstances. If there is a perceived need to give medication covertly, serious thought must be given to the ethics of this, and local protocols must be followed (see 📖 Chapter 18, Restraint, pp. 323–324).

Advance care planning

- Advance care planning can prevent many crises, build confidence and reduce strain in carers, and allow a rational response to crises that do occur. It can also allow patients' own wishes to be translated into reality.
- Advance care planning has to include a number of aspects:
  - Assessment with an eye to possible problems.

- Ascertaining patient's and family's wishes.
- Prescription and provision of emergency drugs.
- On-call arrangements.
- Provision of appropriate equipment (see 📖 Chapter 11, Physical disabilities, pp. 212–220).
- Decisions re resuscitation and hospital transfer.

Ascertaining patient and family wishes
- If a patient is still able to communicate, their wishes regarding care should be established as far as possible.
- If they are unable to formulate or express their wishes, one needs to determine if they have granted anyone LPA (📖 Chapter 18, The legal framework in the UK, pp. 313–322). If not, in the UK the doctor is legally bound to act in the patient's best interest, after consultation with the family.
- Families can provide clues as to the likely preferences of the patient, as well as expressing their own views and wishes. Families' wishes must be listened to very carefully and seriously, but this does not absolve one from acting in the patient's best interest. Good communication will usually produce agreement between professionals and family members as to the desirable course (📖 Chapter 16).
- It can be helpful when there has been much discussion to reach a consensus over a complex issue to set this down in writing and circulate it to all involved in the discussion and execution, so that clarity is shared.

Prescription and provision of emergency drugs
- Anticipatory prescribing is a key factor in allowing people to stay at home.
- Try to anticipate potential complications, considering the underlying condition and comorbidities, any functional risks, e.g. of falls, drugs the patient is already on for possible interactions with emergency drugs, and metabolic status, especially renal and hepatic function.
- For patients with advanced dementia, antipsychotics, analgesics, anti-emetics, anticholinergic drugs to dry up respiratory or other secretions, sedatives, and occasionally anticonvulsants are often needed, but the requirements must be judged case by case. Such medication may need to be in injectable form (📖 Chapter 14, Management of syringe drivers (SDs), pp. 270–271). A case can also be made for oral antibiotics to be available at home for people who are highly susceptible to infection.
- It is prudent to review such prescriptions regularly, e.g. monthly, to renew them or alter them if need or drug metabolism have changed.
- A prescription and administration form is needed to record drug use and allows later review.
- It is sensible to provide the prescribed drugs either in a pre-prepared pack or in a box, possibly with equipment such as a SD with a spare battery, syringes, needles, and cannulas. This avoids time wasting and highly stressful hunting around for drugs or equipment in a crisis. Relatives have been known to miss somebody's last hours of life because they were out looking for prescribed medication in the middle of the night.
- Clear local arrangements regarding out of hours provision of emergency drugs need to be made, e.g. will the drugs be supplied by the hospital pharmacy, a local pharmacy or pharmacies, or the deputizing doctors' service?

- Once prescribed, drugs are the patient's responsibility. There is no legal requirement for opioids to be kept under lock and key, but it is imperative to encourage safe storage of drugs, even more so when children or people with a history of drug abuse may obtain access.
- After somebody dies, or if drugs are no longer needed, remaining drugs need to be disposed of safely. This would usually mean taking them back to a chemist for safe destruction.

Resuscitation and hospital transfer

- Should a patient suffer from a cardiac arrest, most emergency services are duty bound to resuscitate unless there is a signed medical order not to resuscitate. This can be highly distressing for family members.
- Each decision must be individualized. Resuscitation of people with advanced dementia is usually unsuccessful, and it may be unethical to resuscitate someone with a very poor quality of life. The BMA, Resuscitation Council (UK), and RCN have drawn up guidelines regarding decisions for CPR.[1]
- A discussion with the patient or family should include:
  - An appraisal of the prognosis and quality of life of the patient.
  - A realistic appraisal of the likelihood of success of CPR.
  - The potential for damage (e.g. further disabling brain damage for people with dementia).
  - An explanation that a 'not for CPR' decision would not mean 'not for other treatment', e.g. antibiotics.
  - An exploration of any previously expressed wish by the patient.
- Documentation of the CPR decision is essential, to prevent, for example, ambulance crews attempting CPR of a patient for whom it has been agreed not to be appropriate. Local ambulance services have their own forms, and clinicians should familiarize themselves with these and local procedures.
- Copies of the paperwork will usually be kept at the patient's home, with the ambulance service, and perhaps the GP and other interested parties.

The message in a bottle scheme

A simple but effective scheme to prevent unwanted resuscitation was sponsored in a number of areas in the UK by the Rotary Club and Lions' Club.

A form is filled out listing illnesses, essential medication, allergies, family contacts, advance decisions regarding CPR, and transfer to hospital in an emergency. The form is put in a special plastic bottle, which is left inside the fridge door at the patient's home. (Since practically everyone has a fridge, the paperwork can be located quickly in an emergency.) A sticker with a small green cross is placed on the outside of the fridge door as a marker to ambulance crew of belonging to the scheme; another similar sticker is placed on the inside of the house's front door. A sticker with emergency telephone numbers (e.g. local specialist palliative care team) is left on the telephone so more information can be obtained by ambulance crews or families.

The bottles are free and are widely available in participating pharmacies and community teams e.g. specialist palliative care teams. See http://www.lions.org.uk/health/miab/index.php.

---

1 British Medical Association (2007) *Decisions relating to cardiopulmonary resuscitation. A joint statement from the British Medical Association, the Resuscitation Council (UK) and the Royal College of Nursing* (http://www.resus.org.uk/pages/dnar.htm).

Carers' needs (📖 Chapters 21 and 22)

- In providing good support at home, care input up to four times a day, and/or a night carer (though this is expensive and rarely available long term) are very helpful. With more advanced dementia, moving will require two people and so this will either be shared between the main carer and paid carers or be done by two paid carers attending simultaneously.
- Some families hire their own carers, e.g. via local newspapers; vigilance is needed to spot those who might not be competent or honest.
- Respite is crucial to maintain carer health and motivation, as looking after someone with dementia can be totally exhausting.
- Regular day respite using day care and sitting services by support agencies such as Crossroads Care allow the main carer time of their own to go out and do shopping, see friends, indulge their interests, etc.
- Inpatient respite in care homes is invaluable, especially if regular. The opportunity can be taken to assess or work on problems the patient is experiencing. Such respite allows carers to go away on holiday or to visit family. Some carers prefer more frequent but shorter periods of respite, e.g. over a weekend, as they feel that longer periods mean that a longer readaptation period is needed by the person with dementia.
- It is also possible to provide fulltime carers within the home for a period of up to 2 weeks to allow the main carer a break away.
- However, a recent systematic review found only limited and weak evidence that respite care helps carers; the RCTs and quasi-experimental work in the study did not show a reduction in carer burden. This is an important area where further evaluation is clearly needed.
- Carers' physical and mental health needs to be safeguarded as much as the patient's. Sometimes they may not avail themselves of support because they are too busy or harassed, or because they do not trust others to deliver good enough care, often following bad experiences.
- In the Hope for Home study in Greenwich, London, UK, all of the 14 carers interviewed qualitatively said they were glad they had provided care and 11 said that they would have been happy to sacrifice their own health to look after their loved one with dementia. Two of the three who said they would not were parents of small children.[2]
- Carer issues may precipitate permanent admission of the person with dementia to a care home if, e.g.
  - There is carer exhaustion despite optimal support including respite admissions.
  - Night time sleep is badly disrupted.
  - The patient has become aggressive or even violent.
  - The health of the carer is precarious.

2 Treloar A, Crugel M, Adamis D (2009) Palliative and end of life care of dementia at home is feasible and rewarding: results from the 'Hope for Home' study. *Dementia* **8**, 335–47.

Care in care homes

Some demographics

- See 📖 Chapter 5, Where is palliative care delivered?, pp. 71–74 for overview of palliative care in care homes.
- A third of people with dementia live in care homes, more if they:
  - Are older.
  - Have inadequate extra care at home (e.g. no carers or carers who are unwell themselves).
  - Have a greater deficit in performing ADLs.
  - Have BPSD.
  - Are depressed.
  - Have reached a late stage of dementia.
- In Europe and the USA, 50–75% of nursing home residents have cognitive impairment. In the UK, dementia is the commonest cause of placement.
- 67% of dementia deaths in the USA occur in nursing homes.
- In the UK, 16% of all deaths occur in nursing homes, compared with 20–24% in the USA. However, 59% of patients certified as dying of Alzheimer's, dementia or senility die in care homes.
- The number of care home places for older people in the UK has been falling after climbing from the mid-1980s to reach an all time high in 1997. Since then it has shown a steady fall, both in residential and nursing home places. The number of places has fallen by 14% since 2004. However, in 2010 there were some indications of an increase in provision again, and the trend was expected to grow for a few years unless it was neutralized by difficult economic conditions. There has been a huge decrease in local authority care home provision over the years.
- However, demographic changes mean more people need institutional care. In 2007 Macdonald estimated that to keep up the present ratio of care home to own home deaths, care home beds in the UK would have to more than double by 2043; yet in the 10 years before the paper was written, the number of nursing home places had fallen by a sixth.
- Despite the fact that almost 3/4 of nursing home patients in the UK have cognitive impairment, only 30% of places are registered for dementia care.
- In a recent Italian study, patients admitted to special AD care units tended to be younger, less functionally impaired, but more behaviourally disturbed than those admitted to traditional nursing homes; they tended to have fewer hospitalizations and less restraint, and were more likely to have their antipsychotics stopped. By contrast, a US study carried out in 2004 found no differences apart from a higher use of antipsychotics in special units. However, this was before the risks of antipsychotic use in dementia became apparent.

Issues for dementia care in care homes

- In the UK, care homes were for a number of years cut off from the rest of the health service. For a time DNs were not permitted to visit care home patients, just one sign of the isolation of these units. There is an urgent need to integrate care homes in a wider health care context, with much greater knowledge of and permeability to the NHS.
- Medical care of care home residents falls to GPs, but fewer than 40% of GPs have training in health of older people and social care needs.

- Many GPs are not paid for their sessions in care homes, so that they cannot provide locum cover to their practice, for example. This leads to reduced contact with patients.
- There is a conflict between providing patients with a GP of their choice, and providing a GP for the whole care home, which increases efficiency, uniformity of care, and makes communication easier. PCTs have different policies on this.
- GPs are often given insufficient information by inadequately trained staff when asked to see nursing home patients who have been unwell, with the result that the assessments they can make are not of good quality.
- A recent survey from the Royal College of Physicians in England[3] showed that only 16% of geriatric departments allocated time specifically to care homes, translating into 1% of consultant geriatrician sessions available. Another 5.6% gave help outside contractual arrangements, in 'goodwill time'. While 52% of PCTs required geriatricians' involvement in admission to care homes or ongoing care home care, only 18% actually funded this.
- This represents a large drop in involvement since the closure of long-stay wards with frequent geriatrician input in favour of private care homes.
- Geriatrics has developed into a predominantly hospital-based specialty, and other specialties too expect patients to be referred to them. It may be time for a more proactive approach, with multiprofessional team members regularly reviewing care home patients to advise and triage and refer for primary care or specialist review as needed.
- Many people in care homes have undiagnosed dementia. Known dementia may not be listed on the referral form due to fear of admission to a dementia unit instead of a general care unit.
- In the UK there is a split in nurse training between general nursing and mental health nursing. Each has only limited exposure to the skills of the other. This has often led to a situation in dementia care where mental health trained nurses miss physical problems as causes of behavioural disturbance, and general nurses fail to appreciate psychiatric problems they encounter in their patients. It would seem that for an illness requiring holistic care like dementia, the current pattern of nurse training is inadequate.
- Care home staff in the UK (and elsewhere) are among the lowest paid members of the community and are poorly trained. Over 95% are women, staying in a care home for a mean of 3 years, although some care homes have a 70–80% annual staff turnover. Staffing shortages are common.
- A US survey found care home workers wanted better pay, more supervision, to be listened to and appreciated, and to be treated with respect.
- Care home staff rarely give their patients the same level of care that informal carers would in their own homes. This is partly due to numbers and partly because they lack the emotional investment of family members or others close to the patient. In residential and nursing care, it is easy to leave a patient with advanced dementia in their room, in bed, or in their chair, and not engage with them for hours at a time.
- However, it must be said that many care home staff achieve a lot with limited resources, and provide their patients with a caring and

3 Steves CJ, Schiff R, Martin FC (2009) Geriatricians and care homes: perspectives from geriatric medicine departments and primary care trusts. *Clin Med* **9**, 528–33.

personalized environment. Many staff members are very willing to learn new ways of giving better care, but may not have enough opportunities or leadership in this.

- A NAO study in Sheffield, UK, showed that the largest number of patients with frailty or dementia die in care homes. Care homes and patients' own homes were the two alternatives judged best able to reduce the number of frail or demented people dying in hospital.

Possible solutions

- See also ⬚ Chapter 20, Care at home, pp. 340–348.
- The recommendation made in 2000 by the British Geriatric Society, Royal College of Physicians, and the RCN that care home admissions need to follow a geriatrician-led multidisciplinary team assessment needs to be implemented more universally.
- Screening patients being admitted to care homes for dementia is highly desirable, given the large proportion of people with this condition in care.
- Notes in care homes need to become more systematic, with greater training in, and application of, instruments to diagnose problems in people unable to communicate well verbally (e.g. pain; see ⬚ Chapters 7 and 8).
- Handovers between shifts must improve as much valuable clinical and personal information is lost.
- Handover of cases to GPs should be more formalized, perhaps utilizing forms with prompts to ensure the right information is communicated to enable a proper assessment.
- Staff should be mentored in dealing with real cases of advanced and end-stage dementia. They need to learn about symptom recognition and management (both psychiatric and physical), alternatives to drug use when appropriate, ethical issues, and communication with relatives and professionals. Mentoring needs to be coupled with formal teaching.
- The GSF framework can be applied in care homes and provides a useful tool-set for perpetuating learning and improvement.
- Proactive regular geriatrician- or psychogeriatrician-led multiprofessional team visits to care homes would seem highly desirable.

Preventing unnecessary hospital admissions

- The NAO study in Sheffield, UK, showed that almost half the care home patients dying in hospital could have died quite appropriately in their own care home. If someone is dying anyway, it is better for them to die in a familiar place, surrounded by staff who are familiar with them, than in a busy hospital with insufficient staff or time to deal with their needs.
- To do this, care planning needs to be put in place (⬚ Chapter 20, Care at home, pp. 340–348). It is essential to have a written plan which all staff are aware of and signed up to.
- Many hospital admissions happen at night, when there may be a single nurse in charge of a care home who panics despite plans and agreements and calls the emergency services. To prevent this, documentation, availability of medication, and sharing the plan with all relevant staff is essential. It is possible to prevent many hospital deaths. For example in the Croydon Project (⬚ Chapter 20, Care at home, pp. 340–348) there were only 12 hospital admissions over 3 years for the first 150 referrals; 90% of all deaths occurred in their normal place of care.

Care in hospital

- Dementia is common in hospitals, though often undiagnosed. A third of people aged >65 have cognitive impairment in their last year of life, a period when they are likely to spend an inordinate amount of time in hospital.
- People with dementia may be admitted because of direct dementia-related problems, such as delirium, or because of concurrent (e.g. cancer) or intercurrent (e.g. chest infection) conditions.
- In a study in Lincolnshire, UK, sponsored by the NAO, almost half of all hospital admissions of people with dementia followed a 999 call (equivalent to 112 in Europe or 911 in the USA). A fifth were admitted following disorientation or loss of consciousness, which in dementia may often not indicate an acute event.

How hospital affects people with dementia

- Acute hospital care is far from ideal for people with advanced dementia.
- Simple care needs are often poorly met. Staff rarely have the training or the time to feed people with dementia properly; the resulting malnutrition may lead to faster deterioration, more complications, and behavioural problems.
- The busy hospital environment, associated with quick turnover and procedure-oriented, can be particularly confusing and disorientating.
- Procedures can be very distressing and feel very invasive as people with dementia may fail to understand their purpose and see them as personal attacks.
- People who are admitted for surgical procedures may be particularly vulnerable. Delirium is more common with pain and infection; understanding may be less and the feeling of threat may be greater; and procedural and post-procedural pain are often poorly treated. In a well-known paper, people with dementia and a hip fracture were shown to have received only a third of the analgesia of similar but non-demented patients; and half of the non-demented patients found their analgesia to be inadequate anyway. p.r.n. analgesia was often not prescribed and rarely given.
- People who are deluded may find admission particularly confusing. They may form instant likes or suspicions of particular members of staff which may be very difficult to shake off and which may complicate care delivery.
- Staff are unfamiliar with the patient, will be less able to interpret their behaviour, and may miss the presence or significance of important symptoms, which may remain untreated.
- Hospital care is far more expensive than care in the community. For people with dementia the costs are even higher. The costs for treatment of hip fractures in people with dementia nationally were reckoned by the NAO to be almost double those of psychiatrically well patients. Yet the care delivered is at best inadequate and often harmful.
- Much of the extra cost comes from longer admission times associated with dementia. The Lincolnshire study suggested that 68% of people with dementia in acute beds no longer had any need to be there. The NAO also calculated that nationally, a patient with dementia and a hip fracture

has a mean length of hospital stay of 43 days compared with 23 days for psychiatrically well patients. There are studies which show that when earlier discharge is enforced, it simply results in early readmission.

- Hospital care is associated with greater morbidity and functional decline.
- Many markers of inadequate care can be found. In one study in London, people with dementia were less likely to have their religion noted in their notes or to have a spiritual assessment before they died; more likely to have blood gases measured, have urinary catheters or NGTs; and less likely to be referred to the palliative care team or to have palliative medication prescribed.
- Hospital admission leads to significantly greater mortality if advanced dementia is present. A recent study by Sampson in a major London teaching hospital found a fourfold increase in risk of dying if advanced dementia was present. In the Croydon study ([] Chapter 20, Care at home, pp. 340–348), ten out of the twelve people admitted to hospital died during that admission.
- Patients with advanced dementia should be managed with the participation of the hospital psychiatry and palliative care teams. Discharge planning has to be carefully worked out to prevent unnecessary readmission, with much thought given to support needs at home and to planning and preparation for potential crises.
- Clearly, efforts to keep people out of hospital whenever possible are worthwhile. To make this viable, money needs to move from acute care to provide better alternatives for this section of the population.

Care in hospices

- Although in some countries with different health and hospice systems dementia patients are commonly referred to a hospice programme, in the UK hospices have tended to exclude people whose primary diagnosis is dementia (see 📖 Chapters 1 and 5).
- In 2007, out of over 100,000 new referrals for palliative care in the UK, 400 were for a primary diagnosis of dementia.
- Projects now under way appear to indicate that inundation with numbers can be prevented, and that specialist palliative care input can make a very big difference to quality of care. For example in the Croydon project (📖 Chapter 20, Care at home, pp. 340–348), no patient required admission to the hospice—almost all patients were cared for in their usual place of care. Only about 2% needed to be under the hospice home care team, and then almost always for less than a week before death, mainly because of difficulties relating to renewing SDs and giving out-of-hours medication in the very last days of life. The key is utilizing the right model of care, which takes into account the differences between dementia and more acute conditions with which specialist palliative care usually becomes involved.
- Apart from training issues, hospices may be poorly designed for the care of people with moderate or advanced dementia. For example, many hospices have numerous doors leading to the outside which could encourage patients who wander to find their way out. One would hope that hospices being built or adapted now will be more dementia-friendly. However, it is often possible to compensate at least partially for these deficiencies, and the provision of calm, good, personal care is likely to be on effective counter-measure.
- Hospice staff clearly need training in handling people with dementia. Even if they do not admit people whose dementia is their primary diagnosis, a large number of hospice inpatients and home care patients will have cognitive impairment, often undiagnosed. In a recent study of 120 consecutive admissions to a hospice inpatient unit, a third were found to be cognitively impaired.[4] Learning how to care for people with dementia is not an optional extra.

Further reading

Hossack Y on behalf of Residents Action Group for the Elderly (RAGE) (2006) *Care homes closures, the law, its practice and the implications*. Available at: http://www.ragenational.com/closure_facts. htm (accessed 27 March 2009).

National Audit Office (2007) *Improving services and support for people with dementia*, p. 72. National Audit Office, London.

Sampson EL et al. (2006) Differences in care received by patients with and without dementia who died during acute hospital admission: a retrospective case note study. *Age Ageing* **35**, 187–9.

Sampson EL et al. (2009) Dementia in the acute hospital: prospective cohort study of prevalence and mortality. *Br J Psychiat* **195**, 61–6.

Shaw C et al. (2009) Systematic review of respite care in the frail elderly. *Health Technol Assess* **13**, 1–224, iii.

Williams J, Netten A (2003) PSSRU Personal Social Services Research Unit. guidelines for the closure of care homes for older people: prevalence and content of local government protocols. Available at: http://www.pssru.ac.uk/pdf/dp1861_2.pdf

4 Henderson M, Hotopf M (2007) Use of the clock-drawing test in a hospice population. *Palliat Med* **21**, 559–65.

The role of the GP in the community

- 2/3 of people with dementia will live and die in the community.
- The majority will be older people with comorbidities whose health care needs (physical, psychological, and palliative), will be addressed in the main within the framework of general practice.
- There is no consistent level of provision of specialist dementia nursing (Admiral Nurses and community psychiatric nurses) in the UK and continuity of care, for many, comes from their GP and DNs.
- Diagnosis of dementia:
  - Only 20–40% of people affected have any formal diagnosis.
  - Only 33% receive any specialist health care.
  - 2 new cases/GP/year.
- Characteristics of a diagnosis of dementia:
  - Late.
  - At a time of crisis.
  - Too late for effective intervention.
  - Too late to prevent harm.
  - Followed by a low level of active management.
- A GP appointment, usually in a busy surgery, is only 10 minutes long, is often a triadic consultation (confidentiality is lost, the needs of the carer may dominate), and addresses other health matters in addition to those arising from dementia. The earlier stages of dementia provide the opportunity to talk about and record views and wishes for care in the future.
- In advanced dementia, home visits are more likely as people affected become increasingly physically frail. A regular home visit by the GP (1–3 monthly depending on need):
  - Supports patient and family.
  - Allows early recognition of problems (psychobehavioural disturbance, swallowing difficulty, recurrent falls, weight loss, carer exhaustion, abuse).
  - Provides appropriate treatment.
  - Makes timely referral to other agencies.
  - Recognizes and plans for care in terminal phase.
- Include the patient on the GSF register. Share information with the primary care team, identify the preferred place of care and death, discuss treatment options, anticipate and plan for likely problems, avoid unnecessary hospital admissions.
- *End of life care in the community.* GP symptom assessment and active management including use of SDs if necessary. Advice from the local palliative care team on drugs and doses in opioid-naive patients. DNs plus Marie Curie nurses or local Hospital at Home teams to support the family day and night in the terminal phase.
- For many, avoidance of institutional care is a priority. The person may have expressed strong views at an earlier stage of dementia. Family carers may feel very guilty if unable to cope. Main carer may be a spouse of advanced years with their own health problems. Well-supported individuals and family are less likely to need institutional care.

Strategies to help people with dementia

What people with dementia experience:
- Loss of immediacy of thought and response.
- High stress if conversations are full of questions.
- Sounds may be jumbled or meaningless.
- Reception and understanding may be intermittent or lost.
- Increasing difficulty finding the right words.
- Tire easily because of the effort involved in communicating.

Strategies to manage:
- Slow measured pace to all encounters.
- Minimizing background noise and motion.
- Using clues and shared reminiscences to identify yourself.
- Allowing time for the answers.
- Looking for anxiety and providing reassurance.

GP role in nursing and residential homes
- Nearly 2/3 of residents in UK care homes have cognitive impairment but many have not had a formal assessment and diagnosis. Possible causes:
  - Depression.
  - Hypothyroidism.
  - Institutionalization and lack of stimulation.
  - Dementia.
- Cognitive impairment should not be viewed as 'expected' but assessed and actively treated or managed depending on the cause.

GP visits
- In inner city areas, individuals tend to remain registered with their GP when entering a care home (nursing or residential) and GP practices may have patients in as many as 18 homes. Care homes may have residents registered with similar numbers of GP practices and be liaising with up to 60 different GPs. The resulting care offered is often reactive in nature. An *aligned system of care* between an individual care home and a lead GP from a single GP practice allows a proactive approach which may bring substantial improvements to the standard of medical care received by residents. There is potential to address workload and financial implications for practices within practice-based commissioning and locally enhanced service agreements with the managing authority (the PCT in UK, although this may be changing) (Table 20.2).
- The GSF (📖 Chapter 4, Identifying the need for palliative care, pp. 63–65) facilitates planning for patients with advanced dementia in care homes. The GP or care home manager can take the lead role, coordinate regular discussions and organize sharing of information with other health professionals and the out-of-hours service provider.

Advance care plan
- An advance care plan considers the following elements:
  - What elements of care are important to you and those close to you as your condition progresses?
  - What would you and those close to you like to happen?

Table 20.2 Reactive versus proactive GP care

Problems of reactive care	Benefits of proactive care
Reactive to an acute problem—'visit when called'	Proactive care—regular weekly visit
GP may have limited knowledge of the patient	GP with knowledge and long-term responsibility for patient
Accompanying staff member may be poorly briefed	Fully briefed supernumerary staff member
Lack of privacy and confidentiality	Private room for discussion
Poor facilities for examination and hygiene	Appropriate facilities for examination and hand washing
At lunchtime (person eating, staff busy)	Visit planned to avoid mealtimes
Brief (GP time constraints, between surgeries)	Adequate time to discuss and assess patients
Meets short-term health needs only	Meets short- and longer-term health needs
Does not address advance planning	Allows for advance planning of care, including end of life care
Ignores potential for staff support and training	Provides adequate support and potential for staff training
Multiple prescribers for each patient	Limits prescribers for each patient

- What would you and those close to you NOT want to happen?
- Preferred place of care and death?
- Any special requests or arrangements?
- Uses knowledge of person's values, wishes and beliefs and views from families and friends to inform 'best interest' decisions about care.
- A values history is worth undertaking. This explores a person's views and values (directly or from close acquaintances) so that subsequent decisions when the person is incompetent can be taken in line with these views. Values are also less threatening and more easily shared than making a formal advance directive. They can be formalized into a document, although this has no legal force[5] (see also Chapter 13, Elements of decision-making, pp. 236–239).
- Identifies patients with an advance directive or appointed attorney re health and welfare.
- Identifies patients needing an independent mental capacity advocate (IMCA).
- Assists the GP and staff in planning for care at the end of life.

5 Doukas DJ, McCullough LB (1991) The values history. The evaluation of the patient's values and advance directives. *J Fam Pract* **32**, 145–53.

- Dynamic document—can be updated at any time.
- May identify dispute between family members.

Medication review
- Primary aim of medication in advanced dementia is symptom control.
- No research evidence to support continued use of drugs to reduce cardiovascular disease risk in patients with advanced dementia.
- Explore alternative formulations (liquid or dispersible) and delivery mechanisms (buccal, TD) for required repeat medication if there are compliance issues related to behavioural symptoms or swallowing problems in advanced dementia.

Some example of medication review

Antihypertensives	Weight loss in advanced dementia, postural hypotension, increased renal impairment	Consider dose reduction or stopping
Potentially toxic drugs	Warfarin, especially if high fall risk, amiodarone, digoxin	Consider stopping
Sedatives and antipsychotics	Often high dose on arrival; aim for short-term use only; monthly review of dose	Consider dose reduction and/or stopping antipsychotics after patient has settled into care home

End of life care

Recognition of the particular difficulties in providing good end of life care for people with advanced dementia has led to the formation of a Palliative Care in Dementia Group in Peterborough, UK. The group includes health professionals from a wide range of disciplines in both primary and secondary care and is dedicated to resolving these difficulties, improving standards of care, and fulfilling a local educational role. The work of the group is cited as an example of innovative practice in the End of Life Care Strategy, 2008.
- Practical tools have been developed with documentation designed or adapted to meet the needs of both residents and nursing and care staff and supported by written protocols. Generic versions of all the documents and associated protocols are available on line.

Palliative Care in Dementia Group, Peterborough (founded February 2005)

- GPs
- Consultant physician, older people
- Lead clinical psychologist, older people
- Consultant psychiatrist, older people
- Macmillan nurse
- Specialist nursing and residential home manager
- Palliative care consultant, Sue Ryder Thorpe Hall Hospice

- Older people's specialist team (OPST) (responsibility for residents in care homes):
  - Senior community dietician
  - Modern matrons
  - Speech and language therapist
  - Community psychiatric nurse

End of life care pathway

Recognition of the terminal phase is difficult in people with advanced dementia. Criteria for entry onto an end of life care pathway have been adapted to accommodate that difficulty. The doctors and the team should have:

- Knowledge of the disease stage/progression.
- Knowledge that there are no other practicable or appropriate medical options available to the patient.
- Awareness that removal from the pathway is an option if spontaneous improvement occurs.

AND

- The patient is:
  - Profoundly weak (bed- or chairbound) (2).
  - Drowsy for extended periods (2).
  - Finding it increasingly difficult to swallow medication (1).
  - Becoming increasingly uninterested in food and drink (1).
- A score of 6/6 is the criterion for commencing the pathway, assuming that remediable measures have been considered and inappropriate sedation is not a significant contributory factor.
- In practice, the inclusion of an option to remove a patient from the pathway if improvement occurs is a reassurance to the GP and team using the pathway. Recognition that the patient has become uninterested in food and drink has proved to be the most important factor in identifying the terminal phase in those patients with advanced dementia who have become totally bedbound and dependent, sometimes for years.

Emergency situations

- GPs can take the lead in educating and empowering staff in decision-making in the acute situation and holding regular *significant event meetings* with care home staff provides a forum in which these issues can be addressed. The potential harm and distress caused by an emergency hospital admission for a person with dementia must always be weighed up against the likelihood of benefit. The out-of-hours service provision is more likely to result in hospital admission in an acute situation. Having a robust advance care plan, holding regular reviews of those patients assessed as requiring palliative care, and having good communication with the out-of-hours service, helps to support staff willing and able to care for patients in the care home setting.
- The GP has a continuing responsibility for any patient with dementia who has been admitted to hospital as a person closely involved in the care of the person who lacks capacity, under the terms of the MCA, e.g. consideration of PEG placement for a patient with advanced dementia who has had a stroke and acute loss of the ability to swallow,

is a decision in which the GP should contribute to discussion about the best interests of the patient.

The future

GPs will be looking after increasing numbers of patients with dementia, in the community and care homes.

Aims

- Work in partnership with those affected, families, care homes and health professionals across primary and secondary care to deliver high-quality holistic care.
- Improve health and ameliorate the course of the disease.
- Remove the stigma of a diagnosis of dementia.
- Maintain a high standard of care when palliative care needs become the priority and at the end of life.
- Ensure that death is peaceful and dignified for patient and families.

A family carer's perspective

Introduction

We asked Barbara Pointon for a personal view of what it is like to care for someone throughout their dementia illness [Eds]

Malcolm, my husband, was an engaging music lecturer, a brilliant pianist, a wonderful husband and father, and his razor-sharp wit could make you laugh until your sides ached. Diagnosed with AD at 51, I cared for him at home (except for 2 years spent in a nursing home in the middle stage) until he died 16 years later from the physical ravages caused by the disease. Living and dying with dementia can take an agonisingly long time.

Pinpointing when palliative care began proves difficult. Total dependency? For Malcolm that was 8 years before he died and the following year he completely lost his mobility and became mute. Problems with swallowing and tonic–clonic seizures (myoclonic jerking having been present from an early stage) arose 4 years before he died, along with steady weight loss which accelerated in the last year of his life. When I brought him home from the nursing home, it was believed that he had only 6 months left, but he lived for a further 7 years. Malcolm always was a nonconformist. But it illustrates how problematical it is to predict the length of the illness, why aspects of palliative care may need to be introduced over a long time, and why artificial time limits to its access are simply not workable. Every individual patient and carer is different.

I freely admit that caring for Malcolm proved both physically and emotionally demanding. He required two people (myself and a live-in carer) to be on duty or on call at all times. I did a 142-hour week, with my 26 hours off-duty covered by replacement care at home; in the later stages we had some extra night cover. Using direct payments (and later NHS continuing care) it was no more expensive than a nursing home placement and less than the cost of a hospital bed. Good-quality care from familiar staff gave Malcolm contentment and I gained peace of mind. Although it was often an uphill struggle for equipment, care personnel, services, and funding, it taught me an important lesson. Palliative care for someone with dementia is not the same as that for those who have all their cognition; it requires special skills and advice which cross over the usual physical/mental health boundaries, sometimes resulting in modification of both medical and nursing procedures.

In the descriptions of aspects of Malcolm's care that follow, I will highlight the lessons I learned, the effects upon me and the family, and where I looked for advice and moral support.

Physical care

Visuo-perceptual problems

The great majority of patients who have AD encounter visuo-spatial problems and have difficulties in processing what they see. Malcolm frequently miscued his environment or other people's actions and did not know where he was in space. This seriously affected three areas of his care.

Moving and handling

When being transferred by hoist, the combination of myoclonic jerking and not knowing where he was in space made Malcolm very fearful. Two people were required at all times, for safety and reassurance. Even when in bed, Malcolm would not know whether he was looking up at the ceiling or down into an awesome bottomless pit.

Changing incontinence pads

After losing mobility, it would be normal practice to change incontinence pads by rolling the patient on the bed. But Malcolm believed that the roll would cause him to fall and desperately fought to return on his back. It took us ages to get the pad in place, and the alternative, to personally support him in a semi-standing position, proved hazardous for all. The Alzheimer's Society outreach worker recommended a standing hoist; job done, quickly, efficiently and with no trauma for Malcolm or for us. It was the best piece of equipment we ever had, but it took 4 months to arrive from the Joint Equipment Service. When equipment is needed, it's needed right away.

Nursing assessments

The nursing assessments had four categories for vision: no problems, wears glasses, visually impaired, or blind. It was impossible to assess the acuity of Malcolm's vision because he could neither read nor speak. So either this box was left blank, or it was based on what was known about his former vision, both completely missing the point that no matter how well or badly Malcolm was seeing, he could no longer accurately process what he saw. The physical and terrifying psychological effect upon him was huge, yet this neurological factor is frequently a major omission in assessment of AD patients, especially for continuing care.

Bowel management

- It is not your usual constipation. The brain has difficulty in interpreting signals from the bowel and may fail to coordinate muscles to effect a conscious bearing down. Giving daily laxatives simply produced faecal leakage and risked breakdown of skin. Later on, even normal suppositories and enemas were ineffective, so, with the continence adviser, we devised a regimen for Malcolm.
- We kept his liquid intake up to a litre a day for as long as possible, put black treacle in his breakfast baby porridge and ensured he had plenty of pureed fresh fruit, especially pears. We allowed the bowel to fill until, on the fourth day, we gave him five pureed prunes and their juice at breakfast, inserted two bisacodyl suppositories after lunch and allowed 4 hours for them to work.

- We then hoisted Malcolm onto a shower-chair/commode (with a horseshoe-shaped padded seat for comfort) and massaged his abdomen, giving plenty of time for gravity to help. If I stood behind and leaned him forward against my body, he would push back against me and the action would start things off.
- In the last stages, we also had to use digital stimulation of the anus. Some nurses and care staff would not do it, calling it abuse, but I felt it was more abusive to leave Malcolm in his discomfort. I understand that the whole regimen is similar to that used for paraplegics, and in reality there is little difference—both cause disruption to nerve pathways.

Tissue viability

- When someone is immobile, it can be tempting to allow them to become bedbound. Malcolm could not even slightly shift himself in bed, so we embarked on a routine of six transfers between bed, recliner chair, wheelchair, and armchair each day to alternate potential pressure points.
- We were immensely grateful to the DNs for early provision of pressure relief—gel mattress (later on, alternating air mattress), gel cushion, and a hospital bed with electrically operated headrest, height, and foot positioning. Its versatility made it easier for us to reposition him (e.g. for feeding) without hauling him about.
- Malcolm believed showers were people hitting him; with the bathroom upstairs inaccessible, he took no harm whatsoever from 7 years of strip-washes in his shower-chair in the kitchen, where there was plenty of space for us and the standing hoist facilitating scrupulous cleansing and drying. Having no access to bathroom or showering facilities need not be a barrier to caring at home.
- At one point, catheterization was suggested, but Malcolm would not have understood the apparatus and may have tugged at it, as well as it presenting a potential source of infection. Providing incontinence pads were periodically reviewed for correct size, absorbency, and snug fit, we used them to the very end. Mountains of daily laundry can become the last straw causing carers to give up.
- We only used pure aloe jelly on Malcolm's skin, and despite being doubly incontinent and immobile for 7 years, he never had a bedsore, let alone an infected one.
- Despite its physical demands, the care workers and I were proud of this aspect of our care, which contributed so much to Malcolm's comfort and contentment.

Pain identification and control

- Malcolm never had a pain assessment, let alone one designed specifically for dementia. His face became mask-like and so the usual signs of screwing up were simply not there—the smallest frown could mean big trouble.
- He was mute, unable to nod or shake his head, and, because of visuo-spatial problems, unable to point to or clutch at the site of the pain. His idiosyncratic sign of infection was a bright red left ear—but we had no idea where the trouble lay and would phone for a GP to call.

- Continuity of live-in care staff in this situation was vital, because they recognized when he was 'not quite himself today'. We all relied on keen observation and the kind of sixth sense you develop when you have a small baby.
- Malcolm developed torticollis; we were unsure whether this caused pain. The physiotherapist advised laying him fairly flat on his back, at odds with other nursing advice on positioning in relation to his swallowing problems. Sometimes specialist nurses only saw their particular bit of the jigsaw.
- Just occasionally, out-of-hours GPs tended to attribute all physical symptoms to AD, and queried why we were bothering. In contrast, our own GP was unfailingly supportive of both of us.

Medication

- I discovered, through the Alzheimer's Society, that medication may in some cases need to be reduced in line with severity of dementia and/or weight loss. In the nursing home, Malcolm had become rigid, could no longer bend in the middle and spent his days miserably confined to bed. His consultant advised reducing his sodium valproate, but it had not been actioned by the home's GP because the nurses felt that Malcolm was 'easier to manage now he's off his feet'. I asked for a meeting, the medication was gradually reduced, and Malcolm was soon walking about again, albeit gingerly. It became the turning point for me to bring him home again.
- Adult doses had the effect on his compromised brain of overdoses. For example, adult antibiotics caused him to be so sleepy that he couldn't take drinks. So, throughout his last 7 years, he was prescribed paediatric dosages or preparations of all medications. Even his final SD had only a half-dose in it. *[Response to medication is a very individual matter, which in many cases is resolved by titrating medication to response and dose reduction may not be as true for antibiotics. If necessary, take microbiological advice. Eds].*
- A small dose of clonazepam, prescribed to hold his epileptic activity at bay during the night, severely depressed his breathing and caused episodes of Cheyne–Stokes respiration. With the agreement of our GP, we gradually reduced it to a quarter of the dosage and Malcolm's breathing returned to normal. Fine adjustment of drugs was often required.
- When swallowing problems began, his sodium valproate was prescribed in liquid form, but its strong taste and aroma caused long spasms of coughing. We found it helpful to mix it with a small amount of yoghurt and administered it before food, rather than after, so that it was not pouched in his cheeks to just dribble out again later. A nurse commented that mixing it into yoghurt could be regarded as covert administration of drugs and therefore constituted restraint. It is at times like these that one feels very vulnerable. Surely restraint should not be defined by the action, but by the intention behind the action?

Food and drink: swallowing problems

I was impressed with the support we received from the speech and language therapist, dietician, and community dentist.

Offering food and drink
- It used to take up to an hour to feed Malcolm a small bowl of pureed home-cooked food and 350mL of thickened fruit juice, served cold, which was more easily controlled in the mouth than warm drinks.
- It is the most trustful thing in the world to open your mouth to be fed; continuity and patience of staff are essential; Malcolm used to refuse to take food from a new care worker for several days—which could be seriously misinterpreted in other settings.
- After being away for a short break, Malcolm refused to accept food from me. I found this emotionally devastating; it was as though he was rejecting me personally. Overcome with guilt for taking a break, I fled the room and burst into tears, illustrating how near to the edge carers can get.

Artificial feeding and regurgitation
PEG feeding is not normally recommended in dementia because of the equal risk of choking on regurgitation; when Malcolm vomited (usually a result of rapid rise in his temperature) he no longer understood to lean forward and open his mouth. Like a small baby, the vomit would appear from down his nose; we had to forcibly hold his mouth open and rapidly tip the bed forwards to prevent choking, all emphasizing the high level of vigilance and quick action required at this stage of dementia care.

Oral hygiene
- Extra care with oral hygiene, once Malcolm lost the natural cleansing actions of speaking and chewing, became a priority and the community dentist visited regularly to advise us. He reassured us that broken-down teeth are not necessarily painful, as the nerve recedes to compensate.
- Malcolm no longer understood to rinse out, so we had to examine labels on toothpastes to confirm that they were safe to swallow, and several were not. We discovered that a pure aloe vera toothpaste was not only safe to swallow but also prevented the recurrence of gingivitis, ulceration, and thrush.

Weight loss
- Despite eating the same amount of food over the last 4 years, Malcolm inexorably lost weight until he became cadaverous. For me, this was one of the most harrowing parts of the illness.
- We kept daily records of food and liquid intake and output. Knowing how much Malcolm ate, and that fortified drinks and powders made no difference, I mused that, in a nursing home, it would be all too easy for relatives to wrongly accuse the staff of neglect. Inevitable weight loss needs to be understood and carefully explained to families.

Tonic–clonic seizures
Complication of being mute
Tonic–clonic seizures began about 4 years before Malcolm died. He obviously had the same aura or 'warning' as anyone else, but could neither tell us nor take action to put himself in a safe position. Sometimes they would occur in the middle of hoisting or feeding him, or when he was in

the wheelchair. The seizures were heralded by a series of head-drops, requiring rapid action to get him into a horizontal position to prevent him hurting his back as it arched.

The value of oxygen therapy

On several occasions we had to call paramedics to get Malcolm out of a prolonged seizure. As oxygen levels drop sharply in seizure, they administered oxygen and eventually one of them suggested that we should have a canister in the house to save callouts. Our GP applied on our behalf, but was stunned to receive the message that Malcolm, incapable of following instructions, would have to go to hospital for a spirometry test before he could be prescribed it. When we eventually received the oxygen, it worked like magic—decreasing both the length and severity of attacks. *[This is an intriguing idea, possibly explicable in terms of brain hypoxia, but there is currently no published evidence for the use of oxygen in this way. Eds.]*

When Malcolm's oral secretions became copious and troublesome, instead of using pharmaceutical methods of drying them up (which would have adverse effects on other bodily functions requiring secretions), we would administer a few minutes of oxygen to successfully clear the mouth.

Chest infections

To treat or not to treat?

- At the beginning, I was of the opinion that a serious chest infection might provide a kindly exit. After all, my parents' generation regarded pneumonia as 'the old man's friend'. But the reality became very different.
- Malcolm had several chest infections in the last 3 years, some of which caused the GP to warn that he may only have days or hours left; he was certainly true to the GSF graph of dying from dementia which bumps along the bottom for a long time. But a curious thing happened. With all rationality gone, an almost primitive instinct for survival took over. If Malcolm was still fighting and showing a desire to live, then I had to support him in that.
- So the GP and I agreed that Malcolm should still be prescribed a paediatric antibiotic, with the full understanding that it may not work, but it would give symptomatic relief and I would feel that I was supporting him.

Some non-pharmaceutical strategies

Changing Malcolm's pads on the standing hoist had an extra benefit; the act of leaning forward in a supported standing position nearly always brought about a good cough and expelling of infected mucus; we also put a few drops each of eucalyptus, lavender, tea tree, and sometimes manuka oils in an oil-burner at night which helped to keep his airways clear and relaxed him (and me!).

Temperature control

Diagnosis of infections was complicated by Malcolm occasionally losing control of his temperature, producing very high readings with no underlying cause. We used well-tried methods: tepid sponging, fans, packets of ice cubes wrapped in tea towels, but one night could not bring the temperature down. He was admitted to hospital, where I told nurses and medical staff that this was a usual effect of his AD and all he needed was plenty of icepacks. But Malcolm was subjected to an i.v. antibiotic drip, had bloods taken, and was admitted to a ward, before it was declared that no infection could be found. The staff were surprised that losing temperature control (such as is found in some brain tumours) could be part of severe dementia. On one hand I was pleased that they had left no stone unturned, but on the other a carer's knowledge of this patient had been disregarded.

Care beyond the physical—a model of self

Reflecting on the way we develop as whole human beings, we enter the world simply as who we are, our very core of identity. As babies we learn to explore the world through our five senses, thereby experiencing emotions; our psychological self begins to take shape, forming a second layer around the core. Then as toddlers, a third layer appears: gaining control of basic physical functions to walk, talk, feed and dress ourselves, eye–hand coordination, and continence. Our large outside layer contains our sophisticated human skills acquired later—the 3 Rs, abstract thinking, advanced motor and intellectual skills, learning about the wider world, and social skills. But dementia attacks this model of self from the outside, stripping away over time the two outer layers—the layers which the world sees and values most—leaving the two inner layers more exposed and therefore more important.

So often, particularly if someone has been aggressive in the middle stage, when they become mute and immobile, care staff say, 'He's no trouble now' (and often downgrade them in continuing care assessments) when nothing could be further from the truth. The greatest gift anyone can give to people with dementia is time. In this severe stage, the patient needs one-to-one attention to fulfil their sensory, psychological, emotional, and spiritual needs. So what contributed to Malcolm's contentment in the palliative stage?

- *Sight*: bright colours (red/yellow spectrum), smiley faces, not looking at the same bit of wall all day.
- *Taste*: strong flavours, not bland invalid food (unless for medical reasons).
- *Smell*: favourite aftershave, flowers, aromatherapy (he found this blissful), smell of cooking.
- *Hearing*: continuing to talk to him—the sound of the human voice is a basic need—even though there was no response. Music got through when all channels were blocked: CDs of his taste, live music (carol singers came in to sing 'Away in a Manger'), and we sometimes hummed while going about his care.
- *Touch*: the most important of all. At night, when Malcolm woke up in fear, I did not run to the medicine bottle, but whispered in his ear, gave him a cuddle and he would sigh, relax into me, and drift off to sleep again. Political correctness did not stand in the way of paid staff also responding similarly to Malcolm's deep psychological need to be physically comforted and feel safe.

In this way, his deeper spiritual needs were met: feeling loved and cherished.

The dying phase

I sensed that Malcolm's final chest infection was very different; he had begun on the paediatric antibiotic but appeared listless and world-weary. A few days later, his swallowing stopped altogether and I had to decide whether to send him to hospital to continue the antibiotic i.v. or to allow nature to take its course.

Making decisions on behalf of another person

Not long after he was diagnosed, Malcolm wrote in his diary: 'So it's Alzheimer's. I hope when the end comes it's not too messy'. Our GP and I had earlier constructed a letter to lie on his file, saying that in the terminal phase, no aggressive interventions except a s.c. SD to ease pain and prevent epileptic seizures. I knew in my head this was still the right path to take, but my heart took a lot of convincing and I spent much of the rest of the day in tears. The finality of the decision weighed heavily.

Receiving and giving support in the end stage

Ten years previously, when nursing Malcolm's mother who was dying from cancer, I greatly appreciated the practical advice and moral support of the palliative care team. So I asked if they could call and advise us, especially on positioning someone who had become almost skeletal. But it was only available for cancer. Patients dying from causes other than cancer can be unnecessarily admitted to hospital (which for Malcolm would have been terrifying after the tranquillity and familiarity of home) because the main carer feels afraid and unsupported. I had to convince our care staff that we were not 'starving Malcolm to death' and that he would feel neither hunger nor thirst provided we kept his lips moist.

He went to the brink and stepped back several times before he died a week later, surrounded by family. As my yoga teacher had recommended, at the very end, I put my fingers in the hollow at the nape of Malcolm's neck and my other hand under his lower back, and each member of the family, including our two young grandchildren (who were not at all fazed) held on to a part of him. She had said that was how Malcolm had entered the world, held securely by the midwife, and it would ease his passing: a return to the imagery of his central core I referred to above (🕮 Chapter 21, Care beyond the physical—a model of self, p. 369). We told him we would always love him and that he was safe while a favourite piece of gentle music played in the background. Coincidence or not, Malcolm's laboured breathing gradually quietened and the gaps between breaths became longer until imperceptibly breathing ceased.

Outside, it had been snowing. A couple of minutes later, the 5-year-old piped up, 'Daddy, can we make a snowman now?'. Which they did, and wrapped Malcolm's treasured old university scarf around its neck—a wonderful reminder that life and death are intertwined.

The death certificate read: (1) broncho-pneumonia (2) AD. But if Malcolm's swallowing and mobility had not been eroded by AD, he would never have died of pneumonia at the age of 66. I look forward to the time when it can be accurately recorded as a joint cause of death.

Effect of Malcolm's illness on me, our family, and friends

Particularly when Malcolm lost normal communication and no longer visually recognized us, some wider family members and friends fell away. But I firmly believe he still recognized my voice and would very slightly turn his head towards the sound. Family and old friends needed reassurance that their visits were still important; in talking to him and holding his hand, even though he could not recognize their faces, nor respond or even smile, their voices would be familiar and comforting. And, selfishly, I wanted their company too.

I was very grateful to those who came regularly to sit companionably with Malcolm, giving me an opportunity to do a household chore, get out in the garden, or simply catch a nap. I realize they sometimes found it emotionally challenging.

The relentless vigilance, broken sleep, and both physical and emotional demands of long-term caring had repercussions on my own health, leaving a legacy of asthma, joint pain, and poor sleep patterns. Caring is all-consuming; I needed the series of battles with officialdom for funding like a hole in the head.

The need for carer support

I appreciated regular visits from our social worker, GP, the Alzheimer's Society outreach worker, and the wisdom of a geriatrician who visited every 2 or 3 months to see Malcolm, reviewed aspects of his condition, and reported back to the GP and DNs. But in terms of nursing advice, what would have helped me most would have been access to a dementia care advisory nurse (with crossover mental and physical expertise, such as an Admiral Nurse) who would also have become a main source of moral support. During the last 2 years, there were 12 professionals actively involved in Malcolm's care, not counting hands-on carers, and I believe one dementia nurse could have covered many of those roles and would have seen the whole picture.

Loss and bereavement

Because I had mourned each loss of an aspect of Malcolm's life over 16 years, the final loss was just the last of many. My initial response at his death was one of relief and release for both of us, and as a result I could not grieve properly. When I thought of him, I could only recall this image of a man broken in mind and body. The celebratory concert in his honour, held 3 months later, where friends played and sang and told hilarious stories about life with Malcolm, proved both healing and cathartic, helping to re-create the Malcolm I knew. Then life became really busy. *Malcolm and Barbara: Love's Farewell*, a programme filmed over Malcolm's last months, was broadcast on UK television in August 2007.[1] It was followed by extensive public speaking and meetings; I did not leave myself enough personal space to reflect and face up to being alone for the first time in my life. Consequently, 18 months after Malcolm died, at a pause in the busy-ness, a delayed bereavement shock hit me, physically and mentally, like a sledgehammer. Apparently, it is common in long-term carers and a case could be made for delayed or staggered bereavement counselling.

Malcolm's real legacy lies in my sharing our experiences of dementia in order to try and enlighten care for those who come after us. Through the pages of this chapter, the losses Malcolm experienced and the huge personal loss of my husband, best friend, and soulmate, are perhaps being turned into gains.

Further reading

Miesen BML, Jones GMM (2006) *Care-giving in dementia – research and applications*, Vol. 4, Chs 1 and 2. Routledge, London.

---

1 This was a follow-up to the film, *Malcolm and Barbara—A Love Story*, portraying the couple facing the earlier stages of Malcolm's AD, which was broadcast on television in 1999.

Chapter 22

Caring for the carers

Who are the carers?

Carers form a very mixed group, of all ages and caring for all manner of disabilities. There are several million carers in the UK. With the number of people with dementia dramatically increasing, the number of carers looking after someone with dementia will also increase steeply. Given the amount of time during which people with dementia require ongoing care, carers face a long and tortuous journey

Although there may be professional or paid assistance going into the home, most of the care for people with dementia at home is provided informally by family and friends. Most carers are close family members, usually spouses or adult children. Less commonly, other relatives or, occasionally, neighbours or friends may be the main carers. Whether the carer resides with the person with dementia will influence contact time and determines the tasks that the carer is required to undertake.

- Spouses are likely to be older than other types of carer and may have physical or mental health needs of their own, which may hamper their ability to provide care.
- Some studies have suggested that wives are more likely to undertake hands-on care tasks, such as personal care, whereas husbands act more 'managerially', concerning themselves mainly with finances and employing paid carers. However, more recent studies have not confirmed this.
- The literature has emphasized the role of adult daughters as carers, with the caregiving often falling to daughters or daughters-in-law, which is the cultural norm in many White Western and other societies. Females are assumed to be nurturing; it is traditional for children to care for elderly members. Women are assumed to be more flexible; and thus to have more free time.
- Spillman and Pezin[1] introduced the concept of the 'sandwich generation', identifying predominantly middle-aged women who have the added stress of employment and are caught between the needs of dependent parents and dependent children. These situations may be further complicated by divorce and remarriage; many women may end up caring for multiple elderly people.
- Recent evidence shows less demarcation between men's and women's roles and assumptions about male and female roles appear less valid than they may have been. Indeed, the Alzheimer's Association in the USA showed that the percentage of male carers had gone up from 19% in 1996 to almost 40% by 2008. The relationship the carer had to the individual prior to the illness still remains. 'Carer' is an additional but not a replacement identity for previous relationships and roles, e.g. husband or son. Indeed, some spouses do not see themselves as carers but see the caring role as part of their bigger identity as wife or husband.
- For some people the acceptance of the new caring element to that relationship is a difficult but crucial step. The changing nature of the relationship as the person with dementia becomes increasingly dependent often requires physical and emotional adjustments and can generate feelings of:
  - Guilt.
  - Depression.

- Resentment.
- Anger.
- Isolation.
- Stress.
- All of these feelings may require individual attention when considering the needs of carers of people with dementia.
- Stress induced by the caring role can manifest itself in many ways:
  - Loss of self-esteem.
  - Lack of concentration.
  - Exhaustion.
  - Irritability.
  - Aggressiveness and even hostility to the person cared for.
  - Sleep problems.
- Providing understanding and emotional support to carers; recognizing the circumstances under which they find themselves, and allowing the opportunity to talk about their situation can give many the space to air their concerns and stressors and can be cathartic. It is an important element of carer support to enable the family member to consider this new and emerging role but also to retain a focus on their previous relationship with the person with dementia.
- There may be times when a carer has mental health problems in their own right, possibly due to their caring role. A survey of 150 family carers in London found that 23% suffered at or above caseness levels for anxiety, and over 10% for depression. A significant proportion of elderly carers suffer from milder dementia themselves.
- Whilst various 'carer supports' may be of benefit in helping the carer to manage their sense of burden and stress, it may be necessary to consider a referral to their GP for physical or psychological problems associated with caring and to specialist services for support in their caring role, e.g. local health and social care services, Alzheimer's Society, Admiral Nursing, etc. The Admiral Nurse service has as its focus the carer of a person with dementia and will target their interventions to address such role and relationship issues at various stages of the dementia journey.

Young-onset dementia (☐ Chapter 3)

- This presents special challenges. The younger person will be more physically robust, making the consequences of any behaviour problems more challenging and difficult for the carer to manage.
- The emotional and practical challenges for carers are also different. As well as a sense of bad luck and earlier bereavement, the youth of spouses, friends, and children also has an impact. Spouses and partners in their 40s and 50s may bring with them a 'get it sorted' mentality and an intolerance of uncertainty and distress that is greater than that which carers in their 70s and 80s will tolerate. Children may still be teenagers or even younger and have huge challenges as a result of caring for Mum or Dad at such a young age. Issues around employment, education, exams, children, and finance, e.g. mortgages etc., will be more prominent. The spouse carer may also be in employment themselves. The financial, emotional, and social consequences may be particularly devastating for this type of carer.

- The presence of young or teenage children provides particular problems. The carer has split loyalties: to the sick person but also an awareness of the need to provide some normality, continuity, and stability for the children. Behavioural problems arising from the dementia, especially if aggressive, may frighten children who witness them. The loss of an important relationship, and the effect on the carer, who is often their only intact parent left, can affect children deeply. This will at times be directly expressed but at others show up in withdrawal, behavioural difficulties, or a fall-off in school performance. Some carers may be too immersed in the caring task to notice the change; others feel under enormous pressure as they try to balance out conflicting demands on their time and energy.

Reference

1 Spillman BC, Pezin LE (2000) Potential and active family caregivers: changing networks and the 'sandwich generation'. *Millbank Quarterly* **78**, 347–74.

Carer burden

- The term carer 'burden' was used from as early as the 1960s when describing the impact of caring for a person with dementia, and it includes several dimensions encountered by the carer:
  - Physical.
  - Psychological.
  - Spiritual.
  - Social.
  - Financial.
- A broader view is now encouraged, encompassing the many positive aspects of caring for a person with dementia:
  - Expression of love.
  - Reciprocity.
  - Satisfaction of a job well done.
  - Enabling dignity to remain intact for the person with dementia.
  - Carrying out to the end a commitment made many years previously.
- A range of approaches can be employed to support carers to explore the positive aspects of caring; it is crucial to facilitate a carer's understanding of the 'world' of the person with dementia.
- Many carers blame themselves if they are unable to understand the communication of the person with dementia, or if the person with dementia becomes ill or they cannot resolve a particular problematic behaviour.
- It is often assumed that when a person with dementia is admitted into a long-term care environment that this largely resolves the carer burden and stress. This is often not the case and may leave the carer with feelings of guilt at 'giving up'. They may feel they have gone against the expressed wishes of their loved one and this may leave them with a sense of failure in that they were unable to continue (📖 Chapter 15, Bereavement in carers of people with dementia, pp. 282–283). This can manifest itself in the carer at times being overly critical of the care provided, but the levels of burden and stress are in danger of going undetected and unsupported. Many carers do not see their caring role as ending when their relative enters residential care—the care tasks may change but the role does not.
- Several scales can be used to assess carer burden. The most widely used is the Carer Burden Inventory[1] which comes in several versions. It covers many contributory aspects of carer burden and stress and a positive finding in many of the assessment points suggests possible need for interventions or support.
- Various mental health assessment scales may be of use where the carer has developed psychological morbidity, e.g. depression or anxiety.
- Carers of people with dementia often remain at high risk of physical and psychological morbidity even after the caring role has ended. During the caring years they may have neglected their own physical health and emotional needs in favour of those of the person with dementia. Often caring for a person with dementia over many years results in social isolation of the carer with a loss of friends and social contact; when they no longer find their days spent caring they may find it difficult to re-establish themselves (📖 Chapter 15).

A carer's view

Grace died peacefully at home after 9 years with VaD. Her husband took her home from the dementia care home 7 years before she died:

'Looking after Grace was never hard work, it was like a person who converts a piece of scrub land into a beautiful garden, he may work very hard but, when he sees the results of his labours he never thinks about how much time and hard work he put into it, his efforts were well worth while. Frankly, I would do the same thing over again except, I would with the experience I have gained do a much better job.'

Jack

Reference

1 Zarit S, Orr NK, Zarit JM (1985) *The hidden victims of Alzheimer's disease: families under stress.* New York University Press, New York.

Carers' assessment

In the United Kingdom regular carers over the age of 16 who help another person to remain at home are entitled to an assessment of their own needs.

- The Carers (Recognition and Support Services) Act 1995 enables carers to request that their needs are assessed at the same time as the assessment of the person cared for.
- In England, Wales, and Northern Ireland the Carers and Disabled Children Act 2000 allows carers to request an assessment of their own needs at any time, even if the person with dementia themselves turns down an assessment for themselves. It also enables local authorities to provide carers with services in their own right. Carers' assessment should include:
  - Their mental and general health.
  - Their level of knowledge and need for information about caring for a person with dementia.
  - Knowledge and understanding of the 'care system' and who is who.
  - Their housing and financial needs.
  - Aids and adaptations to help them care.
  - Their living arrangements and the impact of caring on their own lives, e.g. interruption of studies for younger carers, or effect on leisure activities due to being a carer.
  - Level of perceived stress and burden, which varies from carer to carer.
  - Personal resources of coping skills and self-care, etc.
- In Scotland the situation is slightly different. The Community Care and Health (Scotland) Act 2002 provides for free nursing and personal care for those aged over 65. Carers are entitled to an assessment of their own needs even if the person with dementia refuses an assessment for themselves, as in England and Wales.
- Several factors have been shown to ameliorate how carers feel as a result of their role. Confidence in problem solving, the ability to reframe problems, help-seeking, and low self blame are all associated with increased well-being in carers, so strategies to promote these should be sought.
- Strength-based assessment is an approach that was initially developed for children with special educational needs but is also relevant here. It focuses on the emotional and behavioural skills and competencies of the person with dementia and his or her carers and uses these to develop a sense of accomplishment and resilience and build better relationships.

Doing a carer's assessment

A carer's assessment can be requested by the carer, a community professional such as a GP or DN, or a hospital professional such as a consultant or social worker. The assessment is carried out by social services, usually by a care manager, who may involve other professionals as necessary. Whenever possible, assessments are carried out at a

(continued)

person's home, as this gives a clearer insight into the circumstances. There is a single assessment process which covers social and health care needs.

Assessment is directed at looking at need as outlined above, eliciting what the carer feels they need and how they would like services to be delivered, and matching this against published eligibility criteria for financing of services. As a result, a care plan is set up, listing needs as assessed, what services will be provided to meet these needs, who will be providing care for these needs, how, and when. The care package can include equipment, home adaptations, alarm systems, professional carers attending up to several times a day, meals on wheels, respite, and day care.

An assessment of the patient's financial resources is made to judge whether and how much those resources can be used to contribute to the social care element of the care package. By law charges must be reasonable. If someone is unable to pay, services are provided free of charge and if someone disagrees with an assessment they can appeal to social services for a review.

Planned reviews of care needs are carried out regularly to assess whether the level of need has changed. Reviews can also be requested by the carer or professionals if they feel that new circumstances prevail.

Carers are also entitled to direct payments to organize the patient's care themselves, which can have relevance to carers' own needs.

Support for carers

Information

- Over the course of the dementia carers may be required to cope with various practical and physical aspects of the illness; dealing with difficult and puzzling behaviours, providing physical care, dealing with financial and legal aspects, etc. Some will adapt to the caring role easily whereas others require more support. A common approach in working with carers involves improving their knowledge, understanding, and problem-solving skills.
- Information and guidance when provided within the context of continuing professional support (as, e.g., in the case of Admiral Nursing) is more successful in supporting family carers and reducing anxiety levels.
- Comprehensive information programmes are available for carers and are often delivered over a period of 6–8 weeks by a wide variety of organisations such as the local mental health service, Alzheimer's Society branches, Admiral Nurse teams, etc. and cover various key themes such as:
  - *Caring for yourself*: time management; stress management; anger management; health promotion; emotional responses to caring; bereavement and grief; anticipatory grief; social support networks, e.g. Alzheimer cafes, carer support groups, male carer support groups (as some men respond better to a single sex support group), etc.
  - *Understanding dementia*: types, signs, symptoms, progression, and prognosis, behaviours that challenge; problem solving; treatments; psychosocial therapies; and interventions.

Financial and legal issues

- Benefits and financial support, eligibility and how to apply, e.g. housing benefits, council tax benefits, carer's allowances, etc.
- LPA and other legal issues.
- The MCA.
- Carers' rights and the carer assessment.

Coping with loss and bereavement

See 📖 Chapter 15.

Case example

Frances' husband, Jonathan, was diagnosed with AD at the age of 53. He was a community care worker and his problems first came to light when he forgot visits or lost his way and called into the office again and again for directions. Over time Frances became unable to care for Jonathan, her two teenage children, and, importantly, continue working. Jonathan was admitted to a dementia unit attached to a local social services care home. He deteriorated rapidly and was soon unable to recognize

(continued)

Frances or the children and would sit with his face screwed up and eyes closed, rarely speaking. Frances felt a huge guilt that she was unable to continue caring for him and felt his behaviour was due to her 'abandonment' of him. She was anxious and tearful during visits and felt he was no longer 'Jonathan' but more distressing, that she had contributed to his rapid decline and that he was 'dead yet alive'. She was diagnosed with depression by her GP.

Further reading

Horowitz A (1985) Sons and daughters as caregivers to older parents: differences in role performances and consequences. *Gerontologist* **25**, 612–17.

Max W, Webber P, Fox P (1995) Alzheimer's disease: the unpaid burden of caring. *J Ageing Health* **7**, 179–99.

OPCS (2001) *Health, disability and provision of care. National statistics: carers.* OPCS, London. http://www.statistics.gov.uk/census2001/profiles/commentaries/health.asp

Rashid T, Ostermann RF (2009) Strength-based assessment in clinical practice. *J Clin Psychol* **65**, 488–98.

Some other therapies

Complementary therapies

- The use of complementary therapies in health care has increased progressively in recent years, in particular their practice within the arena of palliative care, with research indicating that 70% of hospice and palliative care units offer complementary therapy. Complementary therapies that might be offered include:
  - Aromatherapy.
  - Massage.
  - Reflexology.
  - Reiki.
  - Hypnotherapy.
  - Acupuncture.
  - Homeopathy.
- Aromatherapy, massage, and reflexology are the most commonly used therapies, and within the context of this chapter, the use of massage and aromatherapy within dementia care will be considered.
- Complementary therapies can be described as therapies that can work alongside, and in combination with, orthodox medical treatment. They complement mainstream medicine by:
  - Contributing to a common whole.
  - Satisfying a demand not met by conventional practices.
  - Diversifying the conceptual framework of medicine.[1]
- The majority of patients use complementary therapies alongside their orthodox treatment as a means of promoting a sense of well-being and to enhance quality of life. They often provide a direct contrast to some of the more invasive treatments a patient might receive, e.g. frequent cannulation for i.v. drug therapy.
- The amount of qualitative and quantitative research conducted into the use of complementary therapies by people with cancer and within the field of palliative care is small.
- However, evidence suggests that user demand and patient satisfaction gained from receiving a complementary therapy session is high and that short-term benefits for psychological well-being are derived
- Therefore if considering the inclusion of complementary therapies in palliative dementia care, both of these issues need consideration. It is also necessary to acknowledge and understand the patient experience of complementary therapy and its role within a structured framework of supportive care, whilst considering the evidence that is available.

What is massage?

- Massage is the manipulation of the soft tissues of the body for therapeutic purposes. It can be used on most parts of the body in a variety of techniques with differing degrees of pressure to bring about a specific outcome .The precise type of massage will depend on where the technique originated from and in what context it will be used, e.g. deep tissue massage to relieve muscular spasm.

---

1 Berman BM (2006) Cochrane complementary medicine field. About the Cochrane Collaboration (fields). Issue 1, Art. No. CE000052.

- Massage techniques for palliative care patients have been specifically adapted to meet the individual's physical and psychological needs. The pressure of massage strokes will be much lighter, the length of treatment shorter, and the massage itself may be carried out through clothing. Similar adaptations will need to be used for a person with dementia.

What is aromatherapy?

- Aromatherapy is the systemic use of essential oils obtained from plants, herbs, trees, or flowers. The essential oil is an aromatic essence and the molecules enter the body through the skin by absorption or inhalation.
- Aromatherapy is most commonly used in combination with massage. Essential oil(s) are added to a carrier oil, e.g. sweet almond oil, and used on the skin during massage.

Complementary therapy in dementia care

The ethos and principles of palliative care have been recognized as a template for developing end of life care for people with dementia. Complementary therapy can be included and integrated into such an approach and used as a non-pharmacological intervention. There are some studies on the use of aromatherapy and massage in dementia day care settings[2] and the use of aromatherapy to trigger conversation and memory.[3]

How might massage and aromatherapy help?

- Massage has been used in various forms for centuries and by many different cultures. The key element of massage is the use of touch and the physiological and psychological effects that touch creates.
- Touch is a basic human need and a method of communication. In dementia, cognitive and communication abilities change and decline and this can be one of the most challenging aspects for patients' families and professionals. A patient may appear locked into their world and carers and professionals can often feel locked out. If given in a gentle rhythmical way, massage can be a calming and nurturing experience demonstrating care with a non-task-orientated outcome.
- When used appropriately, it can help to create a means of non-verbal, tactile communication enabling a reconnection between the patient and the person giving the massage.
- Combining massage with essential oil enables the aroma to be simultaneously inhaled and absorbed through the skin.
- Using an aroma the person likes and derives pleasure from smelling, can create a positive association and may trigger pleasant memories. Selecting essential oils that are familiar or known aromas such as floral or citrus oils may therefore be useful.
- The chemical composition of an essential oil will influence the properties or effects it has. Some oils will potentially have a relaxing or sedative effect, e.g. lavender (*Lavandula augustifola*). Others may be used for their stimulating or uplifting properties, including geranium (*Pelargonium graveolens*) or mandarin (*Citrus nobilis*).

2 Kilstoff K, Chenoweth L (1998) New approaches to health and well-being for dementia day-care staff. *Int J Nurs Pract* **4**, 70–83.
3 Henry J (1993) Dementia. *Int J Aromatherapy* **5**, 27–29.

Benefits
- Relaxation.
- Therapeutic touch.
- Skin-to-skin contact.
- Inclusion of carer.
- Non-pharmacological intervention.

Precautions
- If using essential oils for the first time on a patient, a 24-hour patch test is recommended to screen for any skin reaction.
- Wash hands before and after carrying out any massage technique.
- Some patients may become express agitation or anxiety in response to massage.

Adaptation of therapies

Appropriate use of aromatherapy and massage and patient safety are paramount. The following adaptations are suggested:
- Trial of using gentle massage through clothing with no oils. This can be a way of introducing the use of touch to patients who have not received massage before, and building up to skin to skin contact if the patient is receptive and responds positively.
- Full body massage may not be appropriate—hands/feet only.
- Massage pressure will be lighter in touch.
- Use a lower percentage of any essential oils when blending with a carrier oil, e.g. 0.5–1% only.
- Length of the session will be shorter; 5–10 minutes of massage may be sufficient.
- Do not carry out therapy if the patient is pyrexial, has a new/acute pain, or on skin that is broken or inflamed.
- Ongoing review and evaluation of the use of aromatherapy or massage with a patient by the multiprofessional team.

Adapting the conventional delivery of a therapy is important, and it should be suitable to the person's individual needs. A specifically adapted massage routine, the 'M' technique®, has been devised by Dr Jane Buckle for use when a conventional massage technique would not be appropriate. The 'M' technique® is a series of stroking movements performed in a set sequence at a set pressure and set pace. It is different from conventional massage and may be suitable when massage is inappropriate. Each movement, identified with a mnemonic name, is repeated three times (see http://www.mtechnique.co.uk\).

Carers' needs

The family and carer of a person with dementia may express a sense of feeling excluded or helplessness at no longer being able to participate in the process of giving care. This can increase as the dementia progresses or when the person starts to die. Keeping carers involved in the caring role may be helped by demonstrating to and teaching them a simple hand massage technique that they can carry out with the patient. Carers may find this helps to restore closeness and intimacy, offering an alternative way to spend time together or to some of the other carer tasks they carry out.

Staff support

Working in the dementia care setting may be emotionally challenging and physically draining. Support for staff enables them to balance feelings of stress and continue to meet the demands of the patient group. Organizations that have a complementary therapy service in place often extend it to include staff sessions. Receiving a complementary therapy can help with release of tension and fatigue and also enables the staff member to experience what a patient will feel. For those unsure of the role massage may have for patients, it can be a beneficial introduction.

Introducing a new therapy

Factors to consider when introducing massage and aromatherapy include the following.

Models of use—who will provide the therapy?

This may be from a qualified complementary therapist, or a nurse or other health professional holding a massage or aromatherapy qualification.

Resource implications

Where the therapy will be provided (designated room or at the bedside), space (for storage of towels, lotions, essential oils), training and continuing professional development (for in-house staff or outside practitioners), and cost of materials are all factors that have to be considered.

Legal implications

Any person holding a complementary therapy qualification requires professional liability and indemnity insurance cover and must belong to a relevant professional body

Policy and procedure

A policy and protocol covering the use of aromatherapy and massage must be developed. This can include storage of oils to meet control of substances hazardous to health (COSHH) standards, issue of consent for dementia patients and criteria/indications for use of the therapy.

Further reading

Royal College of Nursing (2003). Complementary therapies in nursing, midwifery and health visiting practice. RCN guidance on integrating complementary therapies into clinical care. Royal College of Nursing, London. Available at: http://www.rcn.org.uk/__data/assets/pdf_file/0008/78596/002204.pdf

Wilkinson S, Barnes K, Storey L (2008) Massage for symptom relief in patients with cancer: systemic review. *J Adv Nursing* **63**, 430–9.

Music therapy

'There are, in fact, no more important communications between one human being and another than those expressed emotionally, and no information more vital for constructing and reconstructing working models of self and other than information about how each feels toward the other.'
John Bowlby

As health care providers need to think more creatively about how we care for older people and the value of supportive and emotional care. With dementia becoming more prevalent we need to focus on individuals' specific needs, seeing 'the person behind the disease'.

What is music therapy?

- Music therapy is based on the fact that everyone can respond to music no matter how ill, disabled, or traumatized.
- It uses improvised music as a basis for relationship between client/patient and therapist to support and develop physical, mental, social, emotional, and spiritual well-being.
- Music therapists are trained at Masters level and are registered with the Health Professions Council.
- Music therapy has been a part of health and social care for over 50 years.
- Music therapists are in a unique position, able to offer individualized and person-centred interventions for adults with dementia (patients).
- These musical interventions can help to preserve patients' unique identity even in advanced dementia.
- Although most people can offer musical experiences for these patients, music therapists focus on the musical relationship that evolves during the creation of musical improvisation.

Who might benefit from music therapy?

- Patients unable to express themselves verbally.
- Patients with language difficulties and disabilities.
- Patients who are isolated and depressed because of behavioural challenges.
- Patients who display anxious or aggressive behaviour.
- Patients who display agitation at meals, bath times, and sundowning.
- Patients who have lost the ability to plan and initiate activities.
- Patients with lack of cognitive and social awareness.
- Patients who wander.

How music therapy works

- Music therapy can alleviate many physical, behavioural, and emotional behaviours attributed to patients suffering with advanced dementia.
- It is achieved through using the specific components of music, i.e. tempo, dynamics, melody, and structure.
- Music therapy mainly uses musical improvisation.

Nordoff and Robbins developed the concept of 'creative music therapy'. They emphasized the central importance of active participation and spontaneity of the music involved and saw that improvised music-making can be a powerful means of making contact.[4] Working with an elderly man

4 Nordoff P, Robbins C (1971) *Therapy in music for handicapped children*. Gollancz, London.

in the late stages of dementia, Nockolds said 'I believe that the core of the human is there and is unaffected … this core of humanity can be created in this positive way'.[5]

Practical help

- Singing can lift the mood and the physical stimulation requires deeper breathing which causes an increase in blood oxygenation. Muscles tense and relax.
- Singing scheduled around certain distressing activities can counteract symptoms of stress.
- Singing in the late stages of dementia can provide stimulation that elicits alert responses, moving the head towards sound, eye blinking, eye movement under the eyelid, movement in the hands and feet, and vocal responses.
- Taped music at bath time can decrease agitated behaviour.
- Light classical music played at a tempo of between 50 and 70 beats per minute at mealtimes may help residents relax.
- Music therapy can motivate exercise.
- Music therapy can give auditory cues that activate neural pathways, supporting and focusing a patient who has great difficulty in moving.
- It can also be used to induce relaxation.
- Music therapy is widely used to reduce isolation for people with dementia. It brings people together in a unique way.
- It offers the potential for togetherness, interaction, to listen to others and be listened to; providing a sense of continuity and support.
- The universality of music means that all cultures and religions can be accepted and acknowledged.
- Singing facilitates periods of arousal which give a sense of awareness, familiarity, comfort, and community.
- It might be challenging for a patient to engage in conversation, but as language deteriorates musical abilities are preserved offering the possibilities of meaningful improvisation.

George was referred to music therapy because he was withdrawn and depressed. He had become socially isolated because he was aggressive when in company. He no longer spoke and was isolated, but was still living an emotional world. The music therapist spent time with him improvising at the keyboard, guitar, and singing to him. She tried to reflect back to him musically and in words how she felt he might be feeling. George innately responded to the music. Music-making formed the basis for communication, a place of human contact giving him a space to express himself emotionally. Through closed doors staff heard this and began to think of him differently. As time has gone by George's ways of vocalizing have become much more flexible and varied. He uses a wider range of colours and dynamics. He seems a little more relaxed and his medication has been decreased. The therapist could see a marked difference, his face is more open and expressive and he is able to spend more time with residents and staff.

5 Nockolds J (1999) *Olive and Jim. Music therapy – intimate notes.* Jessica Kingsley Publishers, London.

Elsa groaned continuously. Unsure what to do the music therapist sang these vocalizations back to her and as time went by she realized that Elsa was making choices about where she pitched her voice, often starting on the note the therapist had just sung. As the therapist introduced new material to her Elsa started to repeat it back to her. By responding to her groaning sounds the therapist was able to relate to her in a unique way. By inhabiting her 'vocal' world they found a space to share.

How music therapy is done

- Work takes place in people's homes, nursing homes, care homes, hospitals, and hospices.
- Music therapy can happen in a lounge, at the bedside, or even up and down the corridor (this is one of its strengths).
- Patients do not need to have to have had musical training in order to receive music therapy.
- It is essential to get permission from the patient, if they are able to give consent, or next of kin before embarking on the work.
- One-to-one sessions and/or group work.
- Short-term and ongoing work both have their benefits.

Relationship in music does not need words. Music offers a context where many things can be experienced. Gestures, movements, and vocalizations are viewed as musical components which can be related and responded to by the music therapist. As Hartley and Payne suggest, music therapy can offer a foundation from which to respond and find your way back into the world. It's certainly the case that adults in the advanced stages of dementia might lose a sense of remembering and reasoning but their emotional world continues, there is something that remains intact, a self that responds. Music therapy offers a place for that self to be heard.

Where do you find a music therapist?

The Association of Professional Music Therapists, 24–27 White Lion Street, London N1 9PD, UK (http://www.apmt.org/)

Further reading

Bonanomi C, Gerosa MC (2002) Observation of the Alzheimer patient and music therapy. *Music Therapy Today* (online), August. Available at: http://musictherapyworld.net

Dehm-Gauwerky B (2002) When the present becomes a mere stage for the past – music therapy in the case of a patient with extreme dementia. *Music Therapy Today* (online) August. Available at: http://musictherapyworld.net

Hartley N, Payne M (2009) *The creative arts in palliative care.* Jessica Kingsley Publishers, London.

Lesta B, Petocz P (2006) Familiar group singing: addressing mood and social behaviour of residents with dementia displaying sundowning. *Aust J Music Ther* **17**, 2–17.

Financial issues

Health and social care

Funding for dementia care comes from the patient's own money, the state, or charity. Most developed countries have some system to provide care when the individual has no money. Many provide free nursing care for those in nursing homes. Far fewer countries pay for predominantly social care in rest homes, etc.

It would be impossible to discuss all the varieties of funding and care sources in all countries, and as a result we present some of the benefits and rules for the UK. We recognize that that is necessarily incomplete, but hope it serves as an example of funding and service structures in a developed country which will have wider relevance.

- In the UK, a distinction is made between health and social care. By law, health care is free at the point of delivery, but social care is partly or fully funded by the person receiving care, if they have the means to pay for it. Social care is therefore means-tested. In Scotland, social care for older people is currently government funded, i.e. free at the point of use for the user.
- Long-term health-funded care in England and Wales is called continuing health care or continuing care.
- Because of the government's legal duty to fully fund care, those eligible are not allowed to top up the care provided through private means.
- In the landmark Coughlan case in 1999, the Court of Appeal in England made a number of key decisions:
  - Nursing care where someone is placed in a care home for health reasons is health care, not social care.
  - Nursing care is only social care in rare cases where it is incidental to the provision of accommodation. To make this judgment one needs to assess the quantity and quality of nursing care provided.
- A number of criteria were proposed to perform this assessment:
  - The *nature of the care needed*: the type of need, how it affects the individual and the care required to manage these needs.
  - The *extent and severity of need*, including the need for continuity of care.
  - The *complexity of need*, how different needs interact and the degree of expertise needed to manage them.
  - The *unpredictability of need*, i.e. if need could be expected to suddenly increase and become complex, so that insufficient timely care might jeopardize the person's health.
- Any one or a combination of these criteria establishes a primary health need, and therefore entitlement to free care funded by the NHS.
- In another key ruling, in the Grogan case in 2006, the High Court in England upheld the complaint that the system of banding according to need then in existence fell far short of the rights set out under the Coughlan judgment. In effect, only those with the very highest levels of need qualified for full health care funding.
- In recognition of the great variability in how the rules were applied across England and Wales (the so-called postcode lottery), a National Framework for NHS-Funded Continuing Healthcare and Nursing Care was published in 2007, and revised in 2009 to bring into effect uniformity and to apply the court judgments alluded to above.

- Assessment of need is carried out by a care manager, usually though not always a social worker, using a Decision Support Tool (DST) published by the Department of Health (Fig. 24.1).

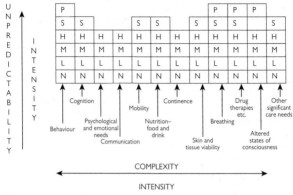

Fig. 24.1 How the different care domains are divided into levels of need (P, S, H, M, L, and N are priority, severe, high, moderate, low, and no need, respectively). As a general rule, it is held that one priority need or two severe needs are likely to be associated with a view that a person is eligible for NHS continuing care funding. Reproduced from Department of Health, *Decision Support Tool for NHS Continuing Healthcare*, July 2009, with permission.

- In making an assessment, carers must be consulted if appropriate.
- The DST assesses a number of domains along the criteria established by the Coughlan case:
  - Cognition.
  - Behaviour.
  - Psychological and emotional needs.
  - Communication.
  - Mobility.
  - Nutrition.
  - Continence.
  - Skin and tissue viability.
  - Breathing.
  - Drug and other therapies.
  - State of consciousness.
  - Other significant needs.
- Each domain is graded across six levels of need going from 'no needs' to 'priority needs'. One 'priority need', two 'severe needs', or a large number of more moderate needs will qualify one for continuing care.
- An application is then made to a PCT panel to consider whether the person is entitled to free (NHS-funded) care, means-tested social care, or a combination of the two. The decision is reviewed after 3 months and then at least annually to see if the level of need and entitlement has changed.
- Carers (or patients themselves) have a right of appeal if they consider the assessment or decision to have been flawed.

- Carers also have a right to assessment of their own needs (📖 Chapter 22, Carers' assessment, pp. 379–380).
- The guidance makes it clear that just because a need is being well met does not stop it being a need, so this should not be used to deny people's eligibility to continuing care.
- There is provision for fast-track assessment for people with a life expectancy of weeks. If they then survive longer than expected, a full assessment will be required.
- Continuing care is funded either in a care home or at home.
- The welfare system is intricate and complex, and difficult for non-professionals to navigate, so it is essential that each person gets good advice and support in this. Obscure benefits can increase the funds available to pay for care. For example in the UK dementia entitles one to a reduction in local taxes as well as a free TV licence.
- The Alzheimer's Society in the UK argues that the current system puts people with dementia at a disadvantage, because except in very complex cases, their needs are adjudged to be social care needs and therefore means tested.
- It is the duty of all welfare systems, in all countries, to be fair and to adapt to remain fair.

Other benefits

- In general benefits are administered by the Department of Work and Pensions; other benefits are administered by local councils.
- The situation regarding benefits differs slightly between the different countries in the UK—see Further reading for country-specific online guidance. At the time of publication, the benefits system in the UK is being overhauled.

Attendance Allowance (AA) and Disability Living Allowance (DLA)

- These allowances are paid to people who have a physical or a mental health need, or both, for which they need help to care for themselves or need supervision for their safety.
- They are not means tested, i.e. do not depend on the income of the recipient. They are not tied to having paid National Insurance (NI) contributions, and they are not taxable.
- To be eligible, the need must have been present for at least 3 months for DLA and 6 months for AA and is likely to continue for at least 6 months, unless one is terminally ill, with a prognosis of six months or less, when special rules apply.
- DLA has to be claimed before one is 65. It is split into two components and one may qualify for either or both parts. One part is a mobility component and the other a personal care allowance. There are different rates for each component depending on the assessed level of need. Over age 65, only the personal care allowance is paid.
- Because needs change as illness progresses, the person's entitlement may change; it is important to keep this under review.
- People with dementia who need some care during the day or cannot cook a main meal for themselves may qualify for the lower rate care component of DLA (This is not available to those newly entitled over age 65.)
- Those who need frequent help or supervision during the day or night may qualify for the middle rate of the care component of DLA which is the same as the lower rate of AA
- Those who need frequent help or continuous supervision day and night for their safety will often qualify for the top rates of either benefit.
- People under 65 qualify for the top mobility rate if their ability to walk out of doors is severely limited by physical disability, or for the lower rate if they can walk but need supervision or assistance so that they are not at risk, including of getting lost.

Employment and Support Allowance (ESA)

- If someone under pensionable age cannot work because of a disability, and can no longer get Statutory Sick Pay, they are entitled to ESA, This replaced Incapacity Benefit (IB) in 2008, although those receiving IB are still entitled to it.
- ESA has two rates. If a medical assessment decides that work capability is limited but with support some work could be managed, one is entered into the Work Related Activity Group. If one is assessed as not being usually capable of any work, they are included in the Support Group which is paid at a higher rate.

- Entitlement is tied to past NI contributions, or is income related and is complex.

Carer's Allowance (CA) and other carer benefits

- Carers are entitled to an assessment of their needs separately from the needs of the person they care for (📖 Chapter 22, Carers' assessment, pp. 379–380).
- Carers aged over 16 who spend more than 35 hours a week caring for someone receiving AA, DLA, or some other similar benefits are entitled to CA. Students in full-time study (more than 21 hours a week) or people earning over £100 a week after deductions are not entitled. CA will affect a number of other benefit entitlements.
- CA is not related to NI contributions, and will pay in NI contributions for most people to preserve their pension rights. However, it is taxable.
- Carers with no other income and/or financially dependent partners or children can claim other benefits to top up their income.
- If the carer leaves their own property to care for someone they may be entitled to council tax exemption. Some carers who share a home with the person being cared for will be ignored for council tax purposes if they are not the spouse or parent of the person being cared for.
- Councils will charge carers for meals, sitting services, and home help, but help filling out forms, occupational therapy visits, and transport to day centres are free. Such charges are means tested.
- Carers who are still working are entitled to reasonable time off in emergencies (such as care breakdown) if they have been with their employer for at least a year.
- Local councils can give direct payments to carers to buy in support for themselves. They cannot be used to meet the needs of the person being cared for.

Other benefits

- A person with dementia or their carer may be entitled to other benefits such as income support, pension credit , Housing Benefit, and Council Tax Benefit to top up their income to basic levels. There are also other benefits they may be entitled to because they have children or have reached pensionable age. The benefits detailed above could allow extra entitlement to these and other benefits.
- Disabled Facilities Grants are given by local councils to enable home adaptations or the provision of equipment to care for a disabled person. They are means tested and will often require a contribution from the recipient.
- The Social Fund administered by the Department of Work and Pensions gives a number of grants including:
  - Cold weather payments: an increase in certain benefits if the temperature falls below freezing for 7 consecutive days.
  - Winter fuel payments: a one-off payment made every year to all people over the minimum women's pension age (currently rising from age 60 to 66 by 2020).
  - Community Care Grants: to enable people receiving certain benefits to live at home, e.g. essential furniture, repairs.
  - Budgeting loans: interest-free loans for essential items for people receiving certain benefits.

- Funeral payments: may be paid to the closest relative of someone who has died if they are on certain benefits. They may be taken out of the estate of the deceased.
- Crisis loans: available in a crisis, e.g. a fire, or loss of money, for essential items. Means tested.

- The Blue Badge scheme allows people with a disability which affects their mobility to park for free in parking bays, or for a certain time on single or double yellow lines (no time limit in Scotland) except in a few areas of central London, where special bays are provided. In London holders are also exempt from the congestion charge . If they apply beforehand they will also be exempt from paying most tolls.
- People over the minimum women's pension age qualify for a free travel pass to cover most local transport. The local council also provides free travel passes for those with a disability which affects their ability to walk.

NHS entitlements

- People over 60 are entitled to free prescriptions, as are those who have any of a number of listed medical condition (e.g. cancer, diabetes needing medication), are on certain benefits, or have a war pension.
- People receiving certain benefits are also entitled to free prescriptions, as well as free dental care, free eye tests, contributions to glasses, free appliances, and transport to hospital.
- People on low income may also be entitled to assistance with health-related costs.

Effect of being in a care home or hospital on benefits

- Prolonged hospital stays and care home stays will affect income from benefits one is receiving. DLA and AA are only paid for the first 28 days of any hospital or care home/nursing home stay. Some people in care homes may also have to pay a substantial part of their benefit income towards the cost of their care.
- The rules are complex—see http://www.direct.gov.uk/en/ CaringForSomeone/CareHomes/DG_10031411

Getting help

Rules regarding benefits and financial entitlements are very complex and ever changing. The above is only a very bare outline, and will certainly change with time. A major review of social care spending is under way. Expert and up to date help is therefore essential if one is not to lose out on often desperately needed help.

- Carers are entitled to free assistance with benefits and form filling.
- Much information can be found on the government public services one stop website http://www.direct.gov.uk/en/index.htm
- Local councils provide information through social services departments; the local PCT will also be a gateway for useful information.
- The Alzheimer's Society produces a series of good factsheets about benefit entitlements and other financial and legal issues—see the list at http://alzheimers.org.uk/site/scripts/documents.php?categoryID=200137
- Other organizations which can help include Age UK, the Citizens Advice Bureau, and Counsel and Care—see 📖 Appendix 1.

Further reading

Alzheimer's Society (2009) *When does the NHS pay for care? Guidance on eligibility for NHS continuing healthcare funding in England and how to appeal if it is not awarded.* Alzheimer's Society, London.

Department of Health (2009) *The national framework for NHS continuing healthcare and NHS-funded nursing care.* Department of Health, London. Available online at: http://www.dh.gov.uk/dr_consum_dh/groups/dh_digitalassets/documents/digitalasset/dh_103161.pdf

Department of Health (2009) Decision Support Tool for NHS continuing healthcare. Department of Health, London. Available online at: http://www.dh.gov.uk/dr_consum_dh/groups/dh_digitalassets/documents/digitalasset/dh_103329.pdf

Citizens' Advice Bureau information on benefits: http://www.adviceguide.org.uk/your_money/benefits.htm. Separate tabs on this page lead to information specific to England, Scotland, Wales and Northern Ireland.

Further information

Admiral Nurses

Specialist dementia nurses, working in the community, with families, carers and supporters of people with dementia. They:

- Work with family carers as their prime focus.
- Provide practical advice, emotional support, information, and skills.
- Deliver education and training in dementia care.
- Provide consultancy to professionals working with people with dementia.
- Promote best practice in person- centred dementia care.

Admiral Nursing DIRECT

Telephone: 0845 257 9406
Telephone information and support line for family carers, people with dementia and professionals.
E-mail: direct@dementiauk.org
Admiral Nursing DIRECT is delivered by experienced Admiral Nurses.

Age UK

The four national Age Concerns in the UK have joined together with Help the Aged to form new national charities dedicated to improving the lives of older people.
Website: http://www.ageuk.org.uk

Alzheimer's Society

Devon House
58 St Katharine's Way
London E1W 1JX, UK
E-mail: enquiries@alzheimers.org.uk
Telephone: 020 7423 3500

Assist UK

Assist UK coordinates a UK-wide network of around 50 locally situated Disabled Living Centres. The website lists all the centres with opening times and other relevant information. Each centre includes a permanent exhibition that provides people with opportunities to see and try products and equipment. Centre staff provide people with expert and unbiased information and advice on disability equipment and ways of managing disability and which products might suit them best.
Website: http://www.assist-uk.org/

Benefit Enquiry Line (BEL)

Benefit Enquiry Line
Red Rose House
Lancaster Road
Preston

Lancashire PR1 1HB, UK
Free helpline: 0800 88 22 00 (8.30 a.m. to 6.30 p.m. weekdays and 9.00 a.m. to 1.00 p.m. Saturdays)
Textphone: 0800 243 544
E-mail: BEL-Customer-Services@dwp.gsi.gov.uk
Website: http://www.direct.gov.uk/en/DisabledPeople/FinancialSupport/index.htm

British Red Cross

British Red Cross
UK Office
44 Moorfields
London EC2Y 9AL, UK
Telephone: 0844 871 11 11
E-mail: information@redcross.org.uk
Website: http://www.redcross.org.uk/
The Red Cross volunteer-led medical equipment service provides short-term loans of equipment to help look after people with dementia at home, including wheelchairs and commodes. There is a network of Red Cross independent living shops which sell more than 1500 products from walking sticks and continence products to mobility scooters. The shopping facility is also available online.

Carers UK

20 Great Dover Street
London SE1 4LX, UK
General enquiries: 020 7378 4999
Free carers line: 0808 808 7777
E-mail: info@ukcarers.org
Website: http://www.carersuk.org/
Charity that aims to help carers recognize their own needs. It provides information, advice, and support for carers and campaigns on their behalf. Leaflets and factsheets are available free to carers.

Citizens Advice Bureau

A network of free, independent, and confidential local services in which trained Citizens Advice advisers offer information and advice on topics such as benefits, housing, employment, debts, family and personal problems, or problems that people experience because they are from a minority group. It can also give details of national and local organizations and services, including support groups.
Website: http://www.citizensadvice.org.uk/

Community Legal Advice

Telephone or check the website to find locations
0845 345 4345 (9.00 a.m. to 6.30 p.m. weekdays)
Website: http://www.clsdirect.org.uk/
A free and confidential service paid for by legal aid, set up to help people tackle their legal problems. It is funded by the Legal Services Commission and delivered in partnership with independent advice agencies and solicitors.

Counsel and Care

Twyman House
16 Bonny Street
London NW1 9PG, UK
General enquiries: 020 7241 8555
Advice line: 0845 300 7585 (weekdays 10 a.m. to 4 p.m. except Wednesdays:
10 a.m. to 1 p.m.)
E-mail: advice@counselandcare.org.uk
Website: http://www.counselandcare.org.uk/
A charity that provides free and confidential advice for people over 60 and
their relatives, friends, and carers on subjects such as welfare benefits or
help at home. The charity has a particular expertise in residential care with a
wide range of factsheets available

Crossroads Association

10 Regent Place
Rugby
Warwickshire CV21 2PN, UK
Telephone: 0845 450 0350
Website: http://www.crossroads.org.uk/
An organization that runs a network of care attendant schemes in England
and Wales and provides a flexible respite care service to carers.

CRUSE Bereavement Care

Telephone helpline: 0844 477 9400
E-mail helpline: helpline@cruse.org.uk
Website: http://www.crusebereavementcare.org.uk/

Dementia UK (previously known as For Dementia)

Dementia UK works in partnership with NHS providers and commissioners,
social care authorities, and voluntary sector organizations to improve the
quality of life for people with dementia and their carers.
Website: http://www.dementiauk.org/

Disabled Living Foundation (DLF)

380–384 Harrow Road
London W9 2HU, UK
Telephone: 020 7289 6111
Helpline: 0845 130 9177 (10.00 a.m. to 4.00 p.m. weekdays)
E-mail: advice@dlf.org.uk
Website: http://www.dlf.org.uk/
The DLF is the London based centre

Help the Hospices

The leading charity supporting hospice care throughout the UK.
Website: http://www.helpthehospices.org.uk/

Hope for Home

A charity that sets out to give advice knowledge and understanding of how
people with dementia can be supported at home to live there until they die.
Website: http://www.hopeforhome.org.uk/

Meals on Wheels/Meals at Home services

Hot, and sometimes frozen, meals can be delivered to your home if you have problems cooking. A 'meals at home' service may be offered to you following an assessment of your needs by your social services department. You should receive a simple 'service agreement' which details the days you will receive meals, the cost, and how to contact the manager of the service. A range of meals is produced taking into account different cultural and religious requirements, personal preferences, and dietary needs. Your GP or social worker will know who to contact or you can visit the Directgov website http://www.direct.gov.uk and go to Home and Community.

Mind

Mind England
PO Box 277
Manchester M60 3XN, UK
Mind infoline: 0845 766 0163 (9.00 a.m. to 5.00 p.m. weekdays)
E-mail: contact@mind.org.uk
Website: http://www.mind.org.uk/
Mental health charity that aims to improve the quality of life for people affected by mental health problems in England and Wales by campaigns, providing advice and information, and producing publications.

Ministry of Justice

Selborne House
54 Victoria Street
London SW1E 6QW, UK
Telephone: 020 7210 8500
E-mail: general.queries@justice.gsi.gov.uk
Website: http://www.justice.gov.uk/
The Ministry of Justice provides a range of useful information online including guidance on the Mental Capacity Act (2005) available at http://www.justice.gov.uk/guidance/mental-capacity.htm

SIFA

10 East Street
Epsom
Surrey KT17 1HH, UK
Telephone 01372 721172
E-mail: sifa@sifa.co.uk
Website: http://www.sifa.co.uk/
Trade association and support group for financial advisers who are partly or wholly owned by solicitors, or accountants who have close links with the professions. It can provide contact details of legal firms that offer financial advice to complement their legal advice.

'M' technique®

E-mail: rjbinfo@aol.com
Website: http://www.mtechnique.co.uk/

Office of the Public Guardian (OPG)

Archway Tower
2 Junction Road

London N19 5SZ, UK
Telephone: 0845 330 2900 (customer services 9.00 a.m. to 5.00 p.m. weekdays)
E-mail: customerservices@publicguardian.gsi.gov.uk
Website: http://www.direct.gov.uk/en/Governmentcitizensandrights/Mental
capacityandthelaw/index.htm
The OPG supports and promotes decision-making for those who lack
capacity or would like to plan for their future, within the framework of the
Mental Capacity Act 2005. The Court of Protection is at the same address.

Parking concessions

The Blue Badge scheme provides a range of parking concessions for people
with severe mobility problems who have difficulty using public transport.
The scheme operates throughout the UK and applies to on-street parking
only. Badge holders may park on single or double yellow lines for up to
3 hours in England and Wales except where there is a ban on loading or
unloading. Badge holders may also park for free for as long as they need at
on-street parking meters and in pay-and-display car parks. Your local
council is responsible for issuing Blue Badge parking permits. There are criteria which are used to assess eligibility to receive a Blue Badge, the one
most likely to apply to people with dementia is 'have a permanent and
substantial disability which means you cannot walk, or which makes walking
very difficult'. For more information visit the Directgov website at http://
www.direct.gov.uk/en/DisabledPeople/MotoringAndTransport/Blue
badgescheme/index.htm

Parkinson's Disease Society

215 Vauxhall Bridge Road
London SW1V 1EJ
Helpline: 0808 800 0303 (9.30 a.m. to 5.30 p.m.)
E-mail: hello@parkinsons.org.uk
Website: http://www.parkinsons.org.uk/

Princess Royal Trust for Carers

142 Minories
London EC3N 1LB, UK
Telephone: 020 7480 7788
E-mail: info@carers.org
Website: http://www.carers.org/

Social services

The Local Government Ombudsman looks at complaints about councils and
some other authorities. It is a free service which investigates complaints in a
fair and independent way. If you have a problem with a council service you
should first complain to the council. If you are not satisfied with the result
the Local Government Ombudsman Advice Team may be able to help.
Information can be provided in a range of languages other than English.
Telephone: 0300 061 0614 (8.30 a.m. to 5.00 p.m. Monday to Friday)
E-mail: advice@lgo.org.uk
Website: http://www.lgo.org.uk/

The Motability Scheme

The Motability Scheme is open to anyone who receives either the Higher
Rate Mobility Component of the DLA or the War Pensioners' Mobility

Supplement. Your mobility allowance is exchanged for a mobility package on the Car Scheme or the Powered Wheelchair and Scooter Scheme. Even if you do not drive yourself you can apply for a car as a passenger and propose two other people as your drivers. Telephone or visit the Motability website for further information.

Telephone: 0845 456 4566

Website: http://www.motability.co.uk/

Uniting Carers (Dementia UK)

Uniting Carers was established in 2005 and is a national network of family carers, former carers, family members, and friends of people with dementia. The aim of the network is to give carers the opportunity to raise awareness and increase people's understanding of dementia. There are over 900 members throughout the country who have joined the network—people who want to use their experience of caring for someone with dementia to make a difference.

Telephone: 020 7874 7225 or 020 7874 7209

E-mail: carers@dementiauk.org

Website: http://www.dementiauk.org/what-we-do/uniting-carers/

Vitalise

Shap Road Industrial Estate

Shap Road

Kendal

Cumbria LA9 6NZ, UK

Telephone: 0845 345 1972

Holiday booking line: 0845 345 1970 (9.00 a.m. to 5.00 p.m. weekdays)

Vitalise was formerly known as the Winged Fellowship Trust. It organizes holidays for people with disabilities and their carers. Four purpose-built centres run special 'Alzheimer's weeks' for people with dementia and their carers. A fifth centre in Cornwall caters for people with dementia and their carers all the year round. Care is provided by qualified staff and volunteers but carers can provide any care they choose.

E-mail: info@vitalise.org.uk

Website: http://www.vitalise.org.uk/

Where to find a music therapist

The Association of Professional Music Therapists

24–27 White Lion Street

London N1 9PD, UK

Telephone: 020 7837 6100

E-mail: APMToffice@aol.com

Website: http://www.apmt.org/

Young person's helpline (RD4U)

RD4U is a website developed by Cruse Bereavement Care's Youth Involvement Project which aims to support young people, after the death of someone close to them.

Telephone: 0808 808 1677

E-mail: info@rd4u.org.uk

Website: http://www.rd4u.org.uk/

Some relevant drug interactions

This appendix lists some relevant drug interactions affecting drugs commonly used in people with advanced dementia. They are grouped by mechanism. Only the more complex mechanisms are listed; pharmacology texts and Appendix 1 of the BNF give fuller lists.

Cytochrome-based interactions (CYP450)

A large enzyme system involved in the hepatic metabolism of many drugs, via oxidation (see 📖 Chapter 8, Common analgesics, pp. 112–115).

CYP1A2

Drugs affected	Inhibitors	Inducers
Antidepressants: amitriptyline, clomipramine, desipramine, duloxetine, imipramine, mirtazapine	Amiodarone, cimetidine, ciprofloxacin*, fluvoxamine*, ketoconazole	Barbiturates, omeprazole, modafinil, tobacco
Anxiolytics: diazepam		
Antipsychotics: haloperidol, olanzapine		
Other: nabumetone, propranolol, ropinirole, theophylline, tizanidine, verapamil, (R)-warfarin		

*Significant inhibitor or inducer.

CYP2C9

Drugs affected	Inhibitors	Inducers
Antidepressants: amitriptyline, fluoxetine	Amiodarone*, clopidogrel, efavirenz, fluconazole*, fluvastatin, fluvoxamine, miconazole, sertraline, sulfamethoxazole, valproate, voriconazole	Barbiturates, carbamazepine, phenytoin, rifampicin
Other: celecoxib, diclofenac, flurbiprofen, glibenclamide, glimepiride, glipizide, ibuprofen, indometacin, losartan, meloxicam, naproxen, piroxicam, phenytoin, tolbutamide, (S)-warfarin		

*Significant inhibitor or inducer.

CYP2C19

Drugs affected	Inhibitors	Inducers
Antidepressants: amitriptyline, citalopram, clomipramine, desipramine, escitalopram, fluoxetine, imipramine, sertraline *Antipsychotics*: aripiprazole, olanzapine *Anxiolytics*: diazepam *Other*: clopidogrel, lansoprazole, omeprazole, pantoprazole, phenobarbital, phenytoin	Cimetidine, esomeprazole, fluconazole, fluoxetine, fluvoxamine, ketoconazole, lansoprazole, modafinil, omeprazole, oxcarbazepine	Carbamazepine prednisone rifampicin St John's wort

CYP2D6

Drugs affected	Inhibitors	Inducers
Antidepressants: amitriptyline, clomipramine, desipramine, doxepin, duloxetine, fluoxetine, imipramine, maprotiline, nortriptyline, paroxetine, venlafaxine *Antipsychotics*: alprazolam, aripiprazole, chlorpromazine, haloperidol, risperidone *Other*: carvedilol, carbamazepine, codeine, dihydrocodeine, metoclopramide, metoprolol, propranolol, timolol, tramadol, trazodone	Amiodarone, bupropion*, celecoxib, cimetidine, citalopram, chlorpheniramine, clomipramine, donepezil, doxepin, duloxetine*, fluoxetine*, haloperidol, methadone, metoclopramide, oxycodone, paroxetine*, promethazine, quinidine*, venlafaxine	Dexamethasone, rifampicin

*Significant inhibitor or inducer.

CYP3A 4,5,7

Drugs affected	Inhibitors	Inducers
Antidepressants: trazodone Antipsychotics: aripiprazole, haloperidol *Anxiolytics*: alfuzosin, alprazolam, diazepam, midazolam *Other*: alfentanil, amlodipine, atorvastatin, chlorphenirmanine, clarithromycin, dexamethasone, diltiazem, domperidone, ergotamine, erythromycin, fentanyl, indinavir, methadone, nifedipine, quinidine, ritonavir, saquinavir, simvastatin, verapamil	Amiodarone, cimetidine, ciprofloxacin, clarithromycin*, diltiazem*, erythromycin*, fluconazole*, fluoxetine, grapefruit juice*, indinavir *, itraconazole*, ketoconazole*, miconazole, norfloxacin, ritonavir*, saquinavir*, verapamil, voriconazole	Carbamazepine, efavirenz, glucocorticoids, modafinil, nevirapine, oxcarbazepine, phenobarbital, phenytoin, pioglitazone, rifampicin, St John's wort

*Significant inhibitor or inducer.

Interactions involving p-glycoprotein (P-gp)

P-gp is a transporter system across cell membranes, playing especially important roles in removing drugs into the intestinal lumen, into the urine, into bile, and out of the brain through the BBB. P-gp inhibitors thus increase serum and brain levels levels of the drug and P-gp inducers reduce such levels.

Drugs affected	Inhibitors	Inducers
Digoxin, morphine, nortriptyline, risperidone	Amiodarone, clarithromycin, erythromycin, ketoconazole, quinidine, ritonavir, saquinavir, verapamil	Carbamazepine, rifampicin, St John's wort

Drugs which prolong QT interval	
Type	Drugs
Psychotropic	Amitriptyline; Amphetamine; Chlorpromazine ; Citalopram; Clomipramine; Clozapine; Desipramine; Doxepin; Droperidol ; Escitalopram; Fluoxetine; Galantamine; Haloperidol; Imipramine; Lithium; Nortriptyline; Paroxetine; Pimozide; Quetiapine; Risperidone; Thioridazine.
Antimicrobial	Azithromycin; Ciprofloxacin; Clarithromycin; Erythromycin; Fluconazole; Itraconazole; Ketoconazole; Levofloxacin.
Cardiac	Amiodarone; Chlorpromazine; Disopyramide; Procainamide; Quinidine; Sotalol.
Other	Alfuzosin; Diphenhydramine; Domperidone; Methadone; Octreotide; Ondansetron; Terfenadine.

For full details see http://www.azcert.org/medical-pros/drug-lists/drug-lists.cfm

Further reading

Flockhart DA. Drug Interactions: cytochrome P450 drug interaction table. Indiana University School of Medicine. http://medicine.iupui.edu/clinpharm/ddis/table.asp. Contains a detailed list of cytochrome drug interactions.

Hansten PD, Horn JR. Current topics in drug interactions. *Hansten and Horn drug interactions* http://www.hanstenandhorn.com/news.htm. A series of articles available online taking a detailed look at various interaction mechanisms.

Appendix 3

Important neurochemical syndromes

Some syndromes due to neurotransmitter excess or lack are frequent or potentially serious in the care of the elderly, and it is important to recognize them. They may be due to illness or to adverse effects of certain drugs. If not recognized many can lead to severe disability and death. Some possible causes in people with dementia/the elderly are briefly mentioned.

Syndromes due to neurotransmitter excess or deficiency

Neurotransmitter	Deficiency	Excess
Acetylcholine	*Anticholinergic effects*: dry mouth and throat, loss of sweating, constipation, blurred vision (loss of accommodation), urinary retention, drowsiness, tachycardia, confusion, poor concentration, occasionally seizures, coma and death *Causes*: e.g. typical antipsychotics, tricyclic antidepressants, anticholinergic drugs for secretions, e.g. glycopyrronium, hyoscine hydrochloride	Sweating, salivation, nausea and vomiting, bronchial secretions, sweating, miosis, abdominal colic, diarrhoea, urinary frequency, negative inotropic effect on heart, bradycardia, possibly heart block, respiratory depression, muscle weakness, seizures *Causes*: e.g. cholinesterase inhibitor toxicity
Serotonin	Depression, anxiety, slowness, tiredness, poor sleep, flushing headaches *Causes*: e.g. reserpine, isotretinoin, phenobarbital	*Serotonin syndrome*: sweating, tachycardia, dilated pupils, nausea, diarrhoea, colic, fever, hyper- or hypotension, shivering, tremor, rigidity, myoclonus, hyperreflexia, hypervigilance, agitation, confusion, hallucinations, seizures, coma and death *Causes*: e.g. MAOI; SSRI, or SNRI alone, but especially with or soon after stopping MAOI; tramadol; 5-HT$_3$ inhibitor

Neurotransmitter	Deficiency	Excess
Dopamine	Bradykinesia, tremor, rigidity. Along with other neurotransmitters, contributes to akathisia (📖 Chapter 10, Psychosis, pp. 185–190) *Causes*: e.g. Parkinson's; typical antipsychotics with extrapyramidal symptoms	Anorexia, nausea, sialorrhoea, hypotension, arrhythmias, disorientation, anxiety, ataxia, headaches, vivid dreams, insomnia, visual and auditory hallucinations, psychoses, dementia, choreiform or dystonic movements, blepharospasm, oculogyric crises, sleepiness *Causes*: e.g. levodopa toxicity
Norepinephrine	Pupillary constriction, loss of sweating, vomiting, postural hypotension, bradycardia, arrhythmias, cardiac arrest. *Causes*: e.g. amyloidosis, diabetes, vitamin B12 deficiency; local, e.g. Horner's syndrome from apical lung tumour	*Sympathetic stimulation*: tachycardia, arrhythmias, hypertension, pallor, vasoconstriction, agitation, anxiety, delirium, seizures, stroke, death *Causes*: unlikely to be found in people with dementia—commonly associated with cocaine or amphetamine toxicity, or catecholamine-secreting tumours
μ-Opioid	*Opioid withdrawal features*: pain hypersensitivity, anxiety, dizziness, sweating, running nose, sneezing, lachrymation, yawning, piloerection (gooseflesh), leg and abdominal cramps, diarrhoea, arrhythmias, seizures *Causes*: unlikely to be seen—precipitated by over-enthusiastic use of naloxone etc. NB: opioid antagonists should only be used if opioids are causing serious respiratory depression, unless by a specialist	Opioid toxicity: drowsiness, nausea and vomiting, pinpoint pupils, postural hypotension, pruritus, delirium, rarely pain hypersensitivity, myoclonus, hallucinations; seizures if pethidine or tramadol particularly, respiratory depression, death *Causes*: unskilled use of opioids, renal failure changing morphine metabolite excretion, genetic intolerance to a particular opioid (see 📖 Chapter 8, Strong opioids, pp. 116–125 for safe opioid use)
GABA	Anxiety, irritability, insomnia, tremor, ataxia, psychotic features, seizures *Causes*: alcohol (Chapter 10, Delirium, pp. 173–177) or benzodiazepine withdrawal	Sedation, respiratory depression, reduced cardiac contractility and vasomotor tone leading to heart failure *Causes*: benzodiazepine or barbiturate toxicity

Neuroleptic malignant syndrome
See 📖 Chapter 10, Psychosis, pp. 185–190.

Body dermatomes

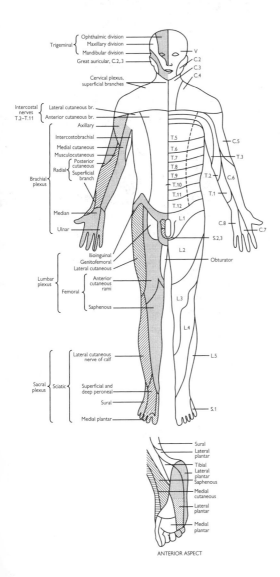

ANTERIOR ASPECT

Ophthalmic division ⎫
Maxillary division ⎬ Trigeminal
Mandibular division ⎭
Mastoid branch, C.2,C.3 ⎫
Great auricular branch, C.2,C.3 ⎬ Superficial cervical plexus
Occipital, C.2 ⎫
Occipital, C.3 ⎬ Dorsal branches
Occipital, C.4 ⎪
Occipital, C.5–C.8 ⎭
Supraclavicular, C.3,C.4
Dorsal rami of thoracic nerves
Cutaneous branch of axillary
Lateral cutaneous branches of intercostal nerves
Medial and lateral cutaneous br. of radial
Medial cutaneous
Intercostobrachial
Musculocutaneous
Anterior branch of radial
Median
Dorsal cutaneous branch of ulnar
Gluteal branch of 12th intercostal
Lateral cutaneous br. of iliohypogastric
Lateral branches of dorsal rami of lumbar and sacral ⎬
Medial branches of dorsal rami, L.1–S.6
Perforating branch of ⎫
Posterior cutaneous ⎬ Pudendal plexus
Lateral cutaneous
Obturator
Medial cutaneous ⎫
Saphenous ⎬ Femoral ⎬ Lumbar plexus
Posterior cutaneous
Superficial peroneal ⎫
⎬ Common peroneal ⎬ Sacral plexus
Sural
Tibial
Lateral plantar

POSTERIOR ASPECT

Reproduced with permission from Longmore et al. (2010). *Oxford Handbook of Clinical Medicine 8e*, Oxford University Press.

Opioid dose equivalence[1]

Approximate equivalent doses of opioid analgesics for adults

Caution should be used when converting opioids in opposite directions as potency ratios may be different.

> **Conversion factors for guidance when converting from one opioid to another**
>
> **Oral morphine to subcutaneous (s.c.) diamorphine**—divide by 3
> e.g. 30mg oral morphine = 10mg s.c. diamorphine
>
> **Oral morphine to oral oxycodone**—divide by 2
> e.g. 30mg oral morphine = 15mg oral oxycodone
>
> **Oral morphine to s.c. morphine**—divide by 2
> e.g. 30mg oral morphine = 15mg s.c. morphine
>
> **Oral morphine to oral hydromorphone**—divide by 7.5
> e.g. 30mg oral morphine = 4mg oral hydromorphone
>
> **Oral oxycodone to s.c. oxycodone**—divide by 2 (suggested safe practice)
> e.g. 10mg oral oxycodone = 5mg s.c. oxycodone
>
> **Oral hydromorphone to s.c. hydromorphone**—divide by 2
> e.g. 4mg oral hydromorphone = 2mg s.c. hydromorphone
>
> **s.c. diamorphine to s.c. oxycodone**—treat as equivalent up to doses of 60mg/24h
> Caution should be used when converting higher doses (suggested safe practice)
> e.g. 10mg s.c. diamorphine = 10mg s.c. oxycodone
>
> **s.c. diamorphine to s.c. alfentanil**—divide by 10
> e.g. 10mg s.c. diamorphine = 1 mg s.c. alfentanil
>
> **s.c. diamorphine to s.c. morphine**—ratio is between 1:1.5 and 1:2, multiply by 1.5
> e.g. 10mg s.c. diamorphine = 15mg s.c. morphine
>
> **Oral tramadol to oral morphine**—divide by 10 (suggested safe practice)[1]
> e.g. 100mg oral tramadol = 10mg oral morphine
>
> *(continued)*

1 Reproduced with permission from Watson M et al. (2009), *Oxford handbook of palliative care*, 2nd edn. Oxford University Press, Oxford.

Oral codeine/dihydrocodeine to oral morphine—divide by 10, e.g. 240mg oral codeine/dihydrocodeine = 24mg oral morphine

1 Limited evidence suggests that when converting from oral tramadol to oral morphine the dose should be divided by 5. However, this may result in too high a dose for some patients, hence locally agreed suggested safe practice is to divide by 10 and ensure appropriate breakthrough dose is available.

Opioid equivalence for transdermal patches—adult use

Transdermal patches are not suitable for patients who require rapid titration of strong opioid medication for severe pain and should be restricted to those diagnosed with stable pain.

Dose equivalence for transdermal fentanyl (Durogesic® DTrans®) andoral morphine

24-hourly oral morphine dose (mg)	Fentanyl patch strength (mcg/h)	4-hourly oral morphine (mg) (also breakthrough medication dose)
<90	25	<15
90–134	37	15–20
135–189	50	25–30

Please note conversion factors may change depending on the direction of conversion.

Note: Transdermal fentanyl patch has a 72-hour duration of action, i.e. changed every 3 days.

Transtec patch® (buprenorphine) conversion guide

Buprenorphine matrix patch/patches (mcg/h)	24-h oral morphine dose (mg)
35	50–97
52.5	76–145
70	101–193

NB: Transtec patch is replaced every 3–4 days

Index